Acquired Neurological
Speech/Language Disorders
in Childhood

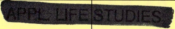

Brain Damage, Behaviour and Cognition
Developments in Clinical Neuropsychology

Series Editors: Chris Code, Scraptoft Campus, Leicester Polytechnic, and Dave Muller, Suffolk College of Higher and Further Education

Acquired Neurological Speech/Language Disorders in Childhood

Edited by
Bruce E. Murdoch

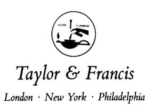

Taylor & Francis

London · New York · Philadelphia

UK	Taylor & Francis Ltd, 4 John St, London WC1N 2ET
USA	Taylor & Francis Inc., 1900 Frost Road, Suite 101, Bristol, PA 19007

First published 1990

British Library Cataloguing in Publication Data

Acquired neurological speech/language disorders in childhood.
1. Children. Speech disorders. Neurophysiological aspects
I. Murdoch, B. E. (Bruce E) II. Series
618.9285507

ISBN 0-85066-490-X
ISBN 0-85066-491-8 pbk

Typeset in 11/13 Bembo
by Chapterhouse, The Cloisters, Formby

Printed in Great Britain by Burgess Science Press, Basingstoke
on paper which has a specified pH value on final paper
manufacture of not less than 7.5 and is therefore 'acid free'.

Contents

Series Preface

From being an area primarily on the periphery of mainstream behavioural and cognitive science, neuropsychology has developed in recent years into an area of central concern for a range of disciplines. We are witnessing not only a revolution in the way in which brain–behaviour–cognition relationships are viewed, but a widening of interest concerning developments in neuropsychology on the part of a range of workers in a variety of fields. Major advances in brain-imaging techniques and the cognitive modelling of the impairments following brain damage promise a wider understanding of the nature of the representation of cognition and behaviour in the damaged and undamaged brain.

Neuropsychology is now centrally important for those working with brain-damaged people, but the very rate of expansion in the area makes it difficult to keep up with findings from current research. The aim of the *Brain Damage, Behaviour and Cognition* series is to publish a wide range of books which present comprehensive and up-to-date overviews of current developments in specific areas of interest.

These books will be of particular interest to those working with the brain-damaged. It is the editors' intention that undergraduates, postgraduates, clinicians and researchers in psychology, speech pathology and medicine will find this series a useful source of information on important current developments. The authors and editors of the books in this series are experts in their respective fields, working at the forefront of contemporary research. They have produced texts which are accessible and scholarly. We thank them for their contribution and their hard work in fulfilling the aims of the series.

CC and DJM
Leicester and Ipswich
Series editors

Contributors

Deborah L. Buttsworth   Doctoral Student
Department of Speech and Hearing
University of Queensland
St. Lucia, Australia

Jill A. Cross   Senior Speech Therapist
Montrose Home
Queensland Society for Crippled Children
Corinda, Australia

Lisa J. Hudson   Doctoral Student
Department of Speech and Hearing
University of Queensland
St. Lucia, Australia

Faye M. Jordan   Doctoral Student
Department of Speech and Hearing
University of Queensland
St. Lucia, Australia

Helen L. Krimmer   Senior Speech Therapist
Royal Children's Hospital
Brisbane, Australia

Bruce E. Murdoch   Head, Department of Speech and Hearing
University of Queensland
St. Lucia, Australia

Anne E. Ozanne   Lecturer in Speech Pathology
Department of Speech and Hearing
University of Queensland
St. Lucia, Australia

Veronica Smyth   Senior Lecturer in Audiology
                          Department of Speech and Hearing
                          University of Queensland
                          St. Lucia, Australia

Lynn M. Woodhouse   Speech Therapist-in-Charge
                          Brisbane North Special Services
                          Resource Centre — Speech Therapy
                          Special Education Resource and
                              Development Centre
                          Brisbane, Australia

Acquired Childhood Aphasia: Neuropathology, Linguistic Characteristics and Prognosis

Anne E. Ozanne and Bruce E. Murdoch

Definition of Acquired Childhood Aphasia

Language disorders occurring in childhood are usually divided into developmental and acquired disorders. In general, the term 'developmental language disorder' is used to describe those language problems which are apparent from the initial stages of language development. In most cases, developmental language disorders in children have an idiopathic origin, although these disorders may also occur secondary to other conditions such as peripheral hearing loss, mental retardation, cerebral palsy, child autism, or environmental deprivation.

In contrast, acquired aphasia in childhood results from brain damage. A variety of definitions of acquired childhood aphasia have appeared in the literature. Some examples of these definitions are shown in Table 1.1. Despite the minor variations evident in these definitions, two major features of acquired childhood aphasia appear to be consistently identified. First, the onset of acquired childhood aphasia is precipitated by some type of cerebral insult. The cerebral insult, in turn, can result from a variety of causes, including head trauma, cerebrovascular accidents, brain tumours, infections and seizure disorders (Miller *et al.*, 1984). Second, most authors agree that acquired aphasia in childhood follows a period of normal language acquisition during which the child commences learning language normally, though some studies of acquired childhood aphasia have included subjects whose cerebral insult occurred before the development of language. In the present book, the demonstrable presence of a cerebral insult is taken as the major feature and discussion is included of subjects where the lesion occurred both before and after language development.

Table 1.1 Definitions of acquired childhood aphasia

Author	Year	Definition
McCarthy	1963	Childhood aphasia is language impairment occurring after language has been acquired in a normal manner
Alajouanine and Lhermitte	1965	Acquired aphasia in children is language disorganization resulting from focal cerebral lesions occurring during childhood
Hécaen	1976	Acquired aphasia in childhood refers only to disturbances of language due to cerebral lesions which have occurred after language acquisition
Carrow-Woolfolk and Lynch	1982	Acquired aphasia results from focal cerebral lesions occurring during childhood, as opposed to suspected injury occurring before or at birth
Miller *et al.*	1984	Children . . . whose normal language-learning progress is disturbed as a direct result of neurological impairment are . . . acquired aphasics

Historical Perspective

Although the first descriptions of acquired aphasia in children were reported in the late 1800s (Bernhardt, 1885; Cotard, 1868, cited in Guttmann, 1942; Freud, 1897), nearly 100 years later, little conclusive information is available to help clinicians in the management of the cases they may find in their caseloads. Little also is understood about the linguistic pathology from which to derive the most effective and efficient treatment strategies.

From the limited number of studies reported in the literature, a traditional description of childhood acquired aphasia has emerged. In the past it has often been stated that acquired childhood aphasia is rare, however, when it does occur it is characterized by an initial period of mutism followed by a non-fluent, motor type of language impairment with no accompanying comprehension deficit or other features of a fluent type of aphasia (e.g. jargon, logorrhea and paraphasia). In addition, acquired childhood aphasia was usually regarded as being transitory in nature, affected individuals making a good recovery. The stated rarity (Cotard, 1868; Denckla, 1979) was in part contributed to by the observation that children who do exhibit aphasia also showed rapid recovery of language skills. Bernhardt (1885) stated that childhood aphasia was not rare but because the aphasia was of a transient nature and rarely permanent it was often not reported. In support of Bernhardt (1885), Nadoreczny (1926, cited in Guttmann, 1942) also noted that most cases of acquired childhood aphasia recover within a few weeks.

The recovery of language in acquired childhood aphasia varies amongst children. Some children go through the normal language development process as they regain their language skills while others skip developmental stages during the recovery process (Basser, 1962; Byers and McLean, 1962). One 8-year-old girl with left hemiplegia, described by Byers and McLean (1962), initially communicated by gestures and within 3 weeks of becoming aphasic was responding verbally to simple sums. Soon after that, with her ability to write letters using her right hand, came the use of automatic speech including counting and reciting poetry. No description, however, was given of her functional language at this time. Within 3 months this child had returned to school, her only reported aphasic symptoms being a word-finding deficit.

Another characteristic of the traditional description of childhood acquired aphasia is a period of mutism immediately post-onset. This has been described as the chief characteristic of childhood aphasia by Branco-Lefèvre (1950) and Alajouanine and Lhermitte (1965). Guttmann (1942) noted an absence of spontaneous speech in 14 of his 16 cases of acquired childhood aphasia, mostly in children less than 10 years of age. Nine of the 15 right hemiplegic subjects (60 per cent) reported by Hécaen (1976) had a period of mutism lasting from 5 days to 3 months. Hécaen (1983) observed that mutism appeared mostly in children with anterior lesions (63 per cent) while only 10 per cent of children with temporal lesions showed mutism.

Some authors have suggested a psychological basis for the initial mutism shown by children with acquired aphasia (Alajouanine and Lhermitte, 1965; Byers and McLean, 1962). Reasons suggested for a psychological basis to the period of mutism include a presence of aspontaneity in written and gestural expression as well as in spoken language. In addition, when speech does return, increased incentives and encouragements are required to get the children to use words they are capable of producing. Furthermore, it has been noted that in general children tend to become silent and isolated at times of conflict or difficulties.

When speech and language do return, the traditional description of the aphasia is of a non-fluent, motor-type (Bernhardt, 1885; Carrow-Woolfolk and Lynch, 1982; Guttmann, 1942). Other features of acquired childhood aphasia reported in the literature include telegraphic speech (Guttmann, 1942) simplified syntax (Alajouanine and Lhermitte, 1965) and hesitation and dysarthria (Byers and McLean, 1962; Guttmann, 1942). Many investigators have noted that paraphasias, logorrhea and jargon are rare, or in the majority of cases, absent (Alajouanine and Lhermitte, 1965; Collignon *et al.*, 1968; Hécaen, 1976). Some authors (Alajouanine and Lhermitte, 1965; Guttmann, 1942; Poetzl, 1926), however, noted that the traditional description of acquired aphasia was most commonly seen in children less than 10 years of age while older children tended to present more like adult aphasics. Hécaen (1976) was unable to confirm this relationship between aphasic type and age, but did, however, postulate a relationship between lesion site and aphasic type. He found that children with acquired aphasia resulting from anterior lesions presented with an initial mutism while those with temporal lobe lesions showed comprehension deficits in the acute stages that resolved within 1 year. Alajouanine and Lhermitte (1965) and Hécaen (1983) also noted transitory comprehension deficits in one-third of their subjects.

Another characteristic of acquired childhood aphasia noted to be present, particularly in the acute stages post-onset, is a naming deficit or poverty of lexical stock (Alajouanine and Lhermitte, 1965; Collignon *et al.*, 1968). Hécaen (1976) noted that naming disorders occurred in 7 of 15 of his left hemisphere-lesioned subjects. In three of these cases this deficit persisted long-term and was often noted in school reports.

Satz and Bullard-Bates (1981: 405) carried out a comprehensive review of the literature to investigate the three aspects of the traditional description of acquired aphasia in children: its rarity, its clinical description and its rapid recovery. Overall, the findings of their review, which are described below, demonstrated a need to re-evaluate the traditional description of acquired childhood aphasia. They took all subjects in published studies who met the following criteria:

1   Some speech reported before the lesion onset
2   Hand preference reported before lesion onset
3   Patient under 16 years of age before lesion onset
4   Evidence that lesion was unilateral only
5   Comparison of presence vs absence of aphasia following unilateral injury

Of 21 studies and 929 reported cases only 68 cases met the above criteria. In many studies handedness data was not provided. In other studies only cases with aphasia were included and therefore could not form part of a review on the incidence of acquired childhood aphasia.

In conclusion, Satz and Bullard-Bates (1981) stated that if the lesion is unilateral and encroaches on the speech areas then childhood aphasias are not rare. They noted, however, a lower prevalence of unilateral vascular disease in children as compared with adults. Furthermore, they concluded that if the left hemisphere is damaged the risk of language impairment is approximately the same in right-handed children as in adults. Regardless of age (at least after infancy), the risk of acquired aphasia is substantially greater following left-sided rather than right-sided lesions. Finally, it was concluded that, although rare, crossed aphasias do exist in left-handed children regardless of age. In particular crossed aphasias are especially rare after 3–5 years of age in right-handed children.

When reviewing the clinical type of aphasia Satz and Bullard-Bates (1981) concluded that the clinical pattern is predominantly non-fluent with rare or absent paraphasias and logorrhea, but disorders of auditory comprehension, naming and writing may co-exist. They stipulated that at that time it was unclear how those clinical patterns related to age and maturational effects or to the lesion, its size, cause, type, site or the time after the lesion.

The third aspect of acquired aphasia in children which Satz and Bullard-Bates

(1981) reviewed was the apparent rapid recovery of the aphasia. They concluded that: in the majority of cases spontaneous recovery is dramatic (i.e. approximately 75 per cent of cases), 25–50 per cent of cases still present with aphasia within 1 year post-onset, the recovery from aphasia is unrelated to the presence/severity of hemiparesis, and that despite recovery from aphasia, intellectual, cognitive or school achievement may still be impaired. Satz and Bullard-Bates (1981) could not identify the factors affecting recovery but suggested that these may include cause, aphasia type, lesion size or age at the time of the lesion.

Satz and Bullard-Bates (1981) did not believe that their findings supported the equipotentiality hypothesis put forward by Basser (1962) and Lenneberg (1967). These authors did state, however, that their findings were in line with studies which have noted a structural asymmetry of the brain at birth (Chi *et al.*, 1977; Galaburda *et al.*, 1978) as well as those which have noted functional asymmetry in non-aphasics (Hiscock and Kinsbourne, 1978; Molfese *et al.*, 1975). Satz and Bullard-Bates (1981) noted that the results of their study, however, do not explain the dramatic recovery rate seen in children with acquired aphasia.

Since the early 1980s, therefore, it has been recognized that childhood acquired aphasia is not as rare as previously thought and despite the rapid recovery seen in some cases, 25–50 per cent of children who develop acquired aphasia still have aphasic symptoms 1 year post-onset. It is these children to whom we will now turn our attention. Several questions still need to be asked. What are the precise linguistic deficits with which children with acquired aphasia present? Do these linguistic deficits relate to specific causes? Do these deficits differ from linguistic impairments seen in children with developmental language impairment? What assessment and treatment strategies are available to clinicians working with these cases? These issues are addressed in the remainder of this chapter and in Chapter 2.

Neuropathological Substrate of Acquired Childhood Aphasia

Although acquired childhood aphasia can be caused by a similar range of disorders of the nervous system as adult aphasia, the relative importance of each of the different causes to the occurrence of language disturbances in children differs from the situation seen in adults. For instance, although in peacetime cerebrovascular accidents are the most common cause of aphasia in adults, the most common cause of acquired childhood aphasia is traumatic head injury.

Head Injury

In the majority of cases of acquired childhood aphasia reported in the literature the cause is head injury. Head injuries can be divided into two major types: closed head injuries and open head injuries. In a closed head injury the covering of the brain remains intact even though the skull may be fractured. An open head injury differs from a closed head injury in that the brain or meninges are exposed. By far the majority of traumatic head injuries in both children and adults in civilian life are closed head injuries.

Damage to the brain following traumatic head injury may be either focal, multi-focal or diffuse in nature. In general, closed head injuries tend to produce more diffuse pathology while open head injuries are associated with more focal pathology. Brain contusions (bruises), lacerations and haemorrhages can be caused at the time of head injury from either the direct trauma at the site of impact on the skull, acceleration of the brain against the bony shelves of the skull (e.g. the sphenoidal ridge) or from contra-coup trauma that occurs when the brain strikes the skull on the side opposite the point of insult. Brain and Walton (1969) identified three different destructive forces which are applied to the brain at the moment of impact: compression or impression which forces the brain tissue together, tension which pulls the brain apart, and shearing produced by rotational acceleration and which develops primarily at those points where the brain impinges upon bony or ligamentous ridges within the cranial vault. According to Adams *et al.* (1977), the primary mechanism producing brain injury following closed head injury is diffuse axonal damage in the white matter occurring at the time of impact and caused by a shearing mechanism arising from rotational acceleration.

It has often been reported that children show a striking rate of recovery following closed head injury. Some authors have suggested that one of the reasons for the good prognosis for recovery in childhood is that the degree of brain damage following head injury is less in children than in adults, due in part to the different nature of their head injuries as well as to differences in the basic mechanisms of brain damage following head injury. Most childhood head injuries result from falls or low speed accidents. Consequently many paediatric head injuries are associated with a lesser degree of rotational acceleration and therefore, presumably, with a lesser amount of brain damage (Levin *et al.*, 1982). Jamison and Kaye (1974) noted that persistent neurological deficits were only present in children injured in road traffic accidents which are, by their nature, likely to yield greater diffuse brain injury. Likewise, a study conducted by Moyes (1980) showed road traffic accidents to be the most common cause of long-term morbidity following childhood head injury. In addition, Strich (1969) suggested that the shearing strains produced by rotational acceleration in head trauma are less pronounced in smaller brains.

Although the rate of spontaneous recovery in children following closed head injury is often described as excellent, persistent long-term language disorders have been reported (Gaidolfi and Vignolo, 1980; Jordan *et al.*, 1988; Satz and Bullard-Bates, 1981) and even when specific linguistic symptoms resolve cognitive and academic difficulties often remain. The speech/language disorders associated with childhood head injuries together with the mechanisms of head injury are discussed in more detail in Chapter 3.

Cerebrovascular Disorders

Several investigators have documented the occurrence of acquired aphasia with vascular disorders in children (Aram *et al.*, 1983, 1986; Dennis, 1980). Cerebrovascular accidents or strokes are spontaneous interruptions to the blood supply to the brain, arising from either occlusion of the cerebral blood vessels (ischaemic stroke) or in some cases from rupture of one of the cerebral blood vessels (haemorrhagic stroke). Although cerebrovascular accidents are much less common in children than in adults, they occur more frequently than is commonly thought and are a significant cause of morbidity and mortality in the childhood population. Banker (1961) reported that of 555 childhood autopsy cases studied by him, death was due to a cerebrovascular accident in 48 (8.6 per cent).

Virtually all the diseases of blood vessels which affect adults may at some time also occur in children (Bickerstaff, 1972; Salam-Adams and Adams, 1988). Despite this, the causes of vascular diseases of the brain in children differ from those in adults. For instance, degenerative disorders such as atherosclerosis affect primarily the middle-aged and elderly and are rare in childhood (Moosy, 1959). Some vascular diseases of the brain, such as embolism arising from subacute or acute bacterial endocardial valvular disease, occur at all ages while others, such as vascular disorders associated with congenital heart disease, are peculiar to childhood.

Acute hemiplegia of childhood is a term used by many paediatricians and neurologists to describe the sudden onset of hemiplegia in children. A wide variety of vascular diseases of the brain, including both occlusive and haemorrhagic disorders, have been described under this heading.

Idiopathic childhood hemiplegia

The most commonly reported and dramatic syndrome resulting from an ischaemic stroke in childhood is idiopathic childhood hemiplegia. This syndrome involves the sudden onset of hemiplegia as a result of a unilateral brain infarct of unknown origin and can affect children from a few months of age up to 12 years of age (Bickerstaff, 1972). According to Bickerstaff (1972), females are affected more than males in a ratio of about 3 : 2.

The cause of idiopathic childhood hemiplegia has been argued for many years and a variety of possible causes proposed including: polioencephalitis (Strumpell, 1884), encephalitis (Adams *et al.*, 1949; Bernheim, 1956; Brandt, 1962), venous thrombosis

(Bernheim, 1956; Brandt, 1962; Norman, 1962), demyelination (Wyllie, 1948), epilepsy (Norman, 1962), and occlusion of the internal carotid artery (Bickerstaff, 1964; Duffey *et al.*, 1957; Goldstein and Burgess, 1958). Although there appears to be some agreement that arterial occlusion is the most common cause of idiopathic childhood hemiplegia the reason for the occlusion is less certain. For reasons indicated above, atheroma cannot be implicated in childhood. Studies using carotid angiograms have demonstrated the presence of thrombosis of either the common or internal carotid arteries in some cases of idiopathic childhood hemiplegia (Salam-Adams and Adams, 1988). Bickerstaff (1964) suggested that roughening of the wall of the internal carotid artery as a result of arteritis secondary to throat, tonsillar or cervical gland infection might be the causal factor in some instances. Further, in some reported cases neither angiography nor post-mortem examination was able to demonstrate the presence of vascular lesions, suggesting that in these cases an embolus may have temporarily blocked a cerebral artery and then later broken up before the angiogram was taken or the post-mortem performed (Salam-Adams and Adams, 1988).

Other vascular occlusive disorders in childhood

A number of other vascular occlusive disorders peculiar to childhood can also cause ischaemic strokes in children. These disorders include: vascular disease associated with congenital heart disease, arteritis (inflammation of an artery) of various types, sickle cell anaemia, vascular occlusion associated with irradiation of the base of the brain, moyamoya, and strokes associated with homocystinuria and Fabry's angiokeratosis.

Ischaemic strokes associated with congenital heart disease occur most frequently in the first 2 years of life, corresponding to the stage when congenital heart disease has its greatest frequency (6 per 1000 live births) (Salam-Adams and Adams, 1988). Banker (1961) reported that of the childhood cerebrovascular accident cases examined by him, 28 per cent were associated with congenital heart disease, making it the single most common cause of cerebrovascular accidents in his study.

Various types of arteritis, including that associated with lupus erythematosus and occurring secondary to infections in the tonsillar fossa and lymph glands in the neck, have also been reported to cause ischaemic strokes in children (Bickerstaff, 1964; Davie and Cox, 1967; Salam-Adams and Adams, 1988). Lupus erythematosus is a diffuse inflammatory disease that involves the kidneys, skin, haematological system, the central nervous system and occasionally the liver. It is more common in females than males with a ratio of about 10 : 1. Although the average onset is around 30 years of age, symptoms can occur in the first decade of life (Bell and Lastimosa, 1980). Neurological complications have been reported to occur in up to 75 per cent of patients (Tindall, 1980), with seizures being the most common single neurological symptom. Hemiplegia secondary to cerebral arteritis, which is either transitory or permanent, occurs in approximately 5 per cent of patients with lupus erythematosus. If permanent neurological loss occurs it is correlated with obstruction of one of the major extracranial or intracranial blood vessels. A case of lymphadenitis (inflammation of the lymph nodes) in the region of the carotid bifurcation and extending to involve the artery was described by Schnüriger (1966, cited in Bickerstaff, 1972). Bickerstaff (1972) reported damage to the carotid artery near its passage past the tonsillar fossa possibly resulting from arteritis due to a throat infection.

Both arterial and venous occlusions leading to cerebral infarction have been observed in children with sickle cell disease, an inherited blood disorder occurring primarily in Negroes (Salam-Adams and Adams, 1988). Likewise, cerebral infarcts have been reported subsequent to cobalt radiation of the base of the brain for treatment of a variety of neoplastic disorders in children, including craniopharyngiomas and pituitary adenomas.

Another vascular disorder of childhood that may cause vascular occlusion of the internal carotid artery is moyamoya disease. Patients with this condition present with headache, seizures, stroke-like episodes, visual symptoms and mental retardation as well as, in some cases, a movement disorder, a gait disturbance and/or a speech deficit. Typically the symptoms are bihemispheric. Moyamoya disease is characterized by the presence of a network of fine anastomotic blood vessels at the base of the brain called a rete mirabile. The aetiology of moyamoya disease is uncertain. There have been some suggestions that the condition is a congenital disorder involving retention of the embryonal rete mirabile. Alternatively, the network of anastomoses may be the consequence of an acquired disorder involving occlusion of the carotid arteries. It is possible, therefore, that several types of arterial disease in childhood may lead to moyamoya.

Complications of certain hereditary metabolic diseases may also occasionally cause occlusive vascular disease in children. Two such conditions where this may occur include homocystinuria and Fabry's disease. Both of these conditions result from enzyme deficiencies and both, amongst other effects, may cause structural damage to the blood vessels leading to thrombosis. Homocystinuria, resulting from a lack of cystathionine-synthetase, manifests as mental retardation. Ischaemic strokes arising from either arterial or venous thrombosis may be experienced by persons with this disorder in late childhood, adolescence or adult life. Likewise, Fabry's disease, a sex-linked disorder affecting males and resulting from a deficiency in galactosyl hydrolase, may also cause structural changes in the blood vessels leading to thrombosis and stroke (Adams and Lyon, 1982).

Brain Haemorrhage in Childhood

Spontaneous intracranial haemorrhage is much less common in children than in adults.

Two major types of cerebral haemorrhage occur in childhood: one type occurring secondary to haematological diseases such as leukaemia, sickle cell disease, haemophilia and thrombopenic purpura, the second type occurring secondary to vascular abnormalities such as arteriovenous malformations. It is noteworthy that haemorrhage resulting from rupture of saccular (berry) aneurysms is rare in childhood (Bickerstaff, 1972). In addition, the majority of arteriovenous malformations manifest as brain haemorrhage or in some other way during the third decade of life. Only approximately 10 per cent of arteriovenous malformations cause haemorrhage or other problems in childhood.

Details of the nature of the linguistic deficits associated with childhood vascular lesions are included in the discussion of the linguistic features of acquired childhood aphasia later in this chapter.

Tumours

Intracerebral tumours are a recognized cause of acquired aphasia in children (Alajouanine and Lhermitte, 1965; Brown, 1985; Carrow-Woolfolk and Lynch, 1982; Hécaen, 1976; Hudson *et al.*, 1989; Rekate *et al.*, 1985; Van Dongen *et al.*, 1985). Neoplasms of the posterior cranial fossa (i.e. those involving the cerebellum, pons, fourth ventricle and cisterna magna) occur more frequently in children than supratentorial tumours (Gjerris, 1978; Matson, 1956; Segall *et al.*, 1985). Cerebellar astrocytoma is the most common type of posterior fossa tumour in childhood, occurring most frequently in children between 5 and 9 years of age (Cuneo and Rand, 1952; Matson, 1969). Fortunately cerebellar astrocytomas are also highly curable and have an excellent prognosis following surgical removal. Next to cerebellar astrocytoma, medulloblastoma is the most frequent tumour type involving structures within the posterior cranial fossa in children. Generally these latter tumours involve children at a younger age than do cerebellar astrocytomas, their maximum incidence being within the age range of 3–7 years (Delong and Adams, 1975). Although initially cerebellar astrocytoma and medulloblastoma may present in a similar manner the prognosis of these two tumours types is quite different. While astrocytoma has a very favourable prognosis medulloblastoma has a poor prognosis for recovery. The third most frequently encountered tumour of the posterior cranial fossa is the ependymoma. These neoplasms grow from the floor of the fourth ventricle and affect children of a similar age to the medulloblastoma, and like the latter tumour type, ependymoma has a poor prognosis with a high proportion of tumours recurring after surgical removal.

Considering their location in the central nervous system (CNS), it would not be expected that posterior fossa tumours would cause language problems. A number of secondary effects, however, are associated with these tumours which can, in some cases, lead to language deficits. Many posterior fossa tumours either originate from or invade the fourth ventricle. As a result hydrocephalus may occur following obstruction to the flow of cerebrospinal fluid (CSF). Subsequent compression of the cerebral cortex can then lead to malfunctioning of the central speech/language centres. In addition, radiotherapy (see Ch. 9) administered after surgical removal of posterior fossa tumours to prevent tumour spread or recurrence, has been implicated in the occurrence of language disorders in both adults and children (Broadbent *et al.*, 1981; Burns and Boyle, 1984; Duffner *et al.*, 1983; Hudson *et al.*, 1989; Meadows *et al.*, 1981).

The effects of intracranial tumours on language functions in children are discussed in further detail in Chapter 8.

Infections

Infectious disorders of the CNS are recognized as a significant cause of acquired childhood aphasia. Van Dongen *et al.* (1985) reported that of 27 children with acquired aphasia referred to their clinic over a 4-year period, 15 per cent had a history of infectious disease. Similarly Van Hout *et al.* (1985) noted that 38 per cent of their child cases with acquired aphasia had an infectious disorder.

Although the brain and its membranous coverings can be infected by the same range of microorganisms as other organs of the body, in the majority of cases of acquired childhood aphasia with infectious disease reported in the literature, the infectious disorder involved has been herpes simplex encephalitis. Two antigenic types of herpes simplex virus (HSV) are now recognized, type 1 (HSV-1) and type 2 (HSV-2). HSV-1 is responsible for almost all cases of sporadic encephalitis in children and adults. HSV-2, which causes congenital herpes, produces aseptic meningitis in the adult and encephalitis in the neonate.

HSV appears to involve primarily the basomedial portion of the frontal and temporal lobes and may present as an intracranial space-occupying lesion. As a result of the destructive nature of the lesions associated with infectious disorders, and in particular herpes simplex encephalitis, the language disorder associated with this disease tends to be more severe than in acquired aphasia resulting from other causes. For instance, Van Hout and Lyon (1986) attributed the severe language disorder they observed in a 10-year-old boy to the destructive bilateral damage to his temporal lobes caused by herpes simplex encephalitis.

Communication disorders resulting from infectious disorders in childhood are discussed in Chapter 4.

Convulsive Disorder

Acquired aphasia with convulsive disorder was first described by Landau and Kleffner (1957). In this condition the child's language deteriorates in association with the epileptiform discharges seen in their electroencephalogram. In some cases the language deterioration is either preceded, accompanied or followed by a series of convulsive seizures (Van de Sandt-Koenderman *et al.*, 1984). Although seizures do occur often, they are not the defining feature of this syndrome.

Onset of the Landau–Kleffner syndrome is usually between 2 and 13 years of age, with the initial loss of language function occurring most frequently between 3 and 7 years of age. Males are affected twice as often as females (Cooper and Ferry, 1978; Msall *et al.*, 1986). Although the cause of Landau–Kleffner syndrome is unknown, several hypotheses on the pathogenesis of this disorder have been proposed. Some authors have postulated that the language regression results from functional ablation of the primary cortical language areas by persistent electrical discharges (Landau and Kleffner, 1957; Sato and Dreifuss, 1973). The characteristics of the language disorder shown by children with Landau–Kleffner syndrome are discussed later in this chapter.

Linguistic Characteristics of Acquired Childhood Aphasia

The presence of methodological limitations in many studies have prevented the identification of definitive profiles of the linguistic characteristics of acquired childhood aphasia. These limitations, often resulting from restrictions on the number of subjects available, include factors such as: the inclusion of a diverse range of causes of acquired aphasia, the use of non-specific methods of lesion localization (e.g. the identification of brain lesions on the basis of the presence of a hemiplegia), the failure to exclude cases with possible bilateral brain damage (e.g. occurring after head trauma or infection), and the inclusion of subjects of different ages before and after the onset of brain damage.

Before the publication of the review by Satz and Bullard-Bates (1981) most reports of the speech and language characteristics of acquired childhood aphasia had been of a descriptive nature with very few standardized speech and language assessments being reported. In the recent studies more objective measures of speech and language performance have been used. In addition, more accurate methods of lesion localization such as computed tomography have also been utilized. Despite this, the problem of groups of mixed pathology and diverse age ranges still exist.

Auditory Comprehension Deficits

As stated earlier, the first reports of acquired childhood aphasia found no auditory comprehension deficits present in any subjects. More recent studies, however, have reported the presence of transitory comprehension deficits. For instance, Hécaen (1976, 1983) and Alajouanine and Lhermitte (1965) observed transitory comprehension problems in one-third of the children with acquired aphasia that they examined. Guttmann (1942) reported 'disturbed auditory comprehension' in two out of his 14 subjects with acquired childhood aphasia. In one of these cases, after a temporoparietal lesion, the comprehension deficit was the major symptom of the aphasia. Guttmann (1942) warned, however, that comprehension difficulties could be 'disregarded' unless expressive language deficits were also present.

Of the 32 children studied by Alajouanine and Lhermitte (1965) only ten were noted to have auditory comprehension deficits. These deficits were 'marked' in only four of the ten cases. In all these cases by 6 months after the lesion, comprehension had returned to 'near normal' with difficulties encountered only on the most difficult tasks. One year post-onset no auditory comprehension difficulties were noted in any of the ten subjects. Alajouanine and Lhermitte (1965) had divided their 32 subjects into two age groups. In the youngest age group (5–9 years old) nearly all (eight out of nine cases) had comprehension deficits in the initial stages, while in the second age group (10–15 years old) only two subjects of the 23 had auditory comprehension deficits. Comprehension deficits from this study, therefore, appear more common in children who acquired a brain lesion before 10 years of age.

Hécaen (1983) reviewed 26 children with acquired aphasia between 3½ and 15 years of age and found no support for the difference between the number of cases with comprehension difficulties in children above and below 10 years of age noted by Alajouanine and Lhermitte (1965). Although Hécaen observed that there were more cases of auditory comprehension deficits in children with left-sided lesions who were less than 10 years of age (i.e. six of 14 cases — 42 per cent) than in children older than 10 years of age (six out of twenty cases — 30 per cent) this difference was not statistically significant. Neither was there any significant difference in the number of cases with comprehension impairments in relation to sites of lesion (i.e. fronto-Rolandic or temporal) nor cause of lesion (i.e. haematoma, trauma or tumour/abscess) in the cases studied by Hécaen, although he noted a trend for more cases of comprehension impairment following an anterior lesion or a rapid onset.

The cause most commonly associated with auditory comprehension disorders in children with acquired aphasia is convulsive disorder (Landau and Kleffner, 1957; Rapin *et al.*, 1977; Miller *et al.*, 1984; Worster-Drought, 1971). The nature of these auditory comprehension deficits will be discussed later in this chapter.

Early studies reporting the nature of comprehension deficits in children with acquired aphasia usually used subjective and/or descriptive notes on the deficits often without reference to the developmental level of competence expected in the child. Later studies, while using objective assessment procedures (usually versions of the Token Test), tended to cite unitary scores. Only in the most recent publications are the descriptive and standardized assessment methods combined in an effort to understand the nature of the auditory comprehension disorders. These early descriptions contained in case studies demonstrate the variable nature of auditory comprehension deficits seen in children with acquired aphasia. Oelschlaeger and Scarborough (1976: 283) described a 10-year-old child who was 'unable to comprehend auditorily any speech stimuli' following a fall from a horse. After therapy, 1 year post-onset she still presented with significantly impaired receptive and expressive language skills but was able to answer questions on current activities appropriately.

Severe comprehension difficulties post-onset (e.g. inability to identify parts of the face) were also described by Pohl (1979) in a 6-year-old child after a suspected occlusion of the middle cerebral artery. Four months post-onset, comprehension had returned to normal while expressive language was at a one to two word level. Visch-Brink and Van de Sandt-Koenderman (1984) described four cases with differing degrees of comprehension impairment immediately post-onset. The first case scored 37 of a possible 61 on the Token Test (De Renzi and Vignolo, 1962) soon after a subdural empyema. This score improved to 44 correct, 6 weeks later and to 53 of 61 correct 5 months post-onset, at which stage the child's expressive language was characterized by mild syntactic difficulties and resolving paraphasias. The second case recovered comprehension and expressive skills within 14 days of a head trauma. Before recovery mild comprehension difficulties, telegraphic speech and paraphasias were evident. The other two cases presented with severe comprehension deficits. One of the two cases also had long runs of unintelligible speech and showed very slow recovery in both areas of language while the other presented with 'empty speech' characterized by strings of disconnected words then periods of adequate speech, paraphasias and paragrammatisms.

Formal assessment results in individual cases of children with auditory comprehension deficits as part of their aphasia, also emphasizes the variable nature of the deficits and the recovery process reported above in the descriptive studies. Van Hout and Lyon (1986) described a 10-year-old boy with a severe comprehension deficit as part of a Wernicke's aphasia following herpes-simplex encephalitis. In the early stages the child scored below five standard deviations from his age-matched test mean on the Gaddes and Crockett (1975) norms of the Spreen-Benton Neurosensory Centre Comprehensive Examination for Aphasia (NCCEA) (Spreen and Benton, 1969). Eight months later he was scoring at a 6-year age level for syntactic comprehension but could only identify an object by name 60 per cent of the time. Another 10-year-old child, described by Dennis (1980), presented on the Identification by Name and Sentence subtests of the NCCEA at below the 6-year age level 2 weeks after a cerebrovascular accident. Three months after the accident, Identification by Name was at an age-appropriate level but Identification by Sentence was still at the original 6-year age level. Descriptive notes stated that 3 months after the cerebrovascular accident the subject understood single words and short commands. Test results indicated that comprehension and expressive skills were developing in parallel.

Two cases with subcortical lesions were reported by Aram *et al.* (1983). Only one of the cases had comprehension deficits. These deficits resolved within 2 months. Initially the subject (7 years old) had exhibited an 18 month delay on the Peabody Picture Vocabulary Test (Dunn, 1965) and a 2½ year delay on the North Western Syntax Screening Test (NWSST): Receptive (Lee, 1971). The authors suggested that the language deficit, including the moderate comprehension impairment noted in one subject but not in the other, was related to the site of the subcortical lesion.

Van Dongen *et al.* (1985), however, described differing degrees of comprehension impairment in three girls with similar lesion sites, all of which involved Wernicke's area. All three subjects presented with a fluent aphasia. The cause in two cases was trauma, and both of these showed rapid recovery. One of the head trauma subjects had normal conversational comprehension 13 days post-onset. The results of her Token Test, however, revealed auditory comprehension deficits as she scored 28 correct of a possible 61 on the test. By 2½ months post-onset, both conversational and test performance comprehension were within normal limits. A faster recovery period was noted in the second head trauma subject. Her Token Test results were 52 of 61 and her conversational comprehension was within normal limits 12 days post-onset. Initially she had presented with marked comprehension impairments both on the test results (i.e. 13 of 61 correct) and in conversation. She also presented as anomic in spontaneous speech. The third subject described by Van Dongen *et al.* (1985) had a suspected haematoma and 2 months later developed convulsions. Although before the onset of convulsions she scored 6 of 10 correct on the easiest part of the Token Test, once the convulsions had commenced this subject could not be assessed using formal test procedures, even though she could understand simple commands. Her expressive language at this stage was described as being comprised of simple words spoken in a telegraphic style. No improvement was noted over the next 2 years.

Studies, using either descriptive or standardized assessment procedures, therefore, have demonstrated a range of auditory comprehension deficits in children with acquired aphasia. These findings are contrary to those of the early reports which either suggested that comprehension disorders did not exist in cases of acquired childhood aphasia or they were of a transitory nature. More recent studies have compared groups of children with acquired aphasia either with a group of non-brain-injured controls or have compared groups of right and left hemisphere-lesioned subjects. Most of these latter studies have served to emphasize the persistent nature of auditory comprehension deficits found in some children with acquired aphasia.

Van Hout *et al.* (1985) studied 16 children with acquired aphasia between 2 and 13 years of age. They reported that the three youngest subjects (all 2 years old) presented according to the classical description of childhood aphasia, while the two oldest subjects (both 13 years old) presented with a Broca's aphasia. The remaining 11 subjects did not fit either pattern. They divided these 11 subjects into three groups based on their recovery from paraphasia. The first two groups whose paraphasias resolved either within days or months presented with moderate comprehension deficits, while the third group who had paraphasias lasting more than 1 year post-onset, presented with severe comprehension impairments. The authors noted that the most common cause in this last group was infection. Decreased receptive language skills or global aphasia were also described as the initial communication deficits in the four children with infections described by Cooper and Flowers (1987). Initial comprehension deficits, however, were also noted in their subjects with anoxia, closed head injury and tumours.

The assessment of Cooper and Flowers' (1987) 15 brain-lesioned children (between 10 and 18 years of age) was carried out 3 to 12 years post-onset. When compared with a control group without brain injury the experimental group performed significantly poorer on all assessments of language comprehension. Despite performing significantly poorer on the assessments than a group of controls, Cooper and Flowers (1987) emphasized the heterogeneity of the group pointing out that one subject showed no impairment on any language test while three subjects showed impairment on all expressive as well as receptive tests. For this reason they gave individual assessment profiles for all 15 brain-injured subjects. Nine subjects scored greater than two standard deviations below the age mean on the Peabody Picture Vocabulary Test-Revised (Dunn and Dunn, 1981). Of these nine subjects two subjects scored more than four standard deviations below the mean while another three subjects scored greater than seven deviations below. On the shortened version of the Token Test (De Renzi and Faglioni, 1978) seven of the 15 subjects scored greater than two standard deviations below the mean; however, Cooper and Flowers (1987) claimed that only one of these could be described as having a moderate comprehension deficit. As a group, the brain-lesioned subjects did not perform significantly different from the controls on Parts 1–5 of the test; however, there was a statistically significant difference between the scores of the experimental and control groups on Part 6 of the test. This would indicate that as a group, the brain-lesioned subjects had no more difficulty than the control group with the increase in syntactical information load but had more difficulty with increased linguistic complexity.

The proposed difficulties with syntactical complexity is supported by the individual case profiles published by Cooper and Flowers (1987) which showed that their brain-injured subjects had most difficulty with the items containing the instructions 'in addition to, if, between' and the item 'touch the blue circle *with* the red square'. Only one subject had difficulty with the earlier parts of the test. Six of the 15 subjects reported by Cooper and Flowers (1987) had difficulties with the Processing Spoken Paragraphs subtest of the Clinical Evaluation of Language Function (CELF)

(Semel and Wiig, 1980). In all cases the authors noted that the subjects appeared to comprehend the questions asked but were unable to recall the appropriate information. Overall three subjects presented with deficits in all three areas of comprehension assessed; two had problems in lexical and auditory language comprehension; two had problems in lexical and comprehension of contextual language while four subjects had one area only of deficit, two in lexical comprehension and one each in auditory language and comprehension of contextual language. No relationships between these results and the side, site, size or cause of the lesion nor of the age at injury or after the lesion could be drawn as the subjects differed too widely on all these variables. The study, however, showed conclusively that after a mean length of time post-onset of 8 years, residual comprehension deficits were still shown by all but three of Cooper and Flowers (1987) 15 subjects.

Another series of studies have investigated the influence of the side of lesion on comprehension abilities in children with acquired aphasia. Most of these studies have included children who received their brain lesions perinatally or within a few months of birth. Therefore any deficits found when brain-lesioned children are compared with a control group would support the notion of persisting deficits of auditory comprehension.

Twenty-eight children with left hemisphere lesions and 25 with right hemisphere lesions were assessed using the Token Test 2 years post-onset (Vargha-Khadem *et al.*, 1985). A significant difference was found between the side of the lesion, with the children who had left hemisphere lesions performing more poorly than those with right-sided lesions. The Token Test scores did not correlate with the WISC-R digit span subtest score, leading the authors to conclude that this was a linguistic not a memory deficit. The scores of the children with right hemisphere lesions did not differ from the control group. Vargha-Khadem *et al.* (1985) also divided the side of lesion groups into three subgroups based on age at the time of the lesions, i.e. prenatal, early postnatal (2 months to 5 years) and late postnatal (5–14 years). There was a trend that the later the injury occurred the greater was the impairment of auditory comprehension.

Significant differences between the auditory comprehension skills of children with right and left hemisphere lesions were also found by Rankin *et al.* (1981). Lexical comprehension measured using the PPVT showed that right hemiplegics performed more poorly than left hemiplegics. This pattern of performance was repeated on the measures of syntactic comprehension using the NWSST:Receptive (Lee, 1971) and the Token Test, i.e. the right hemiplegics performing less well than the left hemiplegics. A closer examination of the components of the Token Test showed that the left hemiplegics showed a progressive decline in correct scores across the five parts of the test while the right hemiplegics showed no errors in Part 1 of the Token Test but their performance deteriorated across Parts 2–4 with the increase in information load. The right hemiplegics, however, improved their performance on Part 5 which showed they did not have difficulty with syntactic complexity *per se*. This is in contrast to the findings of Cooper and Flowers (1987).

Aram *et al.* (1985) compared the comprehension skills of children with right and left unilateral brain lesions. Each group of brain-lesioned children was matched to an appropriate control group. Some children had acquired their brain lesions in the first few months of life while others were 18 months to 6 years of age at the time of the lesion. On the PPVT all left-lesioned children scored within the normal range but five of eight scored lower than their control subjects. Similarly, the right-lesioned subjects performed more poorly than their controls. As a group, the left-lesioned subjects performed higher than the right-lesioned subjects. On the NWSST:Receptive the left-lesioned subjects performed less well than their controls while there was no difference between the right-lesioned group and their controls.

In another study using the Revised Token Test (McNeil and Prescott, 1978), Aram and Ekelman (1987) assessed the effect of unilateral brain lesions on auditory comprehension skills. In addition they also assessed the effect of the site of lesion and the age at lesion onset on those skills. Seventeen children with left lesions and 11 children with right-sided unilateral lesions between 6 and 17 years of age were assessed. Significant differences between the right- and left-lesioned groups and their respective controls were found for all ten subtests of the revised Token Test. As a whole the left-lesioned group performed similarly to their controls on subtests one to three and subtest nine. In subtest ten the left-lesion group appeared to use a memory strategy to enable them to remember the instructions. Aram and Ekelman (1987) concluded that the left-lesioned group presented with memory difficulties which affected their performance as the information load increased. The right-lesioned group, however, made more errors than their controls but there was no difference in the number of errors with the increase in information or linguistic loading. The authors suggested that this reflected the more impulsive nature of the right-lesioned group. In relation to site of lesion, there was a trend for more errors on the Token Test in the children with left retro-Rolandic rather than pre-Rolandic lesions. No difference in performance was noted in the site of the right hemisphere lesions or the presence or absence of subcortical lesions. In general, the earlier the left hemisphere lesions occurred (i.e. less than 1 year of age) the poorer the performance on the Revised Token Test. The reverse was true, however, for right hemisphere lesions. The results for the left hemisphere lesions were in contrast to the results of Vargha-Khadem *et al.* (1985) who found greater deficits the older the child was at the time of the lesion.

In conclusion, auditory comprehension deficits do exist in children with acquired aphasia, particularly when the brain-lesioned subjects are compared with a group of matched controls. These deficits, while of a subtle nature, occur even when the lesions are acquired at an early age. The extent of the comprehension impairment is variable, as is its recovery. The differences found between right and left hemisphere-lesioned subjects would suggest that side of lesion may influence the level and type of impairment. Further research into the aetiology of acquired aphasia is required to determine the influence of cause, size and site of lesion and time post-onset. Certainly, the evidence to date does not support the historical description of auditory comprehension deficits being rare and only of a transitory nature in children with acquired aphasia.

Production Deficits

Syntax

In the traditional description of acquired childhood aphasia, as mentioned previously, the aphasia was described as being of a non-fluent type with simplified syntax (Alajouanine and Lhermitte, 1965) or telegraphic speech (Guttmann, 1942), Alajouanine and Lhermitte (1965) noted that children with acquired aphasia tend to use simplified syntax rather than producing syntactical errors *per se*. Consequently, they stated that the syntax used by children with acquired aphasia does not resemble the agrammatism seen in adults. Despite the description of simplified syntax from the earliest reports (Bernhardht, 1885) few studies have given detailed descriptions of the syntax used by children with acquired aphasia.

Cooper and Flowers (1987) examined 15 brain-injured children who had acquired neurological damage between 2 and 12 years of age and were at least 1 year post-onset at the time of the study. As a group these brain-injured children scored significantly poorer than a matched control group on the Producing Formulated Sentences subtest of the CELF (Semel and Wiig, 1980). Cooper and Flowers (1987), however, observed a wide variety of language skills within the brain-injured group. Of the 15 subjects, only one achieved a score greater than two standard deviations below the test mean. By examining the case descriptions supplied by Cooper and Flowers (1987) it appears that most syntactical errors were made on the items which required complex sentence structures (i.e. 'because', 'if', 'herself'). Cooper and Flowers (1987) also provided examples of syntactically correct complex sentences produced by these same subjects. These correct sentences, however, tended to have a more stereotypic quality (e.g. 'If I tell you, do you promise to keep it a secret? I'll tell my parents about what has gone on at school. I will tell her I'm hungry'). Some acquired aphasia subjects produced agrammatical sentences (e.g. 'Himself and herself is a boy or is a gal'.) while others produced simple or incomplete sentences (e.g. 'Because today is rainy and wet') perhaps suggesting a semantic rather than syntactic impairment.

A series of studies by Aram and co-workers are the only ones reported which have systematically looked at productive syntactic skills in children with unilateral brain lesions. It should be noted, however, that most of Aram's subjects acquired brain lesions early in life, before they began talking. It was claimed by Aram and her co-workers that children who suffer left hemisphere lesions shortly after birth are at risk for syntactical impairment. Their reasons for this claim was the observation of significant differences between the syntactical abilities of appropriately matched controls and children with left hemisphere lesions and between children with either left or right hemisphere lesions.

Rankin *et al.* (1981) found three right hemiplegic children to be markedly below three left hemiplegic children on the NWSST. A later study by Aram *et al.* (1985) comparing eight children with right hemisphere lesions and eight with left hemisphere lesions and two appropriate control groups showed that the children with right hemisphere lesions did not differ from their controls on any syntactic measure except for mean length of utterance. The children with left hemisphere lesions, however, differed from their controls on all measures of syntactical skill including the NWSST and measures based on a spontaneous language sample (e.g. Mean Length of Utterance (MLU) and a Developmental Sentence Score (Lee, 1974)). Examination of individual scores of the children with left hemisphere lesions showed that no subject in this group scored higher than the 18th percentile on the NWSST:Expressive.

An extension of this study by Aram *et al.* (1986) undertook more detailed analyses of the spontaneous language samples by the eight left- and eight right-lesioned subjects. These analyses showed that the left hemisphere-lesioned subjects performed more poorly than their controls on most measures of simple and complex sentences while the right-lesioned group were similar to their controls in most measures of syntactical ability. The two lesioned groups differed from each other on measures of MLU, mean number of interrogative reversals and 'wh'- questions, the percentage of complex sentences attempted, the percentage of complex sentences correct, the number of embedded sentences attempted and the percentage of embedded sentences correct. The right-lesioned subjects differed from their controls on MLU, percentage of all sentences correct, the percentage of simple sentences correct, the total number of main verbs used, the mean number of negatives used and the grammatical markers in error (GME). The only syntactical measures on which the left-lesioned subjects did not differ from their controls were the total number of negatives used, and the use of pronouns or conjunctions. In addition it was noted that while the left-lesioned group performed more poorly than their controls on most measures of syntax, they did use more simple sentences reflecting their reduced use of complex sentences. Aram *et al.* (1986) suggested that these findings are indicative of a developmental immaturity on the part of the left-lesioned subjects. At the same time the right-lesion group produced a small percentage of their simple sentences correctly when compared with their controls, even though they attempted the same number of simple sentences. Both of these counts were different between the left-lesion group and their controls. The obviously poorer performance on the left-lesioned subjects when compared with their controls and when compared with the right-lesioned group and their controls is indicative of a susceptibility for expressive syntactic impairments in children with unilateral left hemisphere lesions.

Semantics

Two outstanding aspects of expressive semantics are commonly noted in the classical description of acquired childhood aphasia. The first of these is the presence and often persistence of naming disorders while the second is the absence or rarity of paraphasias, jargon and logorrhea. As Carrow-Woolfolk and Lynch (1982: 334) state 'once speech re-emerges children may have name-finding difficulties but they do not display the paraphasic or misnaming symptoms characteristic of adults'. (Receptive semantics has been discussed under comprehension.)

Naming disorders in children with acquired aphasia have been described by Hécaen (1983) as frequent and persistent, and are often noted in school reports. He found 15 of his 34 subjects with acquired aphasia (i.e. 44 per cent), between $3\frac{1}{2}$ and 15 years of age, to have naming disorders. No significant difference was found in the number of subjects with naming disorders when examined for site or cause of lesion or for the age of the subject. In an earlier study of 15 subjects, Hécaen (1976) found naming disorders in seven cases, three of which showed persistent problems.

Cooper and Flowers (1987) reported a significant difference between the scores achieved by children with acquired aphasia (between 10 and 18 years of age) and those achieved by a non-brain-damaged group on the Boston Naming Test (Kaplan *et al.*, 1976), including latency of response, and the Producing Word Associations subtest of the CELF. As their subjects were assessed between 3 and 12 years post-onset their findings support the fact that naming difficulties can be of a persistent nature in children with acquired aphasia.

Van Dongen and Visch-Brink (1988) also reported severe naming disorders in their six left hemisphere-lesioned children with acquired aphasia in the initial stages. The recovery from the naming disorder, however, differed between a head-injured group and a non-head-injured group. In the head-injured group recovery was complete within 6 months while the non-head-injured group could not complete a naming test 1 month post-onset and recovery was still not complete 1 year post-onset. Meanwhile six subjects with a right hemisphere lesion had scores on the Boston Naming Test within normal limits immediately post-onset. The complete recovery of naming abilities in the head-injured population is in contrast to the findings of Jordan *et al.* (1988, 1990) (see Ch.3).

Differences in naming abilities between subjects with right and left hemisphere lesions and control groups have been investigated by several other authors. Also using the Boston Naming Test, Kiessling, *et al.* (1983) found that the mean scores for their right and left brain-lesioned children were lower than those for a sibling control group.

This difference, however, was not statistically significant, neither was the difference between the Boston Naming Test scores achieved by children with right compared with left brain lesions. Two studies using the Oldfield and Wingfield Object Naming Test (Oldfield and Wingfield, 1964) did, however, find significant differences between controls and brain-lesioned children. Woods and Carey (1979) reported lower scores for children sustaining a left-sided brain lesion after 1 year of age when compared with a non-lesioned control group. Although a difference between children sustaining a brain lesion before 1 year of age, when compared with controls, was not found by Woods and Carey (1979), such a difference was found by Vargha-Khadem *et al.* (1985) who also used the Oldfield and Wingfield Naming Test. This difference was evident in Vargha-Khadem *et al.* (1985) prenatal, early postnatal (i.e. the lesion occurring between 2 months and 5 years of age) and late postnatal (i.e. 5–14 years of age) left hemisphere-lesioned groups as well as the early postnatal right hemisphere-lesioned group. The results of their study also indicated that the naming disorders were more marked the later the age at which the lesion occurred.

Rankin *et al.* (1981) compared the language abilities of three right and three left hemiplegic children between 6 and 8 years of age and found no differences between the two groups on the Naming Fluency subtest of the Boston Diagnostic Aphasia Examination (Goodglass and Kaplan, 1972). Two studies by Aram and co-workers, however, found slightly different results. Using the Expressive One-Word Picture Vocabulary Test (EOWPVT) (Gardner, 1979), Aram *et al.* (1985) found that both right and left hemisphere-lesioned children between 18 months and 8 years of age performed more poorly than their appropriate controls; however, this difference was only statistically significant for the left-lesioned subjects. Aram *et al.* (1985) noted the wide variation in individual scores in both the lesioned groups. A greater number of subjects with unilateral brain lesions ($n = 32$) between 6 and 17 years of age were assessed by Aram *et al.* (1987) to try to clarify the results of the previous studies. Two measures of lexical retrieval were used: the Word Finding Test (Wiegel-Crump and Dennis, 1984) and the Rapid Automatized Naming Test (RAN) (Denckla and Rudel, 1976). The results indicated that children with left hemisphere lesions required a longer latency to respond than their controls. The type of lexical access on the Word Finding Test affected the results. For example, rhyming cues produced more errors and longer latencies than semantic or visual cues, however, this was also the general pattern seen in children developing normally and the control groups used in the study. The left hemisphere-lesioned group were also slower to respond for the RAN, having greater difficulty naming objects and colours than letters and numbers. The right hemisphere-lesioned subjects, on the other hand, produced more errors than their controls but did not require a longer latency. In fact the right-lesioned group responded faster than their controls on all access conditions of the Word Finding Test. Aram *et al.* (1987) suggested that a speed-accuracy trade-off occurred with the right-lesioned group. In addition, the right hemisphere-lesioned subjects had more errors that could be attributed to visual processing difficulties. These results lead Aram *et al.* (1987) to postulate that left hemisphere-lesioned subjects have lexical retrieval problems while the errors seen in the right-lesioned group could be attributed to impulsivity or visual processing difficulties. Aram *et al.* (1987) also looked at the effects of lesion site and age at time of lesion on naming disorders and concluded that various sites of lesions in the left hemisphere can produce word access problems and that there was no clear relationship between degree of lexical retrieval impairment and age at lesion onset.

The second issue relating to expressive semantics arising out of the classical descriptions of acquired childhood aphasia is the absence or rarity of logorrhea, jargon and paraphasias. Generally this stems from the notion that the aphasia seen in children is of a non-fluent motor type. Several authors, however, have documented fluent aphasias in children (Van Dongen *et al.*, 1985; Van Hout *et al.*, 1985; Van Hout and Lyon, 1986; Visch-Brink and Van de Sandt-Koenderman, 1984). Initially it was felt that these fluent aphasias were only shown by children who had received their brain injury after 10 years of age (Alajouanine and Lhermitte, 1965; Guttmann, 1942).

Visch-Brink and Van de Sandt-Koenderman (1984) disputed the term 'rare' being applied to paraphasias shown by children with acquired aphasia. They approached the problem of rarity from two perspectives; first that paraphasias are not observed in many subjects with acquired childhood aphasia, and second that individual cases of children with acquired aphasia who do show paraphasias produce only a small number of these errors. Both uses of the term 'rare' did not apply to children with acquired aphasia they claimed. Visch-Brink and Van de Sandt-Koenderman (1984) pointed out that despite Guttmann's (1942) claim that paraphasias do not exist, two cases described in his article did show paraphasia. They also noted that Hécaen (1983), who had also described paraphasias as rare, had identified three children using paraphasias. In all cases, Hécaen claims the paraphasias resolved. The three children who did show paraphasias represented 8 per cent of the subjects with left hemisphere lesions. (It should be noted that the other aphasic symptoms described by Hécaen were present in 35–63 per cent of subjects.) There was no difference in the number of subjects showing paraphasias based on lesion site or cause, however, the paraphasias were only shown by children less than 10 years of age. Seven subjects showing phonemic paraphasias were present in Alajouanine and Lhermitte's (1965) study of 32 subjects. In contrast to Hécaen's group all these latter subjects were older than 10 years of age. No examples of logorrhea, verbal stereotypes or perseverations were noted in any subjects. These earlier reports of low incidence of paraphasia are in marked contrast to the findings of Van Hout *et al.* (1985) which showed positive semiology in all 11 subjects studied by them. (Five subjects had been previously excluded as they presented with non-fluent type of aphasia.) All 11 subjects examined by Van Hout *et al.* (1985) between 4 and 10 years of age showed verbal or phonemic paraphasias. In addition, perseverations and stereotypes were also frequently produced.

The types of paraphasic errors seen in children with acquired aphasia have been documented by several authors. For instance Cooper and Flowers (1987) noted the types of errors made on the Boston Naming Test by their subjects. Eight of 15 of their subjects scored more than two standard deviations below the mean on the test. Four of these subjects made semantically related, phonological or descriptive errors, one of them making comments about his difficulty in retrieving the words. Two other subjects made only semantically-related errors while another made phonological and descriptive errors. One subject with a left hemiplegia after anoxic encephalopathy also, at times, misinterpreted the picture (e.g. bat/paddle). As all these subjects were at least 2 years post-onset these errors would indicate persistent paraphasias. Other authors have also noted long-term paraphasic errors. In fact Van Hout *et al.* (1985) divided their 16 subjects between 2 and 13 years of age into three groups based on the rate of recovery of their paraphasias. In the first group recovery from paraphasias was noted within days. Initially the incidence of paraphasias was low (i.e. 3 per cent semantic paraphasias and 22 per cent phonemic). The resolution of the two types of paraphasias in the first group was either synchronous or the semantic ones disappeared before the phonemic. The second group whose paraphasias resolved within months of the brain lesion differed from the first group in that the two kinds of paraphasias did not resolve simultaneously, the semantic paraphasias always resolving first. Also this group was slightly older in age. The third group, whose paraphasias persisted, had a higher incidence of paraphasias (40 per cent) and the phonemic errors resolved before the semantic. The duration of the coma for this group also appeared longer and their comprehension skills were more severely affected.

Van Hout *et al.* (1985) also noted perseveration and stereotypes in their subjects with acquired aphasia. They further felt that the semiology of some of the child cases and the anatomical correlations appeared to be similar to those observed in adults. The major differences between child and adult cases were: first the rapid rate of recovery in most child cases, and second the development of negative symptoms (e.g. lack of spontaneity and the presence of naming difficulties which became more apparent as the positive signs of paraphasias decreased). Van Dongen and Visch-Brink (1988) also charted the resolution of the paraphasic errors in their head-injured and non-head-injured groups of aphasic children. For the head-injured group neologisms were always present on the Boston Naming Test in the acute stages. The neologisms decreased with every succeeding examination (up to approximately 18 days post-onset). This decline, however, was not evident for the literal or verbal paraphasias, although all errors had disappeared by 6 months post-onset. In contrast, for the non-head-injured group, one case never used neologisms and the distribution of neologisms and paraphasias were irregular over time. This low and irregular occurrence of paraphasias was despite a more severe form of aphasia than seen in the head-injured group.

Rapid recovery of paraphasias was also reported in a 9-year-old girl after a stroke (Dennis, 1980). At 2 weeks post-onset this subject showed phonemic and semantic paraphasias and some random misnamings on visual and tactile naming tasks placing her at an age equivalency of 6 years on the NCCEA (Gaddes and Crockett, 1975). Three months after the stroke, naming difficulties had resolved to a mild level of impairment. Similarly, encephalitis in a 10-year-old produced a Wernicke's aphasia (Van Hout and Lyon, 1986) with speech limited to a few stereotyped utterances 2 weeks post-onset. Three weeks after emergence from coma, 15 per cent of this latter subject's spontaneous speech consisted of neologisms. This rose to 45 per cent 10 days later. Meanwhile, verbal paraphasias were evident in 20–30 per cent and phonemic paraphasias in 3 per cent of his utterances. Van Hout and Lyon (1986) suggested that recovery, which showed an increase in semantic paraphasias and then the development of circumlocutory speech, was consistent with that described in cases of adult sensory aphasia (Buckingham and Kertesz, 1974).

There is considerable evidence, therefore, to suggest that naming difficulties do persist in children with acquired aphasia. Examples of fluent aphasia containing neologisms and paraphasias are also more common than first thought (e.g. paraphasias were observed in all of Van Hout *et al.*'s (1985) 11 subjects). The recovery from this fluent type of aphasia, however, can vary. It may resolve totally, paraphasias may persist, or as the paraphasias decrease there may be an increase in aspontaneity of speech and word-retrieval problems.

Many different reasons have been postulated, especially by Van Hout *et al.* (1985), for the inconsistency between the incidence of paraphasias in recent studies when compared with the traditional descriptions of acquired aphasia in childhood. One reason relates to the time after the lesion as paraphasias often resolve quickly (i.e. within days) and if the child is not assessed during that period paraphasias will not be noted. Second, since earlier reports based the presence of a brain lesion in children on the presence of a hemiplegia, an unusually high number of children with anterior lesions could have been described. Third, the method of assessment may affect the identification of paraphasias. If brain-injured children are reluctant to speak then paraphasic errors may only be elicited on formal assessments such as confrontation naming.

Pragmatics

To date, no study has systematically assessed the pragmatic skills of children with acquired aphasia. The reason for the lack of research in this area is partly historical in that pragmatics is an area of language that has only recently been recognized as an important area of research. A suggestion of the presence of pragmatic problems, however, can be gleaned from earlier writings which suggested that soon after the onset of aphasia or in connection with the mute phase, children with acquired aphasia are reluctant to communicate (see Historical Perspective). For instance, Cooper and Flowers (1987) noted that one of their subjects (10 years 3 months old) did not initiate any conversation and only rarely spoke during testing when assessed 6 years post-onset of anoxic encephalopathy.

Cooper and Flowers (1987: 259) also described one other child with acquired aphasia who had 'unusual or inappropriate usage of language'. This subject, a 15: 6-year-old male, often focused on inappropriate topics such as sex, bathrooms, marriage or death. Irrelevant statements on the above topics often occurred when he was attempting to respond to a task. This was the only subject studied by Cooper and Flowers (1987) who was intellectually impaired following encephalitis 11 years previously. Therefore, it is unclear in this case whether the observed pragmatic problem resulted from a linguistic deficit or whether it was a problem related to the presence of a broader cognitive impairment.

Dennis (1980) reported an in-depth study of a nine-year-old girl 3 months after she had acquired expressive and receptive aphasia with a right hemiparesis due to an arteriopathy of the left cerebral hemisphere. Her comprehension and expressive language skills were developing in parallel. At the time of testing she was still non-fluent but was able to produce and comprehend short sentences. It was noted that this subject often avoided speech situations. Through the use of puppets, Dennis was able to encourage this subject to tell three fairy tales which were subsequently analyzed using Mandler and Johnson's (1977) story grammar procedure. From this analysis it was noted that the subject used semantically impoverished and simplified propositions and also failed to include the various episodes of the story, just giving an overall view of the plot. Dennis (1980) stated that in story retelling younger children emphasize settings, motivation for and outcomes of actions. All of these components of the story, however, were omitted by Dennis's subject, indicating that she did not follow the normal developmental pattern for the acquisition of narrative abilities.

Phonology

Again the traditional description of acquired aphasia in children makes reference to the presence of concomitant speech disorders often in the form of a dysarthria or sometimes a dyspraxia (see Ch. 10).

A study by Rankin *et al.* (1981) comparing three right hemiplegic and three left hemiplegic subjects found no difference between the scores achieved by the two groups of subjects on the Templin Sound Discrimination Test (Templin, 1957) but the right hemiplegic group performed more poorly on the Templin–Darley Screening Test of Articulation (Templin and Darley, 1969). Most of the errors made were later developing sounds, thereby leading the authors to suggest that the speech disorder represented an articulation delay rather than dysarthria. The trend of more articulation disorders occurring in children with left unilateral brain lesions than right unilateral brain lesions was supported by Aram *et al.* (1985). They assessed eight left-lesioned and eight right-lesioned children and two groups of appropriate controls. While differences between the two lesioned groups and their appropriate controls were not significant, more children in the left-lesioned group were reported to have articulation scores greater than one standard deviation below the test mean on the Photo Articulation Test (PAT) (Pendergast *et al.*, 1969). Examination of the individual articulation profiles of all children in the study showed that the children with left hemisphere lesions also presented with the greatest number of individual articulation errors. While subject numbers used by Aram *et al.* (1985) were small and no significant differences were apparent their findings do suggest that the left hemisphere-lesioned group have more articulation errors than right-lesioned subjects. These speech errors reported by Rankin *et al.* (1981) and Aram *et al.* (1985) must be assumed to be articulation errors rather than speech errors associated with dysarthria or dyspraxia by the omission of such statements to the contrary in the two studies. The occurrence of articulatory/phonological disorders in left-lesioned subjects could be anticipated from the syntactic deficits also found in this group (see earlier this chapter) and the close association between syntactic and phonological disorders seen in children with developmental language impairment (Rapin and Allen, 1987; Wolfus *et al.*, 1980).

Written Language Impairments

Written language problems in children with acquired aphasia were described by Hécaen (1976) as the most frequent but the most variable of all aphasic symptoms seen in children in the acute stages. He also claimed that written language disorders tended to be the most persistent symptom, at times being of a permanent nature. He reported written language disabilities in 13 of his 15 subjects, seven of them having persistent problems. Similarly, Alajouanine and Lhermitte (1965) claimed that written language is always disturbed in the period soon after the brain injury is sustained. They found that written language disorders were often more severe than oral language impairments, and that expressive disorders were more frequent than receptive disorders of written language. Their longitudinal study (more than 12 months post-onset) of 32 children between 6 and 15 years of age showed that no subject could follow the normal school progression even though 23 of the 32 subjects were currently attending school. The most difficult subjects for the children with acquired aphasia were those involving language skills (e.g. history, English and foreign languages rather than mathematics). Despite their oral language skills being within normal limits, Alajouanine and Lhermitte's (1965) subjects were unable to learn new information. Byers and McLean (1962), however, attributed the poor academic performance seen in six of their ten subjects with acquired childhood aphasia to visuomotor and visuospatial impairments as all the children's language skills had spontaneously improved. Recently Cooper and Flowers (1987) assessed the academic performance of 15 brain-injured subjects between 10 and 18 years of age, 3–12 years post-onset and found the majority of subjects to be experiencing academic difficulties. Seven of the 15 subjects were in full-time special education programmes, three were receiving additional resource instruction, while of the remaining five in regular classrooms, only one was at a state school in an age-appropriate grade. The academic assessments used by Cooper and Flowers (1987) were the Wide Range Abilities Test (WRAT) (Jastak and Jastak, 1965) for Reading Recognition, Spelling and Arithmetic and the Peabody Individual Achievement Test (PIAT) (Dunn and Markwardt, 1970) for Reading Comprehension.

In contrast to Alajouanine and Lhermitte (1965), the subjects examined by Cooper and Flowers (1987) had most difficulty with the arithmetic subtest. Thirteen of the 14 subjects given the arithmetic subtest scored more than one standard deviation below the test mean, while eight scored below the test mean on spelling, five on reading comprehension and three on reading recognition. Only one subject scored below the test mean on all four academic areas and he was the only subject in the study who had cognitive skills within the intellectual handicapped range. Approximately equal numbers of subjects had impairments in one, two or three of the academic areas assessed. No descriptions of the nature of the arithmetical or reading difficulties experienced by these subjects were given by Cooper and Flowers (1987); however, six subjects with spelling difficulties made phonetic errors while one subject (following a left cerebrovascular accident) had difficulties with phoneme-grapheme relationships. Hécaen (1983) had also noted acalculia as a major symptom often associated with language impairments in children with acquired aphasia. Recent reviews (e.g. Zubrick, 1988) have emphasized the relationships between linguistic and mathematical skills, which may provide an explanation for the findings of Cooper and Flowers (1987) and Hécaen (1983).

In Hécaen's (1983) study of 56 children aged between $3\frac{1}{2}$ and 15 years of age he found writing disorders to be the most frequent language disorder, occurring in 63 per cent of the 34 subjects with left hemisphere lesions. Reading problems, however, were only evident in 40 per cent of the subjects with left hemisphere lesions. Hécaen (1983) further investigated the relationship between the number of subjects presenting with reading or writing disorders and the cause, localization of the brain injury and the age of the subject. No significant differences were found for reading disorders but a higher number of subjects under 10 years of age had writing problems (i.e. 90 per cent) than those over 10 years (45 per cent). Hécaen (1983) noted that reading disorders tend to be very common in the early stages post-onset but then tend to disappear rapidly and completely, while writing disorders may persist.

Alajouanine and Lhermitte (1965) also noted the difference in written language disorders relating to the age of the subjects. All subjects less than 10 years of age presented with severe writing impairments. Although 10 subjects (of 23) over 10 years of age had written language comprehension problems, only three of the 10 had severe impairments. Ten subjects also had writing disorders but only four had jargon orthography. Alajouanine and Lhermitte (1965) went on to describe the nature of the written language disorders and their recovery. Eighteen of their 32 subjects presented with alexia (i.e. being totally unable to read letters, syllables or words), a further five subjects could read but had severe difficulties, while a further four subjects could read words but not letters. The authors noted the difference between these reading problems and those seen in adults, with only four subjects (all over 13 years of age) presenting with adult-type symptoms. The writing problems of the subjects examined by Alajouanine and Lhermitte (1965) showed a wide range of impairments, with some subjects displaying quite rapid recovery while others continued to have severe writing difficulties. Nineteen subjects presented with severe writing impairments in spontaneous writing, writing to dictation or copying. Eight further subjects were unable to copy, while a further five children were capable of dictation and spontaneous writing; however, their attempts showed a dysorthographia. These errors were generally of a phonetic nature. Another five subjects (all between 13 and 15 years of age) had jargon distortions in their written work. Six months later, half the 22 subjects assessed by Alajouanine and Lhermitte (1965) had shown improvement in their alexia while the other half still showed severe disorders in, or total lack of, reading. The recovery process seen in the subjects less than 10 years of age showed the reacquisition of written language skills that followed the normal developmental progression. Of the 22 subjects, five children who had initially had severe problems now had writing skills within normal limits while 14 still showed dysorthographia, but only seven of these cases were severe. Another three subjects had no written language abilities. In all cases, Alajouanine and Lhermitte (1965) noted that the written language skills were delayed when compared with the child's oral language skills. As noted earlier, none of these 32 subjects coped with normal school progression 12 months after their brain injury.

Similar variations in the nature of the reading and/or writing disturbances and their recovery have been noted by several other authors. Severe written language problems were described by Byers and McLean (1962) in their eight children with acquired aphasia. Immediately post-onset, when their medical condition had stabilized, none of the eight children could match names and objects or write simple words to dictation, although they could copy. All were able to write letters in alphabetical sequence or numbers in numerical sequence if the sequence was started. However, they could not write or recognize letters out of context nor could they write numbers such as one hundred and twenty-three (i.e. 123). Soon after onset, some subjects could read or write everything except difficult words while others could only spontaneously read a few familiar words. No explanation was given for the rapid recovery or non-recovery of particular subjects. Variability in this recovery process can be seen in individual case studies reported in the literature.

Reading impairments have been described in three of the 11 children (between 2 and 13 years of age) studied by Van Hout *et al.* (1985). One 9-year-old subject was totally unable to read and his writing consisted only of repetitive letters, while another subject had reading retardation as his major aphasic symptom. The third subject was described as paralexic in both reading and writing 1 year post-onset. Another two subjects were described as having writing disabilities (together with naming difficulties) 3 months post-onset. No further details about the nature of the written language problems were given.

Another 9-year-old subject described by Dennis (1980) presented with written language problems which quickly resolved. Two weeks after a cerebrovascular accident the subject was able to write names to objects, read names and sentences for meaning and write simple sentences to dictation; however, her impaired oral skills severely affected her reading skills, even to the point where the subject confused herself by reading instructions aloud. The poorer oral than written language skills are in contrast to those noted by Alajouanine and Lhermitte (1965). Three months post-onset, Dennis's (1980) subject achieved age-appropriate scores on subtests for oral reading of simple sentences, reading names and short sentences for meaning, visual-graphic naming and writing to dictation and copying. Generally Dennis felt that the subject's written language skills were relatively well preserved in contrast to her oral skills which were at the level of telegraphic utterances and comprehension of simple commands. This pattern of recovery is in contrast to the persisting problems with written language noted by Hécaen (1976, 1983).

Rapid recovery of written language skills was described as unusual by Van Hout and Lyon (1986) when they reported on a 10-year-old boy presenting with a Wernicke's aphasia after herpes simplex encephalitis. Six days after the coma the subject was only able to make perseverative attempts at writing. Two days later he was able to read words in isolation with rare literal substitutions, however, matching words to objects was not possible. The subject's ability to read text was adequate for four to six lines only, after which perseveration started to interfere. His speed of reading was high. He was unable to tell anything about what he had read and appeared unaware of his problems. One week later his oral reading/decoding skills were normal but comprehension of the text was poor. He was able to match objects to written words better than to oral words. When the subject encountered difficult passages he would comment on the orthographical features of the words (e.g. the subject said 'there is a /p/, one must say /sap/' when he was reading the word 'camp' (field)). His writing skills also showed rapid improvement. On day 6 after the coma he was only able to write simple over-learned words, however, there was perseveration of letters. Six days later he was able to write a few sentences to dictation with a few surface or grammatical errors. The legibility of his writing was good. His written naming was slightly better than his oral. In contrast to his written language skills his arithmetical abilities through the written mode was never impaired; however, he had problems writing numbers such as three hundred and four. As this was written 3-100-4, Van Hout and Lyon (1986) concluded that these errors were of a syntactical nature.

Three other children with fluent aphasia described by Van Dongen *et al.* (1985) showed evidence of written language problems. A nine-year-old suffering a haematoma was only able to read four words aloud immediately post-onset. No information was available for later stages. A ten-year-old showed rapid improvement in his writing to dictation skills following a craniotomy after a closed head injury. Previously his writing had contained numerous, paraphasias. Two months after craniotomy his only aphasic errors were spelling errors when he wrote to dictation. These errors persisted over 8 months but had resolved by 18 months after the injury. Another subject, an 11-year-old, also had normal school performance 18 months after the closed head injury; immediately after the injury, she was able only to write simple words. Her reading initially was unintelligible because of neologisms.

Case studies reported in the literature also describe written language problems associated with subcortical lesions in children. Ferro *et al.* (1982) described literal errors in reading 46 days after a right subcortical infarct in a 6-year-old left-handed child. Writing showed spatial dysgraphia and poor handwriting skills. Another subject who presented with oral language deficits and written language problems following a subcortical cerebrovascular accident was reported by Aram *et al.* (1983). Six and a half months after the accident this 7-year-old was achieving at a level one grade lower than her age-equivalent in spelling and written language. Her reading comprehension, word attack and mathematical skills, however, were age-appropriate even though she had missed several months of schooling.

Therefore, like oral language skills, varying degrees of written language impairment are seen in children with acquired aphasia and individual cases show individual patterns of deficit and recovery. As a group, however, it would appear that these deficits are more severe in children under 10 years of age (Alajouanine and Lhermitte, 1965; Hécaen, 1976, 1983) and that school performance is affected by the persistent nature of written language and mathematical difficulties (Alajouanine and Lhermitte, 1965; Byers and McLean, 1962; Cooper and Flowers, 1987; Hécaen, 1976, 1983).

Prognosis of Acquired Childhood Aphasia

A variety of opinions have been expressed in the literature on the prognosis for recovery from acquired childhood aphasia. These opinions range from declarations of complete recovery or near complete recovery (Alajouanine and Lhermitte, 1965) to more guarded predictions of only partial recovery, when the influence of other factors such as site and extent of lesion are taken into account. For many years it has been generally accepted that one of the major differences between acquired childhood aphasia and adult aphasia is the more rapid and complete recovery of language function in children (Carrow-Woolfolk and Lynch, 1982; Lenneberg, 1967), the excellent recovery of language in children frequently being cited as indicative of the 'plasticity' of the immature brain. Some authors (e.g. Van Hout *et al.*, 1985), however, do not agree with the assertion that children recover more completely and rapidly than adults. Woods and Carey (1979) for instance went as far as to state that any child over the age of 1 year who receives an aphasia-producing lesion in the left hemisphere is likely to have their performance on verbal tasks permanently impaired. Hécaen (1983) also recommended caution before concluding that complete recovery is to be expected in cases of acquired childhood aphasia.

One reason for the controversy is that many authors, when describing the recovery of language function in children with acquired aphasia, make reference only to 'clinical recovery'. Despite apparent 'clinical recovery', however, some authors suggest that subtle language deficits may persist in the long-term, even in cases where the injury to the left hemisphere occurred at an early age (Alajouanine and Lhermitte, 1965; Rankin *et al.*, 1981; Vargha-Khadem *et al.*, 1985).

The literature relating to the prognosis of acquired childhood aphasia was reviewed by Satz and Bullard-Bates (1981). They concluded that although the majority of children with this condition showed spontaneous recovery, it by no means occurs in all cases. In 25–50 per cent of the cases they reviewed in the studies remained unremitted 1 year post-onset. A recovery period extending up to 5 years in cases of acquired childhood aphasia was suggested by Carrow-Woolfolk and Lynch (1982). Importantly, even in those cases where recovery is reported to occur, serious cognitive and academic difficulties often remain and a majority of children with acquired childhood aphasia, even after apparent recovery, have difficulty following a normal progression through school (Chadwick, 1985; Hécaen, 1976; Satz and Bullard-Bates, 1981). According to Alajouanine and Lhermitte (1965), these children find school subjects requiring the use of language (first language study, foreign languages, history, geography, etc.) more difficult than subjects such as mathematics.

A number of different theories have been proposed to explain the mechanism of recovery in children with acquired aphasia. As indicated earlier, the often-reported good recovery shown by children with acquired aphasia is taken by some investigators as indicating the 'plasticity' of the immature brain whereby language function is assumed by non-damaged areas of the brain, including the non-damaged portions of the left hemisphere and/or the intact right cerebral hemisphere. Alajouanine and Lhermitte (1965) believed that a child's brain has anatomical-functional plasticity such that the neural networks of the injured hemisphere and more so of the sound hemisphere take part in a new functional organization to compensate for the damaged area. Van Hout *et al.* (1985) also suggested that the plasticity of the young brain probably accounts for the rapid disappearance in some cases of the positive signs of aphasia. The authors, however, were of the opinion that the process is limited when the lesion is located in the left temporal lobe and some additional right hemisphere damage impedes the right hemisphere taking over the language functions. As evidence against the theory of transfer of language function, Satz and Bullard-Bates (1981) suggested that the speed of recovery sometimes witnessed in children with acquired aphasia is incompatible with a transfer of language to and the learning of language by the right hemisphere.

Another theory proposed to explain the difference in the prognosis of aphasia in children and adults is what Zangwill (1960) called the 'equipotentiality hypothesis'. According to this theory, at birth each cerebral hemisphere has the same potential to develop language function and that speech and language functions are progressively lateralized and cerebral dominance established as the child matures (Lennenberg, 1967). If the equipotentiality hypothesis is true, it could be expected that aphasia would occur more commonly in children with right cerebral lesions than adults with right cerebral lesions. In recent years, however, support for the equipotentiality hypothesis has declined in that several studies have shown that the frequency of aphasia from right cerebral lesions in right-handed children is similar to that in right-handed adults (Carter *et al.*, 1982; Satz and Bullard-Bates, 1981).

One explanation for the good recovery shown by some children with acquired aphasia is that favoured by some authors and known as the 'displacement phenomenon' (Satz and Bullard-Bates, 1981). According to this theory both cerebral hemispheres contain mechanisms for language. Consequently the right hemisphere (minor hemisphere) has for a time the capacity to subserve speech and language function if the left (dominant) hemisphere is damaged in early life. It is proposed that under normal circumstances the language mechanisms in the right hemisphere are inhibited by those in the left such that only the left hemisphere develops complex language function. When the left hemisphere is damaged, however, the right hemisphere is released from inhibition, allowing it to assume a greater role in language function. The critical period for this release may be only up to 2–4 years of age.

A number of different factors have been identified by various authors that may influence the prognosis of acquired childhood aphasia. These factors include: the site of lesion, the size and side of lesion, the cause, the associated neurological disturbances, the age at onset, the type and severity of the aphasia, and the presence of electroencephalographic abnormalities. The wide diversity of causes, severities of aphasia and length of follow-up in the various studies of acquired childhood aphasia, make it difficult to determine which of these factors are the most important in determining the final outcome of the aphasia (Van Dongen and Loonen, 1977).

The factor most frequently implicated as influencing the prognosis of acquired childhood aphasia is the age at onset. A number of authors have claimed that the prognosis of aquired aphasia becomes poorer as the age at onset increases (Carrow-Woolfolk and Lynch, 1982; Lenneberg, 1967; Penfield, 1965; Vargha-Khadem *et al.*, 1985). It has been stated that any aphasia incurred after the age of puberty does not recover entirely (Lenneberg, 1967). Oelschlaeger and Scarborough (1976) considered the upper limit for complete language recovery following cerebral damage to be 10 years of age, cerebral lesions incurred after that time causing a persistent language deficit. Likewise, Penfield (1965) believed that children under 10 years of age with acquired aphasia have a good chance of re-acquiring their lost verbal skills within 1 year of injury, even though such recovery may occur at the expense of other non-verbal skills. These suggestions are based on an unconfirmed premise that by 10 years of age, cerebral plasticity is lost as a result of the development of cerebral dominance or lateralized specialization of language function.

In contrast to the support provided by the above studies that age at onset is an important prognostic determinant in acquired childhood aphasia, Hécaen (1976) reported three cases of children who showed excellent recovery from acquired aphasia even though the onset occurred at 14 years of age. Further, Alajouanine and Lhermitte (1965) were unable to find a significant difference in the speed of recovery exhibited by a group of acquired aphasic children less than 10 years of age and a similar group greater than 10 years of age. Similarly, no direct relationship between the age at onset and the rate of disappearance of paraphasic errors in children with acquired aphasia could be demonstrated by Van Hout *et al.* (1985). In view of the contradictory nature of the data presented in the literature, it appears that, as yet, the relationship between age at onset and recovery in acquired childhood aphasia is uncertain.

The type of aphasia shown by children in the acute stage post-onset has also been reported to be of prognostic significance (Assal and Campiche, 1973; Guttman, 1942; Van Dongen and Loonen, 1977). Mixed aphasia has been reported to have a poor prognosis (Assal and Campiche, 1973; Van Dongen and Loonen, 1977) while a purely motor aphasia has been reported to have a good prognosis (Guttmann, 1942). Five of six children with an initial amnesic aphasia were observed by Van Dongen and Loonen (1977) to show good recovery.

In relation to causation, children with acquired aphasia resulting from head trauma have been reported to have a better prognosis for recovery than those with vascular disease (Guttmann, 1942). In contrast, consistent with the destructive nature of lesions associated with infectious disorders (e.g. herpes simplex encephalitis), infections have been linked to the occurrence of severe aphasias and persistent language problems (Van Hout *et al.*, 1985). The prognosis for recovery from acquired aphasia associated with convulsive disorder has been reported to be much worse than for other acquired childhood aphasias (Miller *et al.*, 1984).

Several authors (Alajouanine and Lhermitte, 1965; Hécaen, 1976, 1983) have suggested that the persistence of aphasic symptoms in children with acquired aphasia is linked to the extent of the cerebral lesion, the larger the cerebral lesion the poorer the prognosis for recovery. Hécaen (1983) found bilateral lesions to be frequently linked with persistent aphasic symptoms. Likewise, Van Hout *et al.* (1985) reported that the acquired aphasic children in their sample who exhibited the most severe and persistent aphasic disorder all had bilateral brain lesions. Other authors, including Collignon *et al.* (1968) and Gloning and Hift (1970), have also stressed that severe bilateral lesions are indicative of a poor prognosis for recovery in acquired childhood aphasia. Although based primarily on the findings of studies published before the 1940s it was for many years believed that there was a higher incidence of aphasia following right cerebral lesions in children than in adults, more recent studies have shown that the frequency of aphasia from right cerebral hemisphere lesions in right-handed children is similar to that in right-handed adults (Carter *et al.*, 1982; Satz and Bullard-Bates, 1981).

The localization of the cerebral lesion has also been implicated as a factor that influences recovery from acquired childhood aphasia. In fact, it has been suggested that the localization of the lesion is a more important prognostic variable than the extent of the lesion (Van Hout *et al.*, 1985). Although Alajouanine and Lhermitte (1965) suggested a relationship between lesion localization and recovery, they did not cite any specific examples to illustrate how the site of the cerebral damage influences the prognosis for recovery.

Contradictory findings have been reported in the literature on the importance of concomitant neurological signs as a prognostic indicator in acquired childhood aphasia. Lange-Cosack and Tepfner (1973) reported minimal or no recovery in traumatic aphasic subjects who had suffered coma for more than 7 days. Hécaen (1976), however, questioned the importance of coma as a prognostic indicator in children with acquired aphasia, because he was unable to demonstrate a clear relationship between the occurrence and duration of coma and the severity and persistence of the language deficit.

Controversy also surrounds the relationship between changes in the electro-encephalographic pattern and recovery in children with acquired aphasia associated with convulsive disorder. While some authors (Shoumaker *et al.*, 1974; Van Dongen and Loonen, 1977) have found that recovery correlates with a disappearance of abnormalities in the electroencephalographic trace, others have been unable to demonstrate ·a link between improved encephalographic patterns and improved language (Gascon *et al.*, 1973; McKinney and McGreal, 1974).

In summary, although a number of different factors have been suggested as having an influence on the recovery of language in children with acquired aphasia, insufficient information is currently available to say which of these factors are definitely indicative of either a good or poor prognosis.

Linguistic Characteristics of Acquired Childhood Aphasia Associated with Specific Causes

In the past, little attention has been paid to the nature of the specific linguistic impairments shown by children with acquired aphasia resulting from different causes. The nature of the linguistic disturbance associated with three major causes of acquired childhood aphasia, namely cerebrovascular disorders, hemidecortication and convulsive disorder (Landau–Kleffner syndrome) are discussed below. Linguistic disturbances associated with other causes of childhood aphasia are discussed in subsequent chapters.

Cerebrovascular Disorders

The only studies that have specifically looked at the linguistic impairments in children who have suffered cerebrovascular disorders are those conducted by Aram and co-workers. These studies form part of a longitudinal project being carried out to determine the linguistic, cognitive and academic effects of unilateral brain lesions of vascular origin. To date, 25 left-lesioned and 15 right-lesioned subjects have been included in Aram's project.

Left hemisphere lesions

Aram and her co-workers have found that children with unilateral left hemisphere lesions, when compared with a non-lesioned control group, have longer latency times and more errors on lexical retrieval tasks (Aram *et al.*, 1987), more errors on most measures of syntactical abilities, both receptively and expressively (Aram *et al.*, 1985, 1986), and more errors on the Revised Token Test (Aram *et al.*, 1987), which appeared to be more related to a poor memory for the increasing information load than to the increased linguistic complexity. In a recent study, Aram *et al.* (under review, b) also found a quantitative and qualitative difference in the number of dysfluencies produced by children with left hemisphere lesions compared with controls matched for age, sex and socio-economic status. In particular, the children with left lesions produced more non-fluencies, which appeared to be due to an increase in the number of stuttering-type non-fluencies. The left hemisphere-lesioned subjects also had a slower rate of speech than their controls, which the authors postulated may be related to the longer latency required by these subjects on word-retrieval tasks.

Overall despite the above noted significantly poorer performance by their subjects with left unilateral brain lesions, Aram and co-workers have stressed the good performance of these subjects on most linguistic tasks. As predicted from the literature, few of these subjects continued to have clinical signs of aphasia 1 year post-onset and performed within normal limits on most of the language tests used in these studies. For example, only one of the left-lesioned subjects reached the level of non-fluencies (i.e 10 per cent) needed to be classified a stutterer, while another two subjects fitted the classification of 'ambiguous' (Adams, 1980). All the remaining 17 left-lesioned subjects had less than 2 per cent non-fluencies. This good prognosis, however, does not appear to hold if there are ongoing seizures or if the brain damage is bilateral.

Trauner and Mannino (1986) also reported a good prognosis for their ten subjects who had a focal cerebrovascular lesion in the neonatal period. They stated that cerebrovascular accidents in the neonatal period are increasingly diagnosed, especially if the presenting symptom is seizures. Aram (1988) also noted a high frequency of cerebrovascular accidents associated with congenital heart disorders in her prelinguistic subjects. Only one of the ten subjects studied by Trauner and Mannino (1986) showed a mild motor and intellectual delay. Four subjects continued to have seizures, while two (including the mildly delayed subject) presented with microcephaly and one had a mild spasticity in the right leg. Trauner and Mannino therefore concluded that children who suffer neonatal cerebrovascular accidents have a relatively favourable prognosis for normal development, but warned that it was possible for these subjects to present with subtle learning disabilities and attentional or cognitive deficits in the long-term which may affect their academic success. Such long-term problems have also been identified by Aram and co-workers in their left hemisphere-lesioned subjects.

Half of the 20 subjects with left hemisphere lesions studied by Aram and Ekelman (1988a) showed difficulties at school as measured by delayed entry to school, grade repetition, special class placement or need for special academic tutoring. Subsequent assessments have failed to satisfactorily identify the reason for these educational difficulties. The 20 subjects were assessed using the Woodcock–Johnson Psycho-Educational Battery: tests of Cognitive Ability and Achievement (Woodcock and Johnson, 1977). Significantly poorer scores were obtained by the left-lesioned subjects than their controls on all clusters except Verbal on Cognitive Ability, all clusters except Knowledge on Scholastic Aptitude, and the Written Language cluster of the Tests of Academic Achievement. Despite the significantly poorer results obtained by all the left-lesioned subjects in these areas, again their overall performance was better than expected from someone having suffered a brain lesion and from what their educational history might indicate. While neither age at time of lesion nor site of lesion (i.e. pre- or retro-Rolandic) appeared to account for differences in linguistic performance, the division between cortical and subcortical involvement in the lesion did account for the differences.

A similar distinction between subjects with left cortical and subcortical lesions could be made based on the results of spelling and reading assessments (Aram *et al.*, 1989, under review, a). Generally, no significant difference was found between left-lesioned subjects and their controls on multivariate results for any of the five reading or spelling domains assessed despite the lesioned subjects scoring more than ten percentiles below the mean of their controls. Univariate results did indicate a significantly poorer performance by the left-lesioned subjects on the total reading comprehension and the inferential reading comprehension scores. Again group performance indicated a high level of performance by the children with unilateral left lesions. Analysis of individual subject scores, however, identified five subjects who had clinical reading or spelling problems. These included children with left subcortical lesions.

In the five children with reading and spelling difficulties of clinical significance one subject had a strong family history of reading difficulties while another had had a mild phonological-syntactical language disorder before his cerebrovascular accident at 6 years of age. This latter subject presented with a global language and reading disorder. Since the collection of the data, magnetic resonance imaging (MRI) also has shown this subject to have bilateral brain damage, including a small white matter lesion in the right frontal lobe which had not been detected previously by a computed tomographic (CT) scan. It is interesting to note that this subject was also the only child examined by Aram and co-workers who still presented with clinical signs of aphasia 1 year after the lesion, and had a marked verbal-performance IQ discrepancy (i.e. VIQ = 79, PIQ = 118). Other subjects with clinical reading and spelling problems also presented with language and verbal memory problems. The language disorders were a moderate global language deficit with a mild dysarthria, and a word-retrieval difficulty associated with a stuttering disorder. There was a trend that suggested the older the child (i.e. the more reading was established) at the time of the lesion the more specific was the resultant reading disorder.

This still leaves six subjects who had been identified as having academic problems who did not present with clinically significant reading disorders. The assessment of mathematical abilities is presently underway, which may identify some of the other under-achieving students.

Memory deficits specific to verbal stimuli and in particular the retrieval of verbal stimuli have been found in this group of left-lesioned subjects which may also account for academic failure (Aram *et al.*, 1988). In addition to the 11 of 20 left-lesioned subjects identified by Aram and Ekelman (1988a) as having educational difficulties, there were two subjects who had been honours students before their lesion and were now average in their performance and one other student who, although he was coping adequately at school and performed within normal limits on the assessments used in the study, had marked spelling difficulties. Therefore, while left unilateral brain lesions without ongoing seizures result in good recovery of linguistic skills, there is data to suggest a poor academic prognosis. The presenting academic difficulties may range from not achieving at pre-lesion potential to marked reading and/or spelling disorders of clinical significance. This appears to be more likely if the lesion includes the subcortical region.

The nature of the language disorders presenting in children with left hemisphere lesions of vascular origin have been documented in a number of case studies. In the acute stages these have included comprehension impairment, neologisms, paraphasias, mutism, non-fluent telegraphic style, difficulties on repetition tasks, reading and writing impairments, naming difficulties, dysarthria, oral dyspraxia, poor metalinguistic judgements of grammatical and agrammatical sentences, and simplified story grammar (Aram *et al.*, 1983; Cranberg *et al.*, 1987 (cases 3–8); Cooper and

Flowers, 1987 (cases 6, 8 and 16); Dennis, 1980; Ferro *et al.*, 1982; Van Dongen and Visch-Brink, 1988 (case 4); Van Hout *et al.*, 1985 (case 1)).

In most cases the clinical signs of aphasia resolved usually within 10 months of the lesion (Aram *et al.*, 1983; Cranberg *et al.*, 1987; Ferro *et al.*, 1982). The long-term problems that do remain include word-retrieval problems (Aram *et al.*, 1987; Cranberg *et al.*, 1987; Van Dongen and Visch-Brink, 1988), difficulty with comprehension of complex syntactic relationships (Cooper and Flowers, 1987; Cranberg *et al.*, 1987) and difficulty producing complex grammatical constructions (Aram *et al.*, 1986; Cranberg *et al.*, 1987). Most of the subjects examined long-term, however, presented with academic difficulties (Aram and Ekelman, 1988a; Cooper and Flowers, 1987; Cranberg *et al.*, 1987).

The type of aphasia seen in the acute stage after a unilateral left vascular lesion was described by Cranberg *et al.* (1987) in terms of the aphasic syndromes used for the classification of adult subjects. They concluded that the focal lesions seen in five of the six subjects with vascular lesions produced the aphasia type expected from a similar lesion in an adult. One child with a posterior cortical lesion, however, displayed a non-fluent (Broca's) type aphasia instead of the fluent aphasia usually exhibited by adults with such lesions. While Cranberg *et al.* (1987) have demonstrated that in the majority of cases the underlying pathology produced similar clinical pictures to adult aphasics in the acute phase, recent studies by Aram and co-workers have shown that the mechanisms underlying the rapid recovery process seen in children with unilateral lesions may differ from those in adults.

Aram and Ekelman (1986) when studying the cognitive profiles of children with unilateral left hemisphere lesions did not find the typical pattern seen in adults where verbal IQ is lower following a left hemisphere lesion. Nor was the performance of the children with left unilateral lesions similar to either adults with left hemisphere lesions or children with developmental language disorders (Aram and Ekelman, 1988b) on the Tallal Repetition Task: a measurement of auditory temporal processing (Tallal *et al.*, 1985). The performance of the lesioned children was also dissimilar to that seen in adults on a probe-evoked potential procedure (Papanicolaou *et al.*, in press). Instead, the left hemisphere showed attenuation for the language tasks and the right hemisphere showed engagement in visuospatial tasks suggesting that the language recovery seen in children with brain lesions and further knowledge development involves intrahemispheric functional reorganization.

In summary, children with unilateral vascular lesions in the left hemisphere usually recover adequate language skills. Long-term problems, however, include difficulties with lexical retrieval, syntax and comprehension as measured on the Revised Token Test. The last area of deficit may be related to a memory deficit, though further research is required. While language skills may recover, a large percentage of children with left unilateral brain lesions have difficulty coping with school. The exact reasons for this still requires investigation.

Right hemisphere lesions

Similar to the children with left hemisphere lesions, children with unilateral right hemisphere lesions show difficulties with school progress. Aram and Ekelman (1988a) found six of their 11 right hemisphere-lesioned subjects showed poor school progress. Four of the children with academic difficulties had repeated a grade, three of these then going into a special placement. One other subject was in a special education placement while another received extra tutoring. As a group, the subjects with right hemisphere lesions performed more poorly than their controls on all the Cognitive, Academic, Achievement and Scholastic Aptitude clusters of the Woodcock–Johnson Psycho-Educational Battery (Woodcock and Johnson, 1977) except for the Verbal (Cognitive) cluster (Aram and Ekelman, 1988a). On measures of reading ability, multivariate analysis showed no difference between the controls and the children with right hemisphere lesions on any of the five spelling or reading domains. Two individual subjects, however, met the criteria specified by Aram *et al.* (under review, a) for a clinical reading disorder. One of these subjects had a family history of reading problems which would predispose him to difficulties. The other subject had a subcortical lesion. Five other right-lesioned subjects, however, had subcortical lesions and no reading and/or spelling disorders. Both children with problems had difficulty in the areas of reading comprehension, phonetic analysis and blending and one also had difficulty with spelling.

While language problems appear to account for some of the difficulties experienced at school by children with left hemisphere lesions (Aram *et al.*, 1989), this does not seem to be so in children with right hemisphere lesions, as they presented with relatively few linguistic deficits when compared with controls. Generally, children with right hemisphere lesions have presented with a short mean length of utterance, a higher number of non-fluencies and a poorer score for expressive and receptive vocabulary (Aram *et al.*, 1985, under review, b).

Other language deficits noted in children with right unilateral brain lesions, however, have been attributed to poor attention and impulsivity noted during testing sessions. These language deficits include those observed during their performance on the Revised Token Test, lexical retrieval tasks, and the poorer but not significantly different performance of the Tallal Repetition Task (Aram and Ekelman, 1987, 1988b; Aram *et al.*, 1986, 1987). Even a greater number of syntactical errors on simple sentences has been postulated to be related to impulsivity (Aram *et al.*, 1986).

This hypothesis relating poor performance to poor attention is supported by Voeller (1986). While Voeller did not stipulate the cause of the focal right hemisphere lesions in his experimental group the reported findings do support the hypotheses proposed by Aram and co-workers and indicate areas of pragmatic deficit which should be further investigated in children with right hemisphere lesions. Fourteen of the 15 subjects (93 per cent) examined by Voeller (1986) presented with an Attentional Deficit

Disorder (ADD) using the DSM-III criteria. This compares with 3–10 per cent for ADD seen in the normal school-age population. Nine of the subjects had atypical prosody described as high pitched with rapid rate, robot-like, or soft and low pitched. Six of these nine subjects also had a gesturing deficit (no more details were given). Teachers commented on lack of eye contact in most subjects. Thirteen subjects had poor peer relationships, seven of these were also described as insensitive while others presented as shy and withdrawn. Voeller (1986) assesssed the subject's ability to interpret the affective states of others using two tests devised by Tallman (unpublished thesis). In one test the subjects had to point to pictures of people expressing emotions (e.g. 'show me the child who is angry') while the other utilized a 20 word sample of speech which had been filtered so only the intonation patterns remained. Again the subjects had to identify the emotion, reflected by intonation. As a group, the subjects with right hemisphere lesions performed more poorly than their peers than would have been expected. Caution should be used when interpreting these conclusions relating to emotional responses as 8 of the 15 families reported a family history of emotional problems. The high incidence of ADD, however, together with the obvious pragmatic difficulties experienced by the children with right hemisphere lesions highlight areas requiring further research. In addition, 13 of the 15 subjects in the study conducted by Voeller (1986) were in special education placements or in private schools.

It appears therefore, that children with unilateral cerebrovascular disorders usually recover their linguistic abilities, although children with left hemisphere vascular lesions do show mild linguistic deficits when compared with appropriately matched controls, and children with right hemisphere vascular lesions often show attentional deficits. Vascular lesions in either hemisphere, however, are associated with a poor school performance.

Hemidecortication

The surgical removal of a total cerebral hemisphere (hemispherectomy) has occasionally been performed as treatment for various diseases of the brain (Basser, 1962; Smith, 1966). Most reported hemispherectomies have been performed in children with intractable epilepsy secondary to a severely damaged hemisphere.

Hemidecortication has been reported to have a vastly different effect on language skills depending on the age at which the surgery was performed. Gardner *et al.* (1955) reported little or no language impairment subsequent to the removal of the left cerebral cortex following infantile hemiplegia, while hemispherectomies for tumour in adult brains result in the loss of most expressive language skills. Some over-learned words including expletives or words of songs may be all that is retained (Smith, 1966). Two cases of dominant hemispherectomy after the development of tumours during adolescence have resulted in the loss of language skills somewhere between these two extremes. A 14-year-old boy, described by Hillier (1954), was said to have retained comprehension skills but to have lost less expressive language than is usually seen in adults after hemidecortication. His reading was also affected. He was unable to read words but could recognize individual letters.

The second case, a 12-year-old girl, had a tumour removed from her lateral ventricle at 8 years of age. Two years later, however, she had her dominant (left) hemisphere removed when the malignancy reappeared. Gott (1973) assessed this subject 2 years after the hemidecortication. At this time auditory comprehension was least affected. She achieved a verbal intelligence score of 70 on the Peabody Picture Vocabulary test (Dunn, 1965). (It should be noted that this subject had been a slow learner prior to the first occurrence of the tumour. She scored 55 on the WISC Verbal Intelligence Score when assessed by Gott (1973).) A memory impairment was postulated for some of her auditory comprehension difficulties as she could not respond to two or more instructions in a command, was unable to answer questions about a paragraph read to her, or remember a choice of five alternative answers provided for her. She was able to remember words of songs, however, and her singing was more fluent than her speech. Her expressive language consisted mainly of single words or short phrases. A score in the dull-normal range on the Vocabulary subtest of the WISC was reported but she had word retrieval problems and sometimes semantic paraphasias. A rhyming task, when she had to identify words rhyming with 'mat', was 100 per cent correct but on a task where she had to produce synonyms and antonyms less than 50 per cent were correct. Written language abilities were impaired when assessed at 12 years of age using the WRAT, and were equivalent to kindergarten level. Gott (1973: 1087) noted that her language skills did not 'represent just a low level of language development as seen in normal acquisition'.

Other studies assessing the language skills in children after hemispherectomy have compared linguistic abilities of right and left hemidecorticates. Basser (1962) compared groups of children who had right or left hemispherectomies and also those children who had sustained their brain lesion before or after the onset of language. Based on a review of 62 cases of hemispherectomy reported in the literature and an examination of 35 of his own hemispherectomy cases, Basser (1962) noted that the majority of hemidecorticates do not develop post-operative aphasia. He concluded that there was no difference in the language skills between left and right hemidecorticates nor was there any difference in language abilities depending on when the lesion occurred in relation to the onset of language.

The findings of a series of studies reported by Dennis and co-workers supported those of Basser (1962). They showed that most hemidecorticates do not develop post-operative aphasia, and that there is no difference between the language skills of right compared with left hemidecorticates when measured on gross assessments such as verbal intelligence scores and the clinical assessments that were available when Basser

(1962) published his findings. When more sensitive assessments of language were used by Dennis and her co-workers, however, differences between right and left hemidecorticates were observed. In all of Dennis' studies none of the subjects had clinical signs of aphasia.

Dennis and Kohn (1975) studied nine subjects between 8 and 28 years of age who had developed a hemiplegia during infancy. There were four right and five left hemidecorticates matched for age of onset of hemiplegia, age of onset of seizures, age at hemidecortication and level of verbal cognitive ability. The subjects were then assessed on an Active–Passive Comprehension of Syntax task. Active/passive affirmative or active/passive negative sentences were assessed. The left hemidecorticates had longer latencies when responding to the passive sentences. They also performed less well than the right hemidecorticates on the percentage correct for the negative passive sentences thereby indicating that the right hemisphere had more difficulty comprehending complex syntactical structures than the left hemisphere.

This finding was confirmed by Dennis and Whitaker (1976) when they carried out a comprehensive assessment of linguistic skills of three hemidecorticates (one right, two left) between 9 and 10 years of age. All three children had had one hemisphere removed before the onset of speech. Using a combination of standardized tests and experimental language assessments Dennis and Whitaker (1976) systematically assessed the various components of linguistic ability in the three children (i.e. auditory discrimination and articulation skills and receptive and expressive semantics and syntax). Even though the three hemidicorticates had not shown a language impairment when assessed using global measures such as verbal IQ or general conversational skills, an assessment using the Illinois Test of Psycholinguistic Abilities (ITPA) (Kirk *et al.*, 1968) indicated an average language delay of 18 months and Composite Psycholinguistic Age mean standard scores (ss) of 29.3, 30.9 and 31.3, which were at the lower limits of the normal range (test mean ss = 36 ± 6). Although all three subjects differed on what subtests were delayed, a pattern of impairment emerged in the right hemidecorticate that was not apparent in either of the two left hemidecorticates. This pattern comprised superior performance on the auditory subtest over the visual subtests on comprehension (reception), association and closure tasks, and a superior auditory memory than visual memory score. No difference was evident in the scaled scores for verbal or manual expression, though Dennis and Whitaker (1976) commented that the presence of a hemiplegia could have deflated the manual expression scores in all subjects.

No difference was found by Dennis and Whitaker (1976) between the performance of the single right hemidecorticate and the two left hemidecorticates on the Wepman Auditory Discrimination Test (Wepman, 1958), the Goldman–Fristoe–Woodcock Test of Auditory Discrimination (Goldman *et al.*, 1970) or the Goldman–Fristoe Test of Articulation (Goldman and Fristoe, 1969). As the performance of all three subjects was within the normal range and no difference was found between the two types of hemidecorticates it was believed by these researchers that phonological skills were not impaired by hemispherectomy and that phonology could be subserved by the right hemisphere as well as the left hemisphere. Similar findings were reported for the area of semantics. This had been assessed using the Peabody Picture Vocabulary Test (Dunn, 1965) and the subtests from Goodglass and Kaplan (1972) of Word Discrimination, Visual Confrontation Naming, Responsive Naming and Naming Fluency. A difference in performance, however, was noted between the two types of hemidecorticates on the tasks assessing syntactic skills. These tasks included the Test of Syntactic Comprehension (Parisi and Pizzamiglio, 1970), the Active-Passive Test (Dennis and Kohn, 1975), the Story Completion Test (Goodglass *et al.*, 1972), the Token Test (De Renzi and Vignolo, 1962) and experimental tasks on Semantic Anomalies and Syntactic Errors, and Sentence Repetition. Specifically, the left hemidecorticates had difficulty with comprehending auditory language dependent on syntactic structure, especially passive constructions, detecting and correcting syntactic errors, producing appropriate tag questions and replacing missing pronouns by integrating semantic and syntactic information, judging word relationships in sentences, and repeating stylistically permutated sentences. Dennis and Whitaker (1976) claimed that the isolated right hemisphere appeared to have difficulties with the organizational, analytical, syntactical and hierarchical areas of language, and as such, the observed linguistic deficits could not be regarded as a general developmental retardation of language skills. Furthermore, the two left hemidecorticate subjects did not perform identically on some of the language assessments. In particular, their performance differed on those tasks relating to auditory memory and the comprehension of passive sentences.

Consequently Dennis and Whitaker (1976) concluded that gross measures of language (e.g. verbal IQ scores or Composite Psycholinguistic Ages on the ITPA) do not differentiate between left and right hemidecorticates, nor do assessments of phonology or semantics. Syntactic skills and patterns of performance on the ITPA subtests, however, do. The isolated right hemisphere, however, appears to develop a number of different processing strategies for coping with the more analytical and hierarchical aspects of language.

The superiority of the left hemisphere in dealing with certain aspects of language has also been demonstrated in relation to written as well as oral language skills (Dennis *et al.*, 1981). In general terms Dennis *et al.* (1981) found left hemidecorticates to be superior in writing skills and in their ability to learn logographic names. The left hemidecorticates did, however, show deficits in blending and segmenting words, applying phonotactic and morphophenomic rules and reading prose. The only right hemidecorticate subject examined by these workers was better at decoding written material accurately, was a more fluent reader, retained more meaning of what he had read and therefore had better reading comprehension than the left hemidecorticates. In addition, when reading errors were made by the right decorticate, the errors were less likely to violate syntactical or semantic rules. Dennis *et al.* (1981) described their right hemicorticate subject as having a 'generative' system which allowed the reading and spelling of unfamiliar words and a faster rate of comprehension. The system, however, became disrupted if textual constraints were removed. Again, Dennis *et al.* (1981) commented on the differing performance between the two left hemidecordicates signifying a less uniform representation of language skills within the right hemisphere.

Therefore, studies into hemicorticates have shown that if the lesion and/or hemispherectomy occurs early in the child's life the isolated right hemisphere is able to sustain language as well as the left. This is particularly true if the linguistic ability is measured on gross assessments such as clinical signs, verbal IQ measures or composite language scores such as those from the ITPA. Language assessments which are aimed at taxing the linguistic system, however, indicate superior performance on syntactical but not phonological or semantic tasks by the left hemisphere. Similarly, the left hemisphere is better able to handle the language aspects of written language such as the use of rules for reading and spelling unfamiliar words and the use of textual cues whereas the right hemisphere is better able to deal with the visuospatial aspects of written language.

Convulsive Disorder (Landau–Kleffner Syndrome)

The Landau–Kleffner syndrome is a subtype of acquired childhood aphasia associated with characteristic paroxysmal electroencephalographic (EEG) recording of spikes and spike-wave complexes. From the first report by Landau and Kleffner (1957), it has been observed to occur both with and without seizures. This type of acquired aphasia is of particular interest to speech and language clinicians because it combines two elements of language development not commonly seen in clinics, that is, a moderate to severe comprehension deficit, while cognitive functions remain intact, and regression of language skills.

Since Landau and Kleffner's (1957) article over 100 cases have been reported in the literature. The characteristics of these children have been reviewed by Beaumanoir (1985), Bishop (1985) and Miller *et al.* (1984), the results of which are outlined below. In most subjects normal hearing and neurological functioning other than EEG abnormalities were found (see Holmes *et al.*, 1981; Rodriguez and Niedermeyer, 1982; Shoumaker *et al.*, 1974 for details of EEG recordings). Seizures were noted in approximately 30 per cent of the cases reviewed; however, no seizures were reported after 15 years of age. A family history of epilepsy was present in 12 per cent of the cases who had seizures but in only 5 per cent of those cases not exhibiting seizures. The initial presenting symptoms of the Landau–Kleffner syndrome differed amongst subjects. Forty-three per cent of cases had seizures before the regression of language skills while in 16 per cent of cases they co-occurred. Aphasic symptoms were present

6 months to 2 years before the occurrence of seizures in 41 per cent of cases.

The onset of the language regression and the recovery of language skills is variable in children with the Landau–Kleffner syndrome. Twenty-five per cent of cases show a gradual onset of the language regression. The regression takes place over a period of more than 6 months. Beaumanoir (1985) reported 18 per cent of cases where the aphasia developed in stages. In the remaining cases, the language regression may occur within hours or days. Often language performance is variable during the periods of rapid language regression. As the period of onset of aphasic symptoms is variable, so is the pattern of language recovery. The language deficit may last from days to years, some children recover completely, while others show a progressive deterioration of language skills. Beaumanoir (1985) reported relapses of language deficits in 76 per cent of cases. Miller *et al.* (1984), however, reported recurring or persistent communication deficits for periods longer than 6 months in 94 per cent of cases. The relationship between the recovery of language skills, changes in EEG recordings and seizures, however, is still unclear. Therefore predicting which children will recover completely their language skills without language intervention cannot be reliably based on changes in EEG data. One prognostic factor, however, emerged from the review of cases by Bishop (1985). That factor was age of onset. Children less than 5 years of age at the time of onset showed a very poor prognosis.

Subgroups of the Landau–Kleffner syndrome

The variability in rate of onset, presence of seizures and recovery prompted Deonna *et al.* (1977) to state that the Landau–Kleffner syndrome is not a homogeneous syndrome. From their own cases and a review of the literature they proposed three subgroups of Landau–Kleffner syndrome. The first group they felt was similar to the cases of epileptic aphasia described in the adult population. The children in this group showed rapid deterioration of language skills or fluctuating performance usually associated with seizures. Likewise the recovery of language in this group is rapid. The second group showed progressive aphasic symptoms after a seizure or repeated episodes of aphasia. Recovery in this group may take months or years. The third group is made up of children who gradually develop marked auditory comprehension deficits. This group has no or few seizures. Deonna *et al.* (1977) noted variable rates and degrees of recovery of language skills in this last group. The differences in onset and recovery of language skills lead them to postulate different mechanisms underlying the aphasic symptoms for the three groups.

Miller *et al.* (1984), however, noted that the recovery of language skills in each of Deonna *et al.*'s groups was still variable and as such their groupings of cases with the Landau–Kleffner syndrome could not be used to predict language recovery. Instead they proposed another method of grouping children with the Landau–Kleffner syndrome based on their language profiles collected over a 2-year period. Again three subgroups emerged. The first group consisted of two children, aged 6;10 and 11;8 years who presented with complete loss of auditory comprehension and expressive language abilities after a period of normal language development. Seizures were present. Non-verbal cognitive functioning was age appropriate. Their ability to discriminate linguistic stimuli and their performance on auditory comprehension tasks was at chance levels. Some ability to discriminate non-speech sounds was evident until these sounds were a less familiar form. This performance on auditory task lead Miller *et al.* (1984) to diagnose a verbal auditory agnosia. No improvement in auditory comprehension was observed over the 2-year follow-up. Better performance on comprehension tasks, however, was noted in both children when signs, gestures, comprehension strategies and written language were used. Expressive language was very restricted on initial assessment in both cases. After 18 months, the 6-year-old subject was using one to two word utterances with good intelligibility. The 11-year-old subject, however, showed little change over a 2-year period. His expressive language consisted of consonant vowel combinations and his voice quality was similar to that of a deaf child. In addition, some apraxic-like movements of the articulators was noted on the production of isolated phonemes.

The second subgroup described by Miller *et al.* (1984) presented with variable comprehension abilities, delayed expressive language and a word finding problem. These children had also had normal language development prior to onset. They also presented with seizures. Receptive language was described as variable because the children responded to the same words or strings of words differently from moment to moment. Particular difficulty was noted in processing conversational speech. Expressive language impairments were demonstrated to be similar to those seen in children with developmental language disorders. Miller *et al.* (1984) reported that this group of children with the Landau–Kleffner syndrome were able to function in a normal educational setting, though spelling and reading problems were encountered. If speech and language skills improved, however, this improvement was rapid.

The third subgroup of children with the Landau–Kleffner syndrome described by Miller *et al.* (1984) never had a history of normal language development. Two of the cases described did not show a regression of language skills. Both of these children presented with language deficits similar to those described above in the second subgroup. In one of these cases a cognitive delay was also present. The third case belonging to this third subgroup did show language regression at 4 years of age. At this stage the subject's language development was delayed, being at a two to three word level. In association with seizures this child's receptive and expressive language as well as cognitive skills regressed to below the 1-year level. The language skills were similar to those described in the children with verbal auditory agnosia (i.e. the first subgroup described above) except that cognitive skills were also affected. Children with the Landau–Kleffner syndrome who have never had a normal language history have also been described by Rapin *et al*. (1977) and Maccario *et al*. (1982) leading to the notion of a developmental form of the syndrome. Therefore, whether based on the onset or recovery of aphasic symptoms or the linguistic profiles shown by children with the Landau–Kleffner syndrome it is clear that a range of speech and language skills are present in this population.

Comprehension deficits

All children diagnosed as having the Landau–Kleffner syndrome show both receptive and expressive language deficits. In some cases the loss of receptive language skills precedes the loss of expressive language. In its most severe form, the comprehension deficit is a verbal auditory agnosia and in some cases even includes an agnosia of non-speech sounds, while in its mild forms the comprehension deficit may cause difficulty in processing spontaneous speech. Cooper and Ferry (1978) found 42 per cent of their subjects had a severe comprehension deficit, 24 per cent had a moderate to mild comprehension impairment while the other 34 per cent recovered their receptive language abilities. One major difficulty in assessing comprehension skills in children with the Landau–Kleffner syndrome is the fluctuating performance of some of these children from day to day or even within one session.

The underlying deficit thought to underlie the difficulties with comprehending is a phonological decoding deficit, i.e. the child has difficulty at the phonemic identification and discrimination levels (Denes *et al*., 1986; Pearce and Darwish, 1984; Rapin *et al*., 1977). The poorer prognosis for children who have not learned language (i.e. those under 5 years of age) is offered as support for a phonemic decoding deficit (Bishop, 1985). The fact that children with the Landau–Kleffner syndrome perform on a comprehension test like hearing-impaired children and not like normal control or children with a developmental expressive language disorder is also presented as evidence for a deficit at the phonemic discrimination level (Bishop, 1982). The comprehension deficits noted in both the Landau–Kleffner and the hearing-impaired subjects were shown to occur whether the input was oral, signed or written. Bishop (1982) hypothesized that both groups of children fail to develop the hierarchical interpretation of sentences because they have had to learn language through a signing system which fosters a more sequential interpretation of sentence meaning.

Comprehension abilities in Landau–Kleffner syndrome cases have also been shown to improve if the rate of presentation is slowed. When the first instruction was presented at a slower rate but a second instruction was presented at a normal rate, both instructions were more readily comprehended. Campbell and McNeil (1985) explained this phenomena in terms of Kahneman's model of attention capacity which would indicate that children with the Landau-Kleffner syndrome may have difficulty decoding rapid speech because of an inefficient allocation of attention from a finite attentional capacity. More research is obviously required before a complete understanding of the comprehension deficits in children with the Landau–Kleffner syndrome and their recovery over time is forthcoming.

Expressive speech and language deficits

Again a wide range of expressive language abilities are seen in children with the Landau–Kleffner syndrome. In its most severe form children will present as mute or just using grunts. In its mildest form, however, the child may present as having a semantic-pragmatic deficit because comments or questions are not understood and inappropriate responses are made. Also related to comprehension difficulties are echolalia. When a child has had a period of normal language development, self-formulated expressive language can be in advance of receptive language skills after the onset of aphasia. For example, one case stated 'my daddy is a plumber'. However, when asked later in that session where her father worked or what he did, the child was unable to answer.

As stated earlier, word finding deficits and syntactic errors similar to those seen in children with developmental language disorders are also reported. Van de Sandt-Koenderman *et al.* (1984) also documented the occurrence of paraphasias in one child with the Landau–Kleffner syndrome. They showed that monitoring of neologisms gave an indication of the status of the child's language skills. During periods of language deterioration most paraphasias were neologisms while during the recovery phase neologisms were a minor part of the total paraphasias, and they quickly disappeared.

Voice quality changes have also been noted in children with the Landau–Kleffner syndrome. Some authors report a 'deaf-like' voice, while others note a high pitch. A case reported by Deonna *et al.* (1987) presented with only a prosodic disturbance after partial complex seizures. The prosodic features observed were marked slowness and irregularity with prolonged pauses and hesitations and lack of intonation and were not due to motor speech disorders or emotional disturbance. Therefore, what is predominantly a phonemic deficit presents as a wide range of expressive speech and language impairments.

Differential diagnosis

In many cases the differential diagnosis of Landau–Kleffner syndrome is difficult. Eighty per cent of children with the Landau–Kleffner syndrome have behavioural disturbances such as aggression, withdrawal, inattention, hyperactivity and temper outbursts. Organic bases and a reaction to sudden loss of comprehension have been put forward to explain these behavioural problems. Whatever the causes, these behaviours together with the loss of communication skills are often thought to reflect a psychiatric problem. Consequently the differential diagnosis of Landau–Kleffner syndrome is crucial. Sometimes the sudden loss of language skills are mistaken for elective mutism. Similarly the sudden or gradual loss of comprehension is often attributed to a hearing loss. The authors warn against using behavioural measures of audiological status because of the nature of the syndrome.

Any regression of language skills should be assessed by a neurologist for if the acquired aphasia is not due to any of the other causes of aphasia (e.g. tumours, vascular lesions, infections or head injury) an EEG is necessary for the diagnosis of Landau–Kleffner syndrome. The gradual regression of language skills makes the diagnosis of the syndrome particularly difficult as it takes longer to identify the loss of language skills and alternative explanations for the observed behaviour may be given. This is even more so if the aphasic symptoms precede seizures or if seizures are not present. Diagnosis is even more difficult in those cases where a period of normal language development was not present. Therefore it would seem important to get EEG information on any child who presents with a moderate to severe developmental receptive language disorder particularly if cognitive skills are age appropriate.

Speech and language management

The object of language intervention in children with the Landau–Kleffner syndrome is to bypass the phonemic decoding deficit by using alternative methods to access the language skills which are still preserved. For children with severe deficits placement in special classes for either the language disordered or the hearing impaired is important to provide a signing environment. Using the visual system either through signing or written language also helps children with less severe impairments. Bishop (1982), however, warns that signing is not to be considered as a 'panacea' for children with the Landau–Kleffner syndrome for the reasons stated earlier. Children who do not have oral language skills still learn to read. The phonic approach to reading, however, is to be avoided in preference for the whole word approach. Some children with the Landau–Kleffner syndrome, however, present only with written language deficits. Therefore the type of speech and language intervention will depend on the child's age at onset and therefore the language skills already developed and the extent of recovery.

Comparison of Acquired and Developmental Language Disorders

Several authors (Basser, 1962; Byers and McLean, 1962) have noted that the recovery of language skills in children after a cerebral insult or injury follows the normal development pattern. In some instances, children with acquired aphasia will make a very rapid recovery and appear to skip developmental stages. Clinicians often comment on this rapid return of language skills in the acute stages especially if the child is not seen for a few days, for example over the weekend. On Friday the child may have a restricted vocabulary of a few words but by the clinician's return on Monday the child may be using complete simple sentences. The recovery path for other children may be at a steady pace through each developmental stage, while other children may make minimal recovery and/or be left with residual problems.

The following discussion, comparing the linguistic deficits observed in children with acquired aphasia and those observed in children with developmental language disorders, will address first, the linguistic skills observed in children with acquired aphasia in the acute stage, second, the mild linguistic deficits observed after language abilities appear to recover and last, those language skills which remain impaired after a brain lesion. In this comparison the developmental language disorder being referred to is one of specific language impairment without the complicating factors of intellectual handicap, hearing impairment or emotional disturbance.

In the acute stages, the mutism commented upon by a number of authors (Alajouanine and Lhermitte, 1965; Branco-Lefèvre, 1950; Guttmann, 1942; Hécean, 1976, 1983), particularly when it is followed by a reluctance to use language skills which have returned, is not seen as commonly in children with developmental language problems. Generally children with developmental language disorders will use gesture to enhance their communications skills unless there are elements of elective mutism or the child has poor self-esteem.

Another aspect of recovering language skills observed in acquired childhood aphasia is the presence of paraphasias (Van Dongen *et al.*, 1985; Van Hout *et al.*, 1985; Van Hout and Lyon, 1986; Visch-Brink and Van de Sandt-Koenderman, 1984). This is also a linguistic symptom which is rarely seen in the initial stages of a developmental disorder as the children generally do not have the vocabulary in their lexicon from which to draw. The occurrence of the paraphasias seen in the acute stages of acquired childhood aphasia tends to decrease as recovery takes place. Van Hout *et al.* (1985) stated that the characteristics of fluent aphasia (i.e. verbal or phonemic paraphasias, perseverations, stereotypes and neologisms) are often replaced by characteristics of a non-fluent aphasia. In children with developmental language disorders it is unlikely that this pattern of change would occur. While longitudinal studies on children with developmental language impairment have only recently being published (Klee, 1987) it is more likely that either a fluent-type aphasia will remain in that form or that the reverse of the pattern of change described by Van Hout *et al.* (1985) occurs (i.e. as a child's syntactical problems resolve, word retrieval difficulties may become more prominent, causing the type of disorder observed to change from a telegraphic non-fluent type to a more fluent disorder characterized by paraphasias and circumlocutions). The only time a developmental disorder would equate to the change observed by Van Hout *et al.* (1985) would be in those few children who present with a large number of stereotypes, described by Crystal *et al.* (1982) as Pattern 10 on the Language Assessment, Remediation and Screening Procedure (LARSP) profile. In this case the change in linguistic type would be directly related to therapeutic intervention. Visch-Brink and Van de Sandt-Koenderman (1984), however, question the meaningfulness of the terms fluent and non-fluent when describing childhood language disorders.

The presence of neologisms in the acute stages of acquired childhood aphasia described by Van Hout *et al.* (1985) and Visch-Brink and Van de Sandt-Koenderman (1984) would be rarely seen in the spontaneous speech in children with developmental language disorders. It has been noted, however, in children who do not know a particular word and therefore do not have its phonological code in their repertoire. The appearance of neologisms in children with developmental language disorders is most commonly seen in the administration of an articulation test where the child does not know the target word, so it is supplied by the clinician and the child is required to repeat it. (This form of neologism differs from the jargon seen in children with poor comprehension skills.)

Those children with acquired aphasia who make an apparent recovery or whose lesion occurred before language onset have been shown to have mild but statistically significant language impairments in specific areas of linguistic abilities when, as a group, they are compared with a group of appropriately matched controls (Aram and Ekelman, 1987; Aram *et al.*, 1985, 1986, 1987; Cooper and Flowers, 1987; Vargha-Khadem *et al.*, 1985; Woods and Carey, 1979). In the recent study by Cooper and Flowers (1987) a group of subjects (between 10 and 18 years of age) who all had had a brain lesion after the onset of language was assessed on a battery of language and academic tests. The subjects were of mixed causes, lesion sites and time since onset. As a group, however, they performed significantly poorer on all the language and academic measures used. Eliminating all the subjects who were currently in full-time special education as they could not be considered as having recovered, we examined the individual scores and performances of the remaining eight subjects to determine the nature of the linguistic deficits present and how they compared with the linguistic deficits seen in children with developmental language impairments. A range of linguistic skills were impaired in this group of eight subjects, including receptive vocabulary (PPVT), expressive vocabulary (Boston Naming Test and Producing Word Associations subtest of the CELF), verbal comprehension (Token Test and Processing Spoken Paragraphs subtest of the CELF), and oral production of sentences (Producing Formulated Sentences subtest of the CELF). In all cases errors made were on the most difficult items of the test, in some cases they were items on which the controls also make errors. On the Boston Naming Test, errors were of the nature of semantically-related or phonetically-related words or descriptions of the target item. All these errors are those seen in children with developmental language impairments (Fried-Oken,

1983; German, 1979); however, the time taken to retrieve the word was longer in the brain-lesioned group as a whole than in the control group.

Subjects, meanwhile, who had unilateral brain lesions before as well as after the onset of language, were investigated in a series of studies by Aram and co-workers. For some language skills assessed in these studies, the children with brain lesions performed less well but in the same manner as their controls, while on other language tasks they appeared to have specific areas of deficit. Generally the poor performance was of a very subtle nature with the lesioned subjects performing within the normal range according to the test norms but below that of the control groups. One area of language where brain-lesioned subjects did perform lower than the test norms was expressive syntax (Aram *et al.*, 1985, 1986). In general, subjects with left hemisphere lesions performed less well than their controls on most measures of syntactic ability (i.e. Mean Length of Utterance, NWSST, Developmental Sentence Score (Lee, 1974) and other measures derived from a spontaneous language sample), while right hemisphere lesions only affected negative constructions and the number of errors in a simple sentence. Aram *et al.* (1986) stated, however, that the errors made by both right and left brain-lesioned subjects resembled those of developmentally younger children. Similar results were true for phonological skills (Aram *et al.*, 1985).

Slower response latency times were reported for left hemisphere-lesioned subjects on the Word Finding Test (Wiegel-Crump and Dennis, 1984) and the RAN indicating a specific word retrieval deficit in this group (Aram *et al.*, 1987). Error analysis on both tests showed that this group of subjects performed similar to their control group and to a group of normal children. This would indicate that the errors made were of a developmental nature, except for a high percentage of associative errors and the presence of unrelated and category-only responses on the Word Finding Test. Aram *et al.* (1987) noted that no category-specific or pronounced lexical retrieval deficits often seen in adult aphasics were evident. For the children with right hemisphere lesions the nature of the disorder appeared to be specific rather than developmental and to be non-linguistic in nature. Some right hemisphere-lesioned subjects made more errors and had shorter response latency times on the two vocabulary tests than their control subjects. This led Aram *et al.* (1987) to suggest a speed–accuracy trade off which they related to general impulsive behaviour. Error analysis showed developmental errors for all accessing conditions except the visual accessing condition on the Word Finding Test. This, together with longer latencies on the RAN, led the authors to propose visual processing difficulties for the subjects with right hemisphere lesions. This had previously been suggested by Aram *et al.* (1985) when the subjects with right hemisphere lesions performed poorly on the PPVT and the EOWPVT. The general impulsive behaviour seen on the Word Finding Test was also noted on the Revised Token Test (Aram and Ekelman, 1987). Mild problems with spatial linguistic concepts were also noted in the right-lesioned group.

Analysis of the errors made by the subjects with left lesions on the Revised Token

Test showed that their scores became progressively worse as the information load increased but improved in the final subtest which was the most linguistically complex. This pattern of errors and the fact that the left-lesioned group performed significantly below their controls on the WISC-R digit span subtest led Aram and Ekelman (1987) to propose that a memory deficit was affecting the scores of the subjects with left lesions. These identified deficits were in spite of all the lesioned subjects performing well on the Revised Token Test as a whole, and the authors suggesting that a more sensitive test may be required to detect auditory comprehension deficits in children with unilateral brain lesions.

Such a poor performance on the digit span subtest, however, was not found by Vargha-Kadem *et al.* (1985), nor was the pattern of errors of 16 left hemisphere-lesioned subjects the same as that observed by Aram *et al.* (1987). Rather, the subjects in Vargha-Kadem *et al.*'s (1985) study performed less well on the subtest with the greatest syntactical complexity. Similar results to this were found by Cooper and Flowers (1987) though their subjects had mixed lesion sides and may have included some with bilateral damage. Results on another test of comprehension, however, used by Cooper and Flowers (1987) would support Aram *et al.*'s (1987) claim of a memory deficit. Brain-lesioned subjects performed poorer than controls on the Processing Spoken Paragraphs subtest of the CELF. In all cases they appeared to understand the questions asked but could not remember the relevant information. While differences in either the subject population or the version of the Token Test used in each study could explain the difference in results described above, it is clear that whether or not children with brain lesions present with a linguistic deficit on the Token Test has not been resolved. If a linguistic deficit is postulated then it appears to be of a developmental nature as it was the subtest with the greatest linguistic difficulty which was most often in error. If a linguistic disorder is not present then the poorer performance by brain-lesioned subjects on the Token Test can be attributed to more cognitive factors such as a memory impairment in children with a left hemisphere lesion and poor attention in those with a right hemisphere lesion. Both of these behaviours are commonly seen in children with developmental language disorders, particularly those children and/or adolescents who present as developmentally language-learning disabled (Hallahan and Reeve, 1980; McKinney *et al.*, 1982; Tarver and Hallahan, 1974; Torgesen and Goldman, 1977).

A number of the problems observed long-term in children with acquired aphasia, whether they be children who have residual deficits or who apparently recover or who have written language deficits, are the same as those described by Simon (1985a,b), Wiig and Semel (1984) and Wallach and Butler (1984) in relation to language-learning disorders. Some of the problem areas that have been described in the literature on acquired aphasia include: word retrieval problems and therefore lack of specificity and accuracy (Aram *et al.*, 1987; Cooper and Flowers, 1987; Hécean, 1983; Vargha-Khadem *et al.*, 1985), syntactical/morphological errors (Aram *et al.*, 1985, 1986;

Cooper and Flowers, 1987; Woods and Carey, 1979), written language impairments (Alajouanine and Lhermitte, 1965; Cooper and Flowers, 1987; Hécean, 1983); arithmetical difficulties (Cooper and Flowers, 1987; Hécean, 1983), and problems with narratives (Dennis, 1980). Other problems encountered long-term in children with acquired aphasia that resemble difficulties seen in children with developmental language-learning disabilities have not yet appeared in the literature but are encountered by clinicians in their caseloads, for example, difficulties with verbal reasoning skills, processing large amounts of auditory information, understanding linguistically-based humour and sarcasm, monitoring discourse over a period of time, understanding figurative language, and critical to any remediation process and poor self esteem (see Ch. 2).

Case studies of children with acquired aphasia who continue to have severe deficits post-onset show a heterogeneous group of children where no commonalities exist. The literature on acquired aphasia notes that generally the aphasia type seen in children is non-fluent. While evidence exists that this is not the only type it still does appear to be the most common type of acquired aphasia. This would be in line with the subtypes of linguistic deficits seen in children with developmental language disorders, for while Rapin and Allen (1987), Aram and Nation (1983) and Bloom and Lahey (1978) all list six subtypes of developmental language disorders it is respectively the subtype of phonological-syntactic, non-specific formulation-repetition deficit, and the disorder of form which is the most common type seen. In all cases these various subtypes could be classified under the broad title of non-fluent.

Therefore, it can been seen that if linguistic deficits occur long-term in children with acquired aphasia then they will be developmental in nature. This is irrespective of the hemisphere which has the lesion. It can be seen that these long-term deficits in children with acquired aphasia fall into three categories. First, the nature of most linguistic deficits is a developmental immaturity (e.g. in the area of syntax), second, in some linguistic areas (e.g. word retrieval) a specific impairment is evident and third, the deficit may not be linguistic in nature (e.g. cognitive factors such as memory or attention deficits). Therefore, even though the last two categories of impairment may be classed as areas of specific deficit rather than a linguistic immaturity, they are impairments commonly seen in children with developmental language-learning disabilities. Therefore, for long-term deficits in children with acquired aphasia it would seem appropriate to use the assessment and remediation procedures used with children with developmental language disorders, especially those that have appeared recently and are being developed for children/adolescents with language-learning disabilities. Even children with severe residual deficits after a brain lesion can be assessed and treated using techniques developed for children with developmental impairments as the major therapy goal will be a functional communication system.

It will only be in the acute stages, therefore, that special assessment procedures may be required. Generally these may take the form of checklists based on developmental language assessments or assessments developed for adult cases of aphasia. Likewise, techniques developed for adult cases may be necessary in handling the concomitant problems seen in some children with acquired aphasia.

Summary

The long-held belief that acquired aphasia in children is primarily of the non-fluent type has been challenged in recent years by studies which have demonstrated that fluent aphasias can be observed in children if language examination is carried out in the early stages post-onset. In addition, it is apparent that children with acquired aphasia have a number of features in common with developmental language-learning disabilities, especially if the linguistic deficits persist long-term.

Although the literature is sparse on the specific linguistic skills of subgroups of acquired childhood aphasia based on causation, the evidence available indicates that the nature of the aphasia varies according to the specific underlying cause. Consequently, instead of describing the linguistic skills of groups of children with acquired aphasia resulting from different causes, as has occurred in the past, further research into the linguistic abilities of children with language disorders should be carried out with them grouped according to their specific pathology. Only then can the characteristics of acquired language disorders occurring in childhood be correctly elucidated. Language problems arising from cerebrovascular accidents occurring in childhood were discussed as part of the material presented in this chapter. A detailed discussion of the childhood linguistic deficits resulting from head injury, infections, cerebral anoxia, neural tube defects, brain tumours and metabolic disorders will be presented in the following chapters.

References

ADAMS, M. (1980) 'The young stutterer: diagnosis, treatments and assessment of progress', *Seminars in Speech, Language and Hearing*, **4**, pp. 289–99.

ADAMS, R. D., CAMMERMEYER, J. and DENNY-BROWN, D. (1949) 'Acute necrotizing hemorrhagic encephalopathy', *Journal of Neuropathology and Experimental Neurology*, **8**, pp. 1–29.

ADAMS, R. D. and LYON, G. (1982) *Neurology of Hereditary Metabolic Diseases of Children*, New York, McGraw-Hill.

ADAMS, J. H., MITCHELL, D. E., GRAHAM, O. T. and DOYLE, D. (1977) 'Diffuse brain damage of immediate impact type', *Brain*, **100**, pp. 489–502.

ALAJOUANINE, T. and LHERMITTE, F. (1965) 'Acquired aphasia in children', *Brain*, **88**, pp. 653–62.

ARAM, D. M. (1988) 'Language sequelae of unilateral brain lesions in children', in Plum, F. (Ed.) *Language Communication and the Brain*, New York, Raven Press.

ARAM, D. M. and EKELMAN, B. L. (1986) 'Cognitive profiles of children with early onset of unilateral lesions', *Developmental Neuropsychology*, **2**, pp. 155–72.

ARAM, D. M. and EKELMAN, B. L. (1987) 'Unilateral brain lesions in childhood: performance on the Revised Token Test', *Brain and Language*, **32**, pp. 137–58.

ARAM, D. M. and EKELMAN, B. L. (1988a) 'Scholastic aptitude and achievement among children with unilateral brain lesions', *Neuropsychologia*, **26**, pp. 903–16.

ARAM, D M. and EKELMAN, B. L.(1988b) 'Auditory temporal perception of children with left or right brain lesions', *Neuropsychologia*, **26**, pp. 931–5.

ARAM, D. M., EKELMAN, B. L. and FLETCHER, J. M. (1988) 'Verbal and non-verbal memory among children with left and right brain lesions', *Journal of Clinical and Experimental Neuropsychology*, **10**, pp. 18.

ARAM, D. M., EKELMAN, B. L. and GILLESPIE, L. L. (1989) 'Reading and lateralized brain lesions in children', in Von Euler, K. (Ed.) *Developmental Dyslexia and Dysphasia*, Hampshire, England, Macmillan Press.

ARAM, D. M., EKELMAN, B. L. and WHITAKER, H. A. (1986) 'Spoken syntax in children with acquired unilateral hemisphere lesions', *Brain and Language*, **27**, 75–100.

ARAM, D. M., EKELMAN, B. L. and WHITAKER, H. A. (1987) 'Lexical retrieval in left and right brain lesioned children', *Brain and Language*, **31**, pp. 61–87.

ARAM, D. M., GILLESPIE, L. L. and YAMASHITA, T. S. (under review, a) 'Reading among children with left and right brain lesions', *Developmental Neuropsychology*.

ARAM, D. M., MEYERS, S. C. and EKELMAN, B. L. (under review, b) 'Fluency of conversational speech in children with unilateral brain lesions', *Brain and Language*.

ARAM, D. M. and NATION, J. E. (1983) *Child Language Disorders*, St. Louis, C. V. Mosby.

ARAM, D. M., EKELMAN, B. L., ROSE, D. F. and WHITAKER, H. A. (1985) 'Verbal and cognitive sequelae following unilateral lesions acquired in early childhood', *Journal of Clinical and Experimental Neuropsychology*, **7**, pp. 55–78.

ARAM, D. M., ROSE, D. F., REKATE, H. L. and WHITAKER, H. A. (1983) 'Acquired capsular/striatal aphasia in childhood', *Archives of Neurology*, **40**, pp. 614–17.

ASSAL, G. and CAMPICHE, R. (1973) 'Aphasie et troubels du langage chez l'enfant après contusion cérébrale', *Neurochirurgie*, **19**, pp.399–406.

BANKER, B. Q. (1961) 'Cerebral vascular disease in infancy and childhood', *Journal of Neuropathology and Experimental Neurology*, **20**, 127–40.

BASSER, L. S. (1962) 'Hemiplegia of early onset and the faculty of speech with special reference to the effects of hemispherectomy', *Brain*, **85**, pp. 427–60.

BEAUMANOIR, A. (1985) 'The Landau–Kleffner Syndrome', in Roger, J. Dravat, C. Bureau, M. Dreifuss, F. E. and Wolf, P. (Eds) *Epileptic Syndromes in Infancy, Childhood and Adolescence*, John Libbey Eurotext.

BELL, R. D. and LASTIMOSA, A. C. B. (1980) 'Metabolic encephalopathies', in Rosenberg, R. N. (Ed.) *Neurology*, New York, Grune and Stratton, pp. 115–64.

BERNHARDT, M. (1885) 'Ueber die spastiche cerebralparalyse im kindersatter (hemiplegia spastica infantalis), nebst einem excurse uber: Aphasie bei kindern', *Archiv für Pathologische Anatomie und Physiologie und für Klinische Medecin*, **102**, pp. 26–80.

BERNHEIM, M. (1956) 'Thrombophlebitis cerebrales', *Annals of Paediatrics* (Basel), **187**, pp. 153–60.

BICKERSTAFF, E. R. (1964) 'Aetiology of acute hemiplegia in childhood', *British Medical Journal*, **2**, pp. 82–7.

BICKERSTAFF, E. R. (1972) 'Cerebrovascular disease in infancy and childhood', in Vinken P. J. and Bruyn, G. W. (Eds) *Handbook of Clinical Neurology: Vascular Diseases of the Nervous System Part II*, Amsterdam, North-Holland Publishing Company.

BISHOP, D. V. M. (1982) 'Comprehension of spoken, written and signed sentences in childhood language disorders', *Journal of Child Psychology and Psychiatry*, **23**, pp. 1–20.

BISHOP, D. V. M. (1985) 'Age of onset and outcome in 'acquired aphasia with convulsive disorder' (Landau–Kleffner Syndrome)', *Developmental Medicine and Child Neurology*, **27**, pp. 705–12.

BLOOM, L. and LAHEY, M. (1978) *Language Development and Language Disorders*, New York, John Wiley.

BRAIN, L. and WALTON, J. N. (1969) *Brain's Diseases of the Nervous System*, 7th ed., New York, Oxford University Press.

BRANCO-LEFÈVRE, A. F. (1950) 'Contribuicao para o estudo da psicopatologia da afasia en criancas', *Archivos Neuro-Psyquiatria* (San Paulo), **8**, pp. 345–93.

BRANDT, S. (1962) 'Causes and pathogenic mechanisms of acute hemiplegia in childhood', *Little Club Clinics in Developmental Medicine*, **6**, pp. 7–11.

BROADBENT, V. A., BARNES, N. D. and WHEELER, T. K. (1981) 'Medulloblastoma in childhood: Long-term results of treatment', *Cancer*, **48**, pp. 26–30.

BROWN, J. K. (1985) 'Dysarthria in children: Neurologic perspective', in Darby, J.K. (Ed.) *Speech and Language Evaluation in Neurology: Childhood Disorders*, New York, Grune and Stratton.

BUCKINGHAM, H. and KERTESZ, A. (1974) 'A linguistic analysis of fluent aphasia', *Brain and Language*, **1**, pp. 43–61.

BURNS, M. S. and BOYLE, M. (1984) 'Aphasia after successful radiation treatment: A report of two cases', *Journal of Speech and Hearing Disorders*, **19**, pp. 107–11.

BYERS, R. K. and MCLEAN, W. T. (1962) 'Etiology and course of certain hemiplegias with aphasia in childhood', *Pediatrics*, **29**, pp. 376–83.

CAMPBELL, T. F. and MCNEIL, M. R. (1985) 'Effects of presentation rate and divided attention of auditory comprehension in children with an acquired langue disorder', *Journal of Speech and Hearing Research*, **28**, pp. 513–20.

CARROW-WOOLFOLK, E. and LYNCH, J. (1982) *An Integrative Approach to Language Disorders in Children*, Orlando, Grune and Stratton.

CARTER, R. L., HOHENEGGER, M. K. and SATZ, P. (1982) 'Aphasia and speech organization in children', *Science*, **218**, pp. 797–9.

CHADWICK, O. (1985) 'Psychological sequelae of head injury in children', *Developmental Medicine and Child Neurology*, **27**, pp. 72–5.

CHI, J. G., DOOLING, E. C. and GILLES, F. H. (1977) 'Left-right asymmetries of the temporal speech areas of the human fetus', *Archives of Neurology*, **34**, pp. 346–8.

COLLIGNON, R., HECAEN, H. and ANGERLERQUES, G. (1968) 'A propos de 12 cas d'aphasie acquise chez l'enfant', *Acta Neurologie et Psychiatrica Belgica*, **68**, pp. 245–77.

COOPER, J. A. and FERRY, P. C. (1978) 'Acquired auditory verbal agnosia and seizures in childhood', *Journal of Speech and Hearing Disorders*, **43**, pp. 176–84.

COOPER, J. A. and FLOWERS, C. R. (1987) 'Children with a history of acquired aphasia: Residual language and academic impairments', *Journal of Speech and Hearing Disorders*, **52**, pp. 251–62.

CRANBERG, L. D., FILLEY, C. M., HART, E. J. and ALEXANDER, M. P. (1987) 'Acquired aphasia in children: Clinical and CT investigations', *Neurology*, **37**, pp. 1165–72.

CRYSTAL, D., FLETCHER, P. and GARMAN, M. (1982) *The Grammatical Analysis of Language Disability*, London, Edward Arnold.

CUNEO, H. N. and RAND, C. W. (1952) *Brain tumors of childhood*, Springfield, Charles C. Thomas.

DAVIE, J. C. and COX, W. (1967) 'Occlusive disease of the carotid artery in children', *Archives of Neurology*, **17**, pp. 313–23.

DELONG, G. R. and ADAMS, R. D. (1975) 'Clinical aspects of tumours of the posterior fossa in childhood', in Vinken P. J. and Bruyn G. W. (Eds) *Handbook of Clinical Neurology: Tumours of the Brain and Skull*, Amsterdam, North-Holland Publishing.

DENCKLA, M. B. (1979) 'Childhood learning disabilities', in Heilman, K. and Valenstein, E. (Eds), *Clinical Neuropsychology*, New York, Oxford University Press.

DENCKLA, M. B. and RUDEL, R. G. (1976) 'Naming of object drawings by dyslexic and other learning disabled children', *Brain and Language*, **3**, pp. 1–15.

DENES, G., BALLIELLO, S., VOLTERRA, V. and PELLEGRINI, A. (1986) 'Oral and written language in a case of childhood phonemic deafness', *Brain and Language*, **34**, pp. 252–67.

DENNIS, M. (1980) 'Strokes in childhood 1: Communicative intent, expression and comprehension after left hemisphere arteriopathy in a right-handed nine-year-old', in Reiber, R. W. (Ed.), *Language Development and Aphasia in Children*, New York, Academic Press.

DENNIS, M. and KOHN, B. (1975) 'Comprehension of syntax in infantile hemiplegics after cerebral hemidecortication: Left hemisphere superiority', *Brain and Language*, **2**, pp. 472–82.

DENNIS, M., LOVETT, M. and WIEGEL-CRUMP, C. A. (1981) 'Written language acquisition after left or right hemidecortication in infancy', *Brain and Language*, **12**, pp. 54–91.

DENNIS, M. and WHITAKER, H. A. (1976) 'Language acquisition following hemidecortication: Linguistic superiority of the left over the right hemisphere', *Brain and Language*, **3**, pp. 404–33.

DEONNA, T., BEAUMANOIR, A., GAILLARD, F. and ASSAL, G. (1977) 'Acquired aphasia in childhood with seizure disorder: A heterogeneous syndrome', *Neuropäediatric*, **8**, pp. 263–73.

DEONNA, T., CHEVRIE, C. and HORNUNG, E. (1987) 'Childhood epileptic speech disorder: Prolonged isolated deficit of prosodic features', *Developmental Medicine and Child Neurology*, **29**, pp. 96–109.

DE RENZI, E. and FAGLIONI, P. (1978) 'Normative data and screening power of a shortened version of the Token Test', *Cortex*, **14**, pp. 41–9.

DE RENZI, E. and VIGNOLO, L. A. (1962) 'The Token Test: A sensitive test to detect receptive disturbances in aphasics', *Brain*, **85**, pp. 665–78.

DUFFNER, P. K., COHEN, M. E. and THOMAS, P. R. M. (1983) 'Late effects of treatment on the intelligence of children with posterior fossa tumours', *Cancer*, **51**, pp. 233–7.

DUFFY, P. E., PORTNEY, B., MAURO, J. and WEHRLE, P. F. (1957) 'Acute infantile hemiplegia secondary to spontaneous carotid thrombosis', *Neurology*, **7**, pp. 664–6.

DUNN, L. M. (1965) *Peabody Picture Vocabulary Test*, Circle Pines, MN: American Guidance Service.

DUNN, L. M. and DUNN, L. M. (1981) *Peabody Picture Vocabulary Test-Revised*, Circle Pines, MN:, American Guidance Service.

DUNN, L. M. and MARKWARDT, F. (1970) *Peabody Individual Achievement Test*, Circle Pines, MN: American Guidance Service.

FERRO, J. M., MARTINS, I. P., PINTO, F. and CASTRO-CALDAS, A. (1982) 'Aphasia following right striato-insular infarction in a left handed child: A clinico-radiological study', *Developmental Medicine and Child Neurology*, **24** pp. 173–82.

FREUD, S. (1897) *Infantile Cerebral Paralysis* (trans. by L. A. RUSSIN, 1968), Coral Gables, University of Miami.

FRIED–OKEN, M. B. (1983) 'The development of naming skills in normal and language deficient children', Doctoral dissertation, Boston University Graduate School.

GADDES, W. H. and CROCKETT, D. J. (1975) 'The Spreen-Benton Aphasia Tests, normative data as a measure of normal language development', *Brain and Language* **2**, pp. 257–80.

GAIDOLFI, E. and VIGNOLO, L. A. (1980) 'Closed head injuries of school-age children: Neuropsychological sequelae in early adulthood', *Italian Journal of Neurological Science* **2**, pp. 65–73.

GALABURDA, A. M., LE MAY, M., KEMPER, T. L. and GESCHWIND, N. (1978) 'Right-left asymmetrics in the brain', *Science*, **199**, pp. 852–6.

GARDNER, M. (1979) *Expressive One-Word Picture Vocabulary Test*, Novato, CA: Academic Therapy Publications.

GARDNER, W. J., KARNOSH, L. J., McCLURE, C. C. and GARDNER, A. K. (1955) 'Residual function following hemispherectomy for tumour and for infantile hemiplegia', *Brain*, **78**, pp. 487–502.

GASCON, G., VICTOR, D., LOMBROSO, C. T. and GOODGLASS, H. (1973) 'Language disorder, convulsive disorder and electroencephalographic abnormalities', *Archives of Neurology*, **28**, pp. 156–62.

GERMAN, D. J. N. (1979) 'Word finding skills in children with learning disabilities', *Journal of Learning Disabilities*, **12**, pp. 176–81.

GJERRIS, F. (1978) 'Clinical aspects and long-term prognosis of infratentorial intracranial tumours in infancy and childhood', *Acta Neurologica Scandanavica*, **57**, pp. 31–52.

GLONING, K. and HIFT, E. (1970) 'Aphasie im vorschulalter', *Zeitschrift Nervenheilkunde*, **28**, pp. 20–8.

GOLDMAN, R. and FRISTOE, M. (1969) *Goldman–Fristoe Test of Articulation*, Circle Pines, MN: American Guidance Service.

GOLDMAN, R., FRISTOE, M. and WOODCOCK, R. W. (1970) *Goldman–Fristoe–Woodcock Test of Auditory Discrimination*, Circle Pines, MN: American Guidance Service.

GOLDSTEIN, S. L. and BURGESS, J. P. (1958) 'Spontaneous thrombosis of the internal carotid artery in a seven year old child', *American Journal of Disorders of Childhood*, **95**, pp. 538–40.

GOODGLASS, H., GLEASON, J. B., BERNHOLTZ, N. A. and HYDE, M. R. (1972) 'Some linguistic structures in the speech of a Broca's aphasic', *Cortex*, **8**, pp. 191–212.

GOODGLASS, H. and KAPLAN, E. (1972) *The Assessment of Aphasia and Related Disorders*, Philadelphia, Lea and Febiger.

GOTT, P. S. (1973) 'Language after dominant hemispherectomy', *Journal of Neurology, Neurosurgery and Psychiatry*, **36**, pp. 1082–8.

GUTTMANN, E. (1942) 'Aphasia in children', *Brain*, **65**, pp. 205–19.

HALLAHAN, D. and REEVE, R. (1980) 'Selective attention and distractability', in Keogh, B. K. (Ed.) *Advances in Special Education* Vol 1., Greenwich, CT:, J.A.I. Press, pp. 141–81.

HÉCAEN, H. (1976) 'Acquired aphasia in children and the otogenesis of hemispheric functional specialization', *Brain and Language*, **3**, pp. 114–34.

HÉCAEN, H. (1983) 'Acquired aphasia in children: Revisited', *Neuropsychologia*, **21**, pp. 581–7.

HILLIER, W. J. (1954) 'Total left cerebral hemispherectomy for malignant glioma', *Neurology*, **4**, pp. 718–21.

HISCOCK, M. and KINSBOURNE, M. (1978) 'Ontogony of cerebral dominance; evidence from time sharing asymmetry in children', *Developmental Psychology*, **14**, pp. 321–9.

HOLMES, G. L., MCKEEVER, M. and SAUNDERS, Z. (1981) 'Childhood aphasia and abnormal EEG', *Epilepsia*, **22**, pp. 631–9.

HUDSON, L. J., MURDOCH, B. E. and OZANNE, A. E. (1989) 'Posterior fossa tumours in childhood: Associated speech and language disorders post-surgery', *Aphasiology*, **3**, pp. 1–18.

JAMISON, D. L. and KAYE, H. H. (1974) 'Accidental head injury in children', *Archives of Diseases of Childhood*, **49**, pp. 376–81.

JASTAK, J. F. and JASTAK, S. R. (1965) *The Wide Range Achievement Test*, Wilmington, DE, Guidance Associates.

JORDAN, F. M. OZANNE, A. E. and MURDOCH, B. E. (1988) 'Long-term speech and language disorders subsequent to closed head injury in children', *Brain Injury*, **2**, pp. 179–85.

JORDAN, F. M., OZANNE, A. E. and MURDOCH B. E. (1990) 'Performance of closed head injury children on a naming task', *Brain Injury*, **4**, pp. 27–32.

KAPLAN, E., GOODLASS, H. and WEINTRAUB, S. (1976) *Boston Naming Test*, Boston VA Hospital.

KIESSLING, L. S. DENCKLA, M. B. and CARLTON, M. (1983) 'Evidence for differential hemispheric function in children with hemiplegic cerebral palsy', *Developmental Medicine and Child Neurology*, **25**, pp. 727–34.

KIRK, S., MCCARTHY, J. and KIRK, W. (1968) *The Illinois Test of Psycholinguistic Abilities*, Urbana, IL, University of Illinois Press.

KLEE, T. (1987) 'Grammatico-semantic development of language disordered children', paper presented at the First International Symposium of Specific Speech and Language Disorders in Children, Reading, UK, 29 March to 3 April.

LANDAU, W. M. and KLEFFNER F. R. (1957) 'Syndrome of acquired aphasia with convulsive disorder in children', *Neurology*, **10**, pp. 915–21.

LANGE–COSACK, H. and TEPFNER, G. (1973) '*Das Hirntrauma im kinder und jugendalter*', Berlin, Springer-Verlag.

LEE, L. (1971) *Northwestern Syntax Screening Test*, Evanston, IL, Northwestern University Press.

LEE, L. (1974) *Developmental Sentence Analysis*, Evanston, IL, Northwestern University Press.

LENNEBERG, E. (1967) *Biological Foundations of Language*, New York, Wiley.

LEVIN, H.S., BENTON, A.L. and GROSSMAN, R.G. (1982) *Neurobehavioural Consequences of Closed Head Injury*, New York, Oxford University Press.

MACCARIO, M., HEFFEREN, S.J., KEBLUSEK, S.J. and LIPINSKI, K.A. (1982) 'Developmental dysphasia and electroencephalographic abnormalities', *Developmental Medicine and Child Neurology*, **24**, pp. 141–55.

MCCARTHY, J.J. (1963) 'Clinical diagnosis and treatment of aphasia: Aphasia in children', in Osgoon, C.E. and Miron, M.S. (Eds) *Approaches to the Study of Aphasia*, Urbana, University of Illinois Press.

MCKINNEY, J.D., MCCLURE, S. and FEAGANS, L. (1982) 'Classroom behaviour of learning disabled children', *Learning Disability Quarterly*, **5**, pp. 305–11.

MCKINNEY, W. and MCGREAL, D.A. (1974) 'An aphasic syndrome in children', *Canadian Medical Association Journal*, **110**, pp. 637–9.

MCNEIL, M.R. and PRESCOTT, T.E. (1978) *Revised Token Test*, Austin TX, Pro-Ed.

MANDLER, J.M. and JOHNSON, N.S. (1977) 'Rememberance of things passed: story structure and recall', *Cognitive Psychology*, **9**, pp. 111–51.

MATSON, D.D. (1956) 'Cerebellar astrocytoma in childhood', *Pediatrics*, **18**, pp. 150–8.

MATSON, D.D. (1969) *Neurosurgery of Infancy and Childhood*, Springfield, Charles C. Thomas.

MEADOWS, A.T., MASSARI, D.J. FERGUSSON, J., GORDON, J., LITTMAN, P. and MOSS, K. (1981) 'Decline in IQ scores and cognitive dysfunctions in children with acute lymphocytic leukaemia treated with cranial irradiation', *Lancet*, **ii**, pp. 1015–18.

MILLER, J.F., CAMPBELL, T.F., CHAPMAN, R.S. and WEISMER, S.E. (1984) 'Language behaviour in acquired aphasia', in Holland, A. (Ed.) *Language Disorders in Children*, Baltimore, College-Hill Press.

MOLFESE, D.L., FREEMAN, R.B. and PALERMO, D.S. (1975) 'The ontology of brain lateralization for speech and non-speech stimuli', *Brain and Language*, **2**, pp. 356–68.

MOOSY, J. (1959) 'Development of cerebral arteriosclerosis in various age groups', *Neurology*, **9**, pp. 569–74.

MOYES, C.D. (1980) 'Epidemiology of serious head injuries in childhood', *Child Care, Health and Development*, **6**, pp. 1–9.

MSALL, M., SHAPIRO, B., BALFOUR, P.B., NIEDERMEYER, E. and CAPUTE, A.J. (1986) 'Acquired epileptic aphasia: Diagnostic aspects of progressive language loss in preschool children', *Neurology*, **25**, pp. 248–51.

NORMAN, R.M. (1962) 'Neuropathological findings in acute hemiplegia in childhood', *Little Clubs Clinics in Developmental Medicine*, **6**, pp. 37–48.

OELSCHLAEGER, M.L. and SCARBOROUGH, J. (1976) 'Traumatic aphasia in children: A case study', *Journal of Communication Disorders*, **9**, pp. 281–8.

OLDFIELD, R. C. and WINGFIELD, A. (1964) 'The time it takes to name an object', *Nature*, **202**, pp. 1031–2.

PAPANICOLAOU, A. C., DI SCENNA, A., GILLESPIE, L. L. and ARAM, D. M. (in press). 'Probe evoked potential findings following unilateral left hemisphere lesions in children', *Archives of Neurology*.

PARISI, D. and PIZZAMIGLIO, L. (1970) 'Syntactic comprehension in aphasia', *Cortex*, **6**, pp. 204–15.

PEARCE, P. S. and DARWISH, H. (1984) 'Correlation between EEG and auditory perceptual measures in auditory agnosia', *Brain and Language*, **22**, pp. 41–8.

PENDERGAST, L., DICKEY, S., SELMAR, J. and SODER, A. (1969) *Photo Articulation Test*, Danville, IL, Interstate Printers and Publishers.

PENFIELD, W. (1965) 'Conditioning the uncommitted language cortex for language learning', *Brain*, **88**, pp. 787–98.

POETZL, T. (1926) 'Ueber sensorische Aphasie in Kindersalter', 2, *Hals N. Ohrenklin*, **14**, pp. 109–18.

POHL, P. (1979) 'Dichotic listening in a child recovering from acquired aphasia', *Brain and Language*, **8**, pp. 372–9.

RANKIN, J. M., ARAM, D. M. and HORWITZ, S.J. (1981) 'Language ability in right and left hemiplegic children', *Brain and Language*, **14**, pp. 292–306.

RAPIN, I. and ALLEN, D. A. (1987) 'Syndromes in developmental dysphasia and adult aphasia', in Plum, F. (Ed.) *Language, Communication and the Brain*, New York, Raven Press.

RAPIN, I., MATTIS, S., ROWAN, A. J. and GOLDEN, G. S. (1977) 'Verbal auditory agnosia in children', *Developmental Medicine and Child Neurology*, **19**, pp. 192–207

REKATE, H. L., GRUBB, R. L., ARAM, D. M., HAHN, J. F. and RATCHESON, R. A. (1985) 'Muteness of cerebellar origin', *Archives of Neurology*, **42**, pp. 697–798.

RODRIGUEZ, I. and NIEDERMEYER, E. (1982) 'The aphasia-epilepsy syndrome in children: Electroencephalographic aspects', *Clinical Electroencephalography*, **13**, pp. 23–35.

SALAM–ADAMS, M. and ADAMS, R. D. (1988) 'Cerebrovascular disease by age group', in Vinken, P.J., Bruyn, G. W. and Klawans, H. L. (Eds) *Handbook of Clinical Neurology: Vascular Diseases Part 1*, Amsterdam, Elsevier Science Publishers.

SATO, S. and DREIFUSS, F. E. (1973) 'Electroencephalographic findings in a patient with developmental expressive aphasia', *Neurology*, **23**, pp. 181–5.

SATZ, P. and BULLARD–BATES, C. (1981) 'Acquired aphasia in children', in Sarno, M. T. (Ed.) *Acquired Aphasia*, New York, Academic Press.

SEGALL, H. D., BATNITZKY, S., ZEE, S., AHMADI, J., BIRD, C. R. and COHEN, M. E. (1985) 'Computed tomography in the diagnosis of intracarotid neoplasms in children', *Cancer*, **56**, pp. 1748–55.

SEMEL, E. and WIIG, E. (1980) *Clinical Evaluation of Language Functions*, Columbus OH, Charles E. Merrill.

SHOUMAKER, R., BENNETT, D., BRAY, P. and CURLESS, R. (1974) 'Clinical and EEG manifestations of an unusual aphasic syndrome in children', *Neurology*, **24**, pp. 10–16.

SIMON, C. S. (1985a) *Communication Skills and Classroom Success: Assessment of Language-Learning Disabled Students*, London, Taylor & Francis.

SIMON, C. S. (1985b) *Communication Skills and Classroom Success: Therapy Methodologies for Language-Learning Disabled Students*, London, Taylor & Francis.

SMITH, A. (1966) 'Speech and other functions after left (dominant) hemispherectomy', *Journal of Neurology, Neurosurgery and Psychiatry*, **29**, pp. 467–71.

SPREEN, O. and BENTON, A. L. (1969) *Neurosensory Centre Comprehensive Examination for Aphasia: Manual of Directions*, Victoria B.C., University of Victoria.

STRICH, S. J. (1969) 'The pathology of brain damage due to blunt injuries', in Walker, A. E. Caveness, W. F. and Critchley, M. (Eds) *The Late Effects of Head Injury*, Springfield, Charles C. Thomas.

STRUMPELL, A. (1884) 'Über die acute encephalitis die kinder', *Deutsch med. Wschr*, **57**, pp. 212–15.

TALLAL, P., STARK, R. and MELLITIS, D. (1985) 'Identification of language-impaired children on the basis of rapid perception and production skills', *Brain and Language*, **25**, pp. 314–22.

TARVER, S. G. and HALLAHAN, D. P. (1974) 'Attention deficits in children with learning disabilities: A review', *Journal of Learning Disabilities*, **7**, pp. 560–9.

TINDALL, R. S. A. (1980) 'Cerebrovascular disease', in Rosenberg, R. N. (Ed.) *Neurology*, New York, Grune & Stratton.

TEMPLIN, M. C. (1957) *Certain Language Skills in Children*, Minneapolis, University of Minnesota Press.

TEMPLIN, M. C. and DARLEY, F. L. (1969) *Templin-Darley Test of Articulation*, 2nd ed., Iowa City, Bureau of Educational Research and Service.

TORGESEN, J. K. and GOLDMAN, T. (1977) 'Verbal rehearsal and short-term memory in reading disabled children', *Child Development*, **48**, pp. 56–60.

TRAUNER, D. A. and MANNINO, F. L. (1986) 'Neurodevelopmental outcome after neonatal cerebrovascular accident', *Pediatrics*, **108**, pp. 459–61.

VAN DE SANDT–KOENDERMAN, W. M. E., SMIT, I. A. C., VAN DONGEN, H. R. and VAN HEST, J. B. C. (1984) 'A case of acquired aphasia and convulsive disorder: Some linguistic aspects of recovery and breakdown', *Brain and Language*, **21**, pp. 174–83.

VAN DONGEN, H. R. and LOONEN, M. C. B. (1977) 'Factors related to prognosis of acquired aphasia in children', *Cortex*, **13**, pp. 131–6.

VAN DONGEN, H. R., LOONEN, M. C. B. and VAN DONGEN, K. J. (1985) 'Anatomical basis of acquired fluent aphasia in children', *Annals of Neurology*, **17**, pp. 306–9.

VAN DONGEN, H. R. and VISCH–BRINK, E. G. (1988) 'Naming in aphasic children: Analysis of paraphasic errors', *Neuropsychologia*, **26**, pp. 629–32.

VAN HOUT, A., EVRARD, P. and LYON, G. (1985) 'On the positive semiology of acquired aphasia in children', *Developmental Medicine and Child Neurology*, **27**, pp. 231–41.

VAN HOUT, A. and LYON, G. (1986) 'Wernicke's aphasia in a 10 year-old boy', *Brain and Language*, **29**, pp. 268–85.

VARGHA–KHADEM, F., GORMAN, A. M. and WATTERS, G. V. (1985) 'Aphasia and handedness in relation to hemispheric side, age and injury and severity of cerebral lesion during childhood', *Brain*, **108**, pp. 677–96.

VISCH–BRINK, E. G. and VAN DE SANDT–KOENDERMAN, M. (1984) 'The occurrence of paraphasias in the spontaneous speech of children with acquired aphasia', *Brain and Language*, **23**, pp. 256–71.

VOELLER, K. K. S. (1986) 'Right hemisphere deficit syndrome in children', *American Journal of Psychiatry*, **143**, pp. 1004–9.

WALLACH, G. and BUTLER, K. (1984) *Language Learning Disabilities in School Age Children*, Baltimore, Williams & Wilkins.

WEPMAN, J. M. (1958) *Auditory Discrimination Test*, Los Angeles, Western Psychological Services.

WIEGEL–CRUMP, C. A. and DENNIS, M. (1984) *The Word-finding Test*, Toronto, The Hospital for Sick Children (unpublished).

WIIG, E. and SEMEL, E. (1984) *Language Assessment and Intervention for the Learning Disabled*, 2nd ed. Columbus, OH, Charles E. Merrill.

WOLFUS, B., MOSCOVITCH, M. and KINSBOURNE, M. (1980) 'Subgroups of developmental language impairment', *Brain and Language*, **9**, pp. 152–71.

WOODCOCK, R. W. and JOHNSON, M. D. (1977) *Woodcock–Johnson Psycho-Educational Battery*, Hingham, M. A. Teaching Resources.

WOODS, B. T. and CAREY, S. (1979) 'Language deficits after apparent clinical recovery from childhood aphasia', *Annals of Neurology*, **6**, pp. 405–9.

WORSTER–DROUGHT, C. (1971) 'An unusual form of acquired aphasia in children', *Developmental Medicine and Child Neurology*, **13**, pp. 563–71.

WYLLIE, W. G. (1948) 'Acute infantile hemiplegia', *Proceedings of the Royal Society of Medicine*, **41**, pp. 459–66.

ZANGWILL, O. L. (1960) '*Cerebral dominance and its relation to psychological function*', Springfield, Charles C. Thomas.

ZUBRICK, A. (1988) 'The language of mathematics', paper presented at the Annual Conference of the Australian Association of Speech and Hearing, Brisbane, Australia.

Chapter 2

Acquired Childhood Aphasia: Assessment and Treatment

Jill A. Cross and Anne E. Ozanne

Introduction

Little has been written, with the exception of some case studies, isolated articles and in recent times the book edited by Ylvisaker (1985), about the assessment and treatment of acquired aphasia in children and adolescents. In the past, it was assumed that if a child made an excellent physical recovery then the recovery of language was also complete. Consequently, persistent cognitive and linguistic deficits were not suspected. However, for some years now clinicians have been aware that many children who were declared fully recovered from their brain lesion have subtle underlying language problems which may affect their later academic performance.

The literature on the course of recovery of acquired aphasia in children refers to either complete recovery of speech and language functions or to persistent problems. Nowhere is it stated that aphasia sequelae may become apparent years later in children who were believed to have made a complete recovery of language functions. Yet, children with acquired aphasia may appear on the school clinician's caseload a few years after the injury. As with some children with developmental language disorders, it seems that when some of the children with acquired aphasia reach higher grades in school their language and learning difficulties become more obvious because the linguistic and cognitive requirements of academic work are more complex at this stage and they are unable to cope with the increased demands.

No one has researched the methodology of assessment and treatment described below nor is there much empirical research reported in the literature to support the use of such methods. However, the suggestions documented here are based on years of clinical experience in a rehabilitation setting.

Language assessment and therapy will be discussed in terms of Comprehension (Reception) and Expression (Production) primarily because the majority of tests used in the assessment of these children present their results in a like manner. While clinicians are aware of the cognitive processes underlying all intervention strategies many clinicians still formulate their treatment goals using a receptive-expressive framework with the cognitive element inherent in their treatment methodology.

Although many treatment ideas used with aphasic adults can be successfully adapted for children, clinicians must remember that the process of rehabilitation in children is entirely different. In both adults and children treatment goals are influenced by the various stages of the recovery process. However, children, unlike adults, are still acquiring speech and language skills. This developmental process with all the environmental ramifications which influence the normal acquisition of language should not be forgotten when planning remediation.

Concomitant Problems

There are a number of concomitant problems associated with acquired aphasia which must be recognized if accurate assessment results are to be obtained and realistic treatment goals formulated. Dyspraxia, dysarthria and occasionally an agnosia may coexist with the asphasia. Visual and hearing acuity should be tested so that the child is not further disadvantaged by being unable to hear or see clearly. It is also important for differential diagnosis that peripheral problems are not mistaken for central difficulties.

Motor problems such as hemiplegia, quadriplegia and paraplegia, along with a variety of dyspraxias, may hinder the child's ability to respond appropriately to assessment instructions, even though the individual's language skill necessary for carrying out the instructions is intact. For example, the quadriplegic child, particularly if there is an accompanying dysarthria or dyspraxia, may have difficulty responding to test stimuli by pointing or moving tokens and is certainly disadvantaged when there is a time limit on the subtest. A child with a limb dyspraxia and a right hemiplegia may have difficulty carrying out instructions if asked to pantomime an action with his left hand. For example, 'Show me what you would do with scissors'. If the child failed to respond, his failure could be interpreted wrongly as a comprehension problem rather than as a motor planning difficulty. Perseveration may also be confused as incorrect responses (e.g. the child continues to point to a picture in the same place on each page).

Many language tests use visual stimuli. If children with visual deficits, such as an homonymous hemianopsia, have not learned to compensate using good visual scanning, then they can miss stimuli placed too far to the right or left of the focal point. Visual perceptual problems may cause an individual to fail because they cannot effectively discriminate between the visual cues. For example, one child seen at our clinic with severe figure-ground problems could not manage any subtest which had a visual stimulus because he could not discriminate the line drawing from the rest of the page. This difficulty also prevented any testing of his reading or writing skills. Double vision and nystagmus may also cloud the child's real linguistic abilities, particularly reading skills. For example, as the child moves from line to line in a paragraph, he may lose his place and then forget the content of the passage in the effort of finding his place again.

Behavioural problems, including personality changes, egocentricity, depression and mood swings, can influence both day-to-day treatment sessions and long-term goals. Also, the child is usually an integral member of a family unit so that the changes in family life and structure brought about by the child's injury must be addressed. For example, one father, who previously had had a close relationship with his daughter found it difficult to make regular hospital visits to his child after her injury. The girl was extremely upset and believed that her father no longer loved her. Consequently, she was unmotivated in therapy and it was not until the situation was rectified that she regained her motivation.

Underlying all assessment procedures and treatment plans must be an awareness of children's cognitive abilities. In particular, memory may mask the child's linguistic skills (e.g. the child cannot remember the instructions and therefore cannot respond correctly). Current neuropsychological literature and other texts (e.g. Pressley and Brainerd, 1985; Wallach and Butler, 1984; Wiig and Semel, 1984; Ylvisaker, 1985), discuss memory and some procedures for assessment and treatment. Therefore, memory will not be covered specifically in this chapter and will be mentioned only where it impinges directly on linguistic skills. Also, children's susceptibility to fatigue and any medical conditions such as seizures which could affect assessment and remediation must be taken into consideration.

Assessment of Acquired Childhood Aphasia

There are two areas which need to be considered when assessing a child with acquired childhood aphasia: (A) relevant information from the medical file, family history, reports from others concerned in the child's care and ward visits, and (B) language assessment comprised of standardized tests, non-standardized tests and observation (Figure 2.1).

Types of Assessment Procedures

Relevant information

For a thorough assessment of the communicative abilities of a child with acquired aphasia all relevant information from other persons involved in the care of the child must be sought (e.g. the existence of concomitant problems as well as the family's attitude towards the disabled child must be obtained). It is especially important for the clinician to have access to any information about the individual's academic abilities. If possible, samples of the child's school work (e.g. creative writing workbook and

ASSESSMENT OF ACQUIRED CHILDHOOD APHASIA

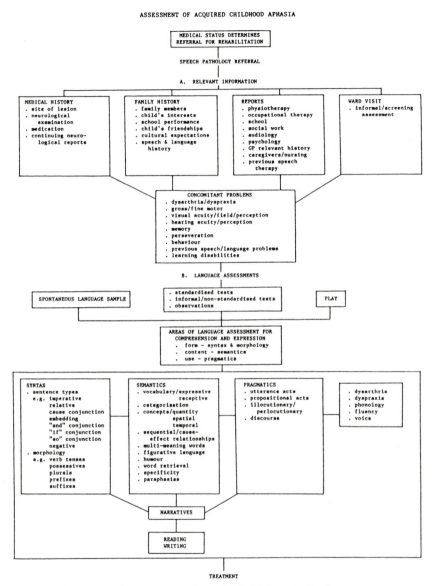

Figure 2.1 Summary of assessment of acquired childhood aphasia

school reports) should be obtained. This information can give an indication of the child's language abilities before the insult, will help the clinician decide on further areas of assessment to probe and will assist them in setting up realistic treatment goals.

Most clinicians use three methods for assessing the communication of the child with a brain lesion: standardized tests, informal procedures (i.e. non-standardized tests) and observation. Each method is important but it is the integration and interpretation of information obtained from all areas which allows the clinician to diagnose the child's difficulties, effect the appropriate treatment and measure subsequent progress.

Language assessments

Standardized tests

Standardized tests play an important role in assessment, especially when progress needs to be measured objectively. In the acute stage of recovery, however, informal testing and observation are usually adopted because these two methods are less threatening to anxious children and their parents. If the clinician persists in using standardized tests and other formal procedures in their entirety when the child is not ready or able to cope with the demands, then the child/clinician relationship and the child's progress in therapy may be put at risk.

There are a number of excellent tests of child language development that can be used in the assessment of children with acquired childhood aphasia (e.g. Clinical Evaluation of Language Fundamentals–Revised (CELF-R) (Semel *et al.*, 1987), Test of Language Development Series-2 (TOLD) (Hammill and Newcomer, 1988; Newcomer and Hammill, 1988), Preschool Language Assessment Instrument (Blank *et al.*, 1978), Porch Index of Communicative Ability in Children (PICAC) (Porch, 1974) and the Reynell Developmental Language Scales-Revised (Reynell, 1977), plus tests which assess specific linguistic abilities (e.g. Peabody Picture Vocabulary Test–Revised (PPVT-R) (Dunn and Dunn, 1981), Token Test for Children (Di Simone, 1978), and Test of Auditory Comprehension of Language–Revised (TACL–R) (Carrow–Woolfolk, 1985). Adult aphasic tests can also provide valuable information when used with the older child or adolescent (e.g. the Boston Naming Test (Kaplan et al., 1983), the Neurosensory Centre Comprehensive Examination of Aphasia (NCCEA) (Spreen and Benton, 1969) or the Communicative Abilities in Daily Living (CADL) (Holland, 1980). The increasing use of these adult tests with children has prompted the development of childhood norms for the Boston Naming Test (Guilford and Nawojczyk, 1988) and the NCCEA (Gaddes and Crockett, 1975). The battery of tests administered by experienced clinicians varies from child to child and the choice of which tests to use is based on careful observation of the child's communicative behaviour. For example, if a child appears to be operating at a younger level than his chronological age then a test for younger children, even though he is outside the age range, may be chosen.

When a child is unable to cope with the entire age-appropriate standardized test then the clinician may have to omit or modify a number of subtests. For example, if the child appears to have significant word-retrieval problems then the subtest involving confrontation naming might not be administered in full or could be adapted to allow the child some success. Modification of standardized tests can include the simplification of instructions for administration, allowing different methods of responding (e.g. written instead of verbal) and the use of a variety of cues to help elicit a response (e.g. semantic or phonemic prompts).

Many standardized test results, unless they are language samples, only yield information about the child's abilities in comparison with his peers. Although this information is important and necessary it is not descriptive enough to assist the clinician with the development of therapy aims. Information gleaned when tests have been modified is mostly descriptive and can contribute greatly to a clinician's understanding of a child's abilities and help in the formulation of treatment goals. For example, what cues best assisted the child to retrieve words or what level of language or linguistic complexity enhanced the child's comprehension or caused a breakdown in understanding? It is important, though, that all modifications of standardized tests be noted and reported. As the child recovers, test modifications are often no longer necessary and this in itself is a measure of progress.

Non-standardized tests

Informal testing may serve a number of functions when working with a child with acquired aphasia. Such testing may be used to: quickly assess children who fatigue easily, measure the rapid recovery of language skills, assess children who fail on standardized procedures because of concomitant problems, follow-up on deficits noted by the child's family or by other professionals, and allows the clinician flexibility of assessment when limited resources of standardized tests are available.

Informal testing, as already stated, is often used in the early stages of recovery. Individual improvement can be so rapid that a test administered on a Friday can be invalid on the Monday (e.g. a child may begin to say single words one day and over a weekend may progress to using sentences). An informal test, devised by the clinician himself/herself can have a similar framework to and be based on a standardized test. An example of an informal test for acquired childhood aphasia is presented in Appendix 1. These informal tests are usually shorter with only a few items used to sample a wide range of semantic and syntactic abilities. They are primarily designed to give the clinician an indication of a child's linguistic and functional abilities soon after onset of the aphasia. It is most often suitable for use at the child's bedside. For example, such a test may be a selection of doll's house furniture with matching photos which can be used receptively and expressively for activities such as naming, functions and associations. Another informal assessment might be a set of 'yes/no' questions specific to the child's environment or a checklist of pragmatic behaviours.

Structured but non-standardized procedures which are often based on the results obtained from standardized tests or suggested from colleagues' comments can be devised for extension testing. For example, the teacher may report that the aphasic child is having problems when the teacher is explaining or discussing school work, thereby indicating the need to assess further the child's ability to recall and retain varying amounts of information presented verbally. In addition, tasks experimenting with different linguistic variables, such as the complexity of semantic content in an utterance or the length of instructions given, can be used to further probe the child's comprehension skills. Although these fore-mentioned tasks are non-standardized they can yield highly specific linguistic information (e.g. the individual's ability to comprehend 'where' questions of varying syntactic difficulty).

Observation

Observation of the child in a number of different settings will yield necessary information on how that child functions in various social situations, such as with his peers in the school playground, in class discussions or with his parents and siblings. Careful note should be taken of how the child receives and gives a message. Did the listener understand? If not, why not? Where did the breakdown occur? Was it the child's inability to encode the message syntactically or his unintelligible speech which appeared to be the main difficulty? If the message was understood, why was it understood? Did the accompanying non-verbal behaviours enable the listener to decode the message?

It is best to have some framework (i.e. a mental or written checklist) from which to base an observation so that the behaviours seen are not random observations and are easily interpreted when all information is gathered and analyzed. (An example of an observational checklist is presented in Appendix 2.) A knowledge of Bloom and Lahey's Content Categories (Bloom and Lahey, 1978), Brown's 14 grammatical morphemes (Wiig and Semel, 1984) or some behaviours from the Pragmatic Protocol developed by Prutting and Kirchner (1987) may form part of such an observation checklist. If possible, audiotape and videotape recordings of these observation and assessment sessions should be made. These can be analyzed later and specific information, which could have been missed during the session, extracted.

During assessment or treatment sessions the clinician may observe children using strategies to help them decode or remember information, for example, mouthing the words after the clinician before giving a response, counting on their fingers or writing letter cues on their legs to help them remember and repeating the instructions. Many children may discover their own strategies and it is important for the clinician to identify them and bring them to the child's awareness. These strategies may be used consistently in later treatment sessions and may become part of the repertoire which the child adopts to assist him in his day-to-day living. Information about those strategies which proved useful in their treatment sessions (e.g. the complexity of language to use with the child when giving instructions) should be made available to other team members.

Areas of Language Assessment for Comprehension and Expression

Language is the knowledge of how content/form/use integrate and this knowledge underlies the behaviours of speaking and understanding (Bloom and Lahey, 1978). Therefore, to assess the language of a child with acquired aphasia, as with any child with a language impairment, it is difficult, if not impossible, to treat semantics, syntax, morphology and pragmatics as discrete areas of language without being aware of the influence each has on the other. There is no doubt that children with acquired aphasia may have greater difficulty in one language area than in another, for example, the child with word-retrieval problems has more difficulty in the semantic area, the child with telegrammatic-type communication may have the greatest difficulty with morphology and syntax, while the child with frontal lobe damage appears to have significant problems with pragmatic language skills. However, the goal of language assessment of a child with a brain lesion is to discover how well that child integrates content/form/use for understanding and speaking. The assessment procedures outlined below are not intended to be definitive but rather to offer suggestions and avenues for the clinician to pursue and explore.

Spontaneous language sample

A spontaneous language sample gives the clinician the best indication of how well the child with acquired aphasia is integrating content/form/use for communication. It provides a detailed description of the child's language abilities, both receptive and expressive, particularly when samples are taken in a number of natural settings (e.g. in the classroom, with a peer in play, with parents or siblings and with the clinician). Each sample can be analyzed semantically, syntactically or pragmatically, the choice of analysis depending on what specific information the clinician may wish to gather. For example, Bloom and Lahey Content/Form analysis (Bloom and Lahey, 1978), Prism-L/Prism-G (Crystal, 1982) for semantics, the Language and Remediation Screening Procedure (LARSP) (Crystal, 1982) for syntax and morphology, and the Clinical Discourse Analysis (Damico, 1985), Graphic Conversational Profile (Wilks and Monaghan, 1988) in the pragmatic area. From analyses of the samples hypotheses may be formed about the child's language skills and these hypotheses then tested using elicited language samples or informal assessment procedures (e.g. asking 'why' questions to test the child's skill at coding and encoding cause-effect relationships). Also, particular formal tests which the clinician thinks best suit the type and level of the child's abilities may be chosen to further explore and test these hypotheses.

In the early stages of a child's recovery, however, it may not be an appropriate assessment tool. The child may have little language to sample or his/her expressive language may be changing so rapidly that by the time a representative sample may be gathered and analyzed it may not truly reflect the child's language abilities. Concomitant problems such as a dysarthria or dyspraxia may also prevent the accurate transcription of the child's expressive language and so limit its use for diagnostic and treatment purposes. It is in such situations that an audiotape or preferably a videotape of the child's communicative abilities should be made. This can serve as a record of the child's recovery or may be analyzed later if the comparison of specific behaviours (e.g. eye contact, turn-taking skills, word retrieval difficulties) in different recovery phases becomes important. As noted in the literature, it is necessary for clinicians to remember, when collecting a language sample, that many children with acquired aphasia are reluctant to communicate and so a representative language sample may not be obtained. However, as trust and rapport grow between the clinician and the child this reluctance may be overcome. Also, much depends on the setting of the language sample. For example, in a play setting with a small group of peers where the emphasis is not on language the child may feel free to communicate.

In the middle and late stages of recovery from acquired aphasia, the spontaneous language sample is a necessary assessment tool, complementing standardized testing procedures. A subtest involving confrontation naming may show that a child is having word-retrieval problems, the language sample then may reveal the types of naming errors that the child uses, which in turn is important for the formulation of treatment goals. Information on children's use and comprehension of complex syntactic structures or their ability to maintain a topic of conversation may also be obtained from the spontaneous language sample. Time constraints in a busy clinic may limit the size and representative quality of the sample but being pressed for time should not be used as an excuse for not taking one. The information obtained from a spontaneous language sample is too valuable for it to be omitted from an assessment battery. Short supplementary observations (hand subscribing of utterances and context) in particular situations, seeking information on one or two language behaviours (e.g. Are the child's responses to 'wh' questions, single words, simple or complex sentences? Does the child use negative structures and if so, what are they?) may enhance or clarify the information already obtained from the spontaneous language sample. The teacher or parent, if given specific instructions, may be the transcriber in such situations.

Comprehension

Most of the standardized tests mentioned previously (e.g. CELF-R, TOLD-2) have subtests which are specifically designed to sample and measure different aspects of auditory comprehension. The literature documenting adult aphasic problems as well as the literature relating to the learning disabled child has relevance to the child with acquired aphasia. The literature on both adult aphasia and learning disabilities detail examples of auditory comprehension non-standardized tasks (Chapey, 1981, 1986;

Simon, 1985; Wiig and Semel, 1984). In some circumstances the tasks used with adult clients may be modified for the child with acquired aphasia (e.g. 'yes/no' questions about school may replace questions about occupations). Often it needs only the topic to be changed for the activity to be suitable for the child (e.g. activities which involve newspaper articles may be changed to information for school projects).

Conversation

The assessment of auditory comprehension in a child with acquired aphasia should include a judgement of the child's ability to understand unstructured spontaneous language such as 'yes/no' questions about the individual's family, school and interests or general conversation among peers and caregivers about what is happening, has happened or will happen in daily living situations. The age and interests of the child should not be forgotten (e.g. a young child may have had difficulty before his brain lesion with certain time concepts).

Word meanings

Assessing the child's knowledge of the meaning of words and their relationship to one another is important. Testing this knowledge may include evaluations of a child's:

receptive vocabulary
semantic categories of words ('lights' may include 'light bulb', 'torch' and 'candle')
antonyms ('big' – 'little')
synonyms ('rabbit' – 'bunny' – 'hare')
homonyms ('blew' – 'blue')
reciprocity ('give' – 'take')
multi-meaning words ('walk' as a verb or as a noun, in expressions such as 'take a walk' meaning 'go away' or 'walk away' 'meaning 'ignore')
spatial terms ('under' – 'next' – 'against')
temporal terms ('first' – 'after' – 'before')
comparative ('bigger' – 'biggest')
familial ('sister' – 'grandmother')
cause-effect relations ('why/because')
relational terms ('if/then' – 'all/except')

Non-standardized testing needs to take into account the child's age and what he/she is expected to know and use in school.

With the older child, the clinician can assess the child's understanding of figurative language such as idioms ('sharp tongued'), similes and metaphors ('the hours creep by'), adages ('still waters run deep') colloquialisms ('pulling your leg') and verbal analogies ('a key is to a door as a dial is to a telephone'). Normal everyday communication abounds with figurative language but for the child returning to high school and who will be studying literature (poetry is full of similes and metaphors) it is of particular importance that these areas are assessed.

Recall of verbal information

When assessing the amount of verbal information that a child can process it is often beneficial to use material from the child's own schoolwork (e.g. science or social studies information which the teacher is likely to use when teaching the subject matter to the class). This may serve a twofold purpose. First, the clinician is able to make an objective judgment of how much semantic content the child can manage and comprehend before his/her understanding breaks down, and second, as a meaningful example to the teacher of his/her comprehension problems. Part of this assessment may include the child's ability to recall detail and make inferences from the information presented. The clinician needs to be aware that with some children memory difficulties may affect their performance as the information load increases.

Morphology and syntax

Assessment should involve the evaluation of a child's understanding of morphology and syntax. Can the child demonstrate comprehension of plurals, tenses, cases, comparatives, superlatives, adjectival and adverbial forms or auxiliary verbs? What sentence structure helps or hinders the child's understanding of language (e.g. questions, negation or passive transformations)? Literature, detailing the normal development of morphology and syntax (e.g. Crystal, 1982) may help in formulating systematic non-standardized tasks to test certain linguistic forms. Much of this information on form may be obtained from a representative spontaneous language sample (e.g. if a child uses plurals consistently, then generally they must understand them).

Pragmatics

A child's auditory comprehension difficulties may influence his/her pragmatic abilities, particularly those skills dependent on linguistic competence (e.g. semantics and syntax must be intact for cohesion, sequencing skills for clarification). Comprehension of a communicative act not only involves the understanding of language but also the ability to perceive situational cues (e.g. facial expressions or the fact that two people are speaking privately and would not appreciate being interrupted). It seems that some children with a brain lesion, particularly frontal lobe damage, have difficulty perceiving or understanding body language and situational cues. They are often the children that people label as 'strange' although these people cannot always describe the specific behaviour that warranted the label. These 'strange' children may be able to respond appropriately given a picture to explain (e.g. What will this girl say when she sees her friend?) but fail to act appropriately when they are in the actual situation. Assessment of pragmatic skills involving the understanding of non-verbal language may be done by using a picture format as in some items of 'Let's

Talk Inventory for Adolescents' (Wiig, 1982), from a videotaped recording of the child's social interactions or from observations.

Extension testing like many of the subtests in standardized tests can take the form of a choice between a number of pictures. However, judgment tasks may prove the easiest to design and can be used to test semantic, syntactic and pragmatic knowledge. For example, the child is shown the picture of a girl running and asked if what the clinician says ('He is running.') is correct or incorrect. As another example the child may be given two sentences, 'I ate an apple and a pear' and 'I ate the fruit' and then asked if the two sentences are the same or different? Alternatively, pictures of a child talking to a teacher and to her friend may be shown and the child asked, 'In which one would she say, "Hi, Jan"?' Individual assessment procedures can be designed. However, it may save time if records of any assessment procedures are kept because parts of them may be relevant for another child. If judgment tasks are stored on computer then it is a simple matter to create new tasks by cutting and pasting from other established files.

Humour

The appreciation of humour and its use by children with acquired aphasia is frequently neglected by researchers and clinicians. Yet parents frequently comment that their brain-injured child does not joke any more, that the good-natured teasing in the family is taken too seriously by the child with acquired aphasia and may lead to outbursts of anger or frustration on the child's part and fights amongst the siblings. For example, one 11-year-old girl's father had a teasing, joking-type of affectionate relationship with his daughter. This relationship suffered after the child's brain lesion and although her difficulty with language was explained the relationship continued to suffer. Two years after the insult the first comment that the father made to the clinician when the child was brought in for a review was, 'She's got her dry wit back again'.

Many verbal jokes are resolved on the basis of lexical, semantic or phonological ambiguity (e.g. 'shaggy dog' stories with the punch line being interpreted two ways: 'The Pirates of Penzance' to 'the pie rates of Penzance'). The riddle also seems to involve an appreciation of jokes as well as a type of problem solving. A question is asked and the answer is incongruous and the listener has the task of solving how the answer does make sense in terms of the original question.

Obviously, humour in the infant and young child is different from that of the older child and adult. Shultz (1976), however, reported findings which suggested that laughter at word plays begins as early as 3 years of age. Humour not only involves appreciation of verbal language but also an awareness of non-verbal and situational cues, in fact, an appreciation of pragmatic, semantic and syntactic areas of communication. Therefore, it would seem valuable to observe how a child with acquired aphasia appreciates and uses humour. Knowledge gained from these observations may help design probes and formulate goals in all areas of communication.

Reading

Children with acquired aphasia, particularly those who have an auditory comprehension problem, often exhibit difficulties with reading, either in recognizing letters and words or in comprehending the written material. The assessment of reading must take into account the level of the child's ability before his/her brain lesion, and the expertise of the occupational therapist, the teacher and the guidance officer/psychologist in the assessment is desirable. Their collective knowledge of perceptual problems, the process of normal reading development and of reading problems in the normal population helps with the differential diagnosis of the reading difficulty.

Assessment of reading may include matching of letters, matching of letters to sounds, matching words and sentences to pictures and graded reading tests. Reading problems appear to reflect deficits apparent in the child's semantic, syntactic and pragmatic systems. Difficulties understanding the meanings of multi-meaning words, complex syntactic structures, figurative language and inferences are problems common to many children with acquired aphasia.

Assessment of the reading abilities of children with acquired aphasia should involve some measure of the amount of written material that the child is able to assimilate and the nature of the details that the child may recall (e.g. names and ages of persons mentioned, directions given or the sequence of events leading to the climax). The recovery of reading ability in a child with acquired aphasia appears to follow similar stages to that of his/her oral language recovery, although this seems to depend on the child's age at the time of his/her brain lesion and its severity. If the child was under school age at the time of the insult then it is possible that the child will have difficulty acquiring the skills of reading. The comprehension of written material often poses the greatest problem for the child with acquired aphasia who has recovered many of his/her other reading skills (i.e. his ability to read words and sentences).

Little has been documented about the problems a child with acquired aphasia has with mathematics but undoubtedly a difficulty often exists. This problem may be language related (e.g. the child is confused with the meaning of mathematical words, 'divide', 'multiply', or is unable to read the instructions which introduce the mathematical problem). The speech and language clinician can assist other professionals by assessing the child's ability to understand the mathematical terms and the underlying concepts related to mathematics (e.g. few, some, many, half etc.) which he/she is expected to know in the classroom.

Expression

Most standardized tests which can be used with the child with acquired aphasia have a number of subtests which evaluate the child's expressive language abilities (see Table 2.1).

Table 2.1 Formal tests and analyses that can be used in assessing children with acquired aphasia

Test	Author(s)
General	
Clinical Evaluation of Language Fundamentals-Revised (CELF-R)	Semel, Wiig & Secord, 1987
Test of Language Development-2 (TOLD-P)	Newcomer & Hammill, 1988
Test of Language Development-2 Intermediate (TOLD-2 I)	Hammill & Newcomer, 1988
Test of Adolescent Language (TOAL)	Hammill, Brown, Larsen & Weiderholt, 1987
Pre-school Language Assessment Instrument (PLAI)	Blank, Rose & Berlin, 1978
Test of Auditory Comprehension of Language-Revised (TACL-R)	Carrow-Woolfolk, 1985
The Token Test for Children (TT)	Di Simone, 1978
Porch Index of Communicative Ability in Children (PICAC)	Porch, 1974
Reynell Developmental Language Scales-Revised (Reynell)	Reynell, 1977
Semantics	
Peabody Picture Vocabulary Test-Revised (PPVT-R)	Dunn & Dunn, 1981
Boehm Test of Basic Concepts-Revised (Boehm-R)	Boehm, 1986
Double Administration Naming Technique (DANT)	Fried-Oken, 1987
The World Test: A Test of Expressive Vocabulary and Semantics (TWT)	Jorgensen, Barrett, Huisingh & Zachman, 1981
Boston Naming Test (Boston)	Kaplan, Goodglass & Weintraub, 1983
Content/Form Analysis	Bloom & Lahey, 1978
Syntax	
Language Assessment, Remediation and Screening Procedure (LARSP)	Crystal, Fletcher & Garmon, 1982
Pragmatics	
Let's Talk Inventory for Adolescents	Wiig, 1982
Clinical Discourse Analysis	Damico, 1985
Communicative Abilities in Daily Living (CADL)	Holland, 1980

Syntax

The literature reports that children with acquired aphasia often used simplified syntax and telegraphic language, as well as being reluctant to communicate. This reluctance to speak may influence the complexity of their language which may in turn affect any spontaneous language sample taken. For example, a 6-year-old girl with acquired aphasia seen in our clinic enjoyed a game after the therapy activities and would ask the clinician, 'Game?' using a rising intonation and appropriate facial expression. In the initial period following her brain lesion, resulting from a cerebrovascular accident, she used telegraphic language but was, at that time, able to produce complex sentences. When the clinician prompted her, 'Kate, can you ask me in a longer sentence?' she would reply, 'Can we play a game now, please?' with no apparent difficulty in generating the sentence structure.

Assessment, then, of morphology and syntax in children with acquired aphasia needs to include information from a spontaneous language sample, standardized tests and elicited tasks. Areas probed may involve activities such as the following:

> plurals (regular and irregular)
> case (use of the possessive 's', nominative pronouns)
> tenses (regular and irregular, past, present, future)
> comparative and superlative forms
> production in a sentence of all parts of speech (nouns, verbs, adjectives, adverbs, prepositions, pronouns, conjunctions)
> noun and adverb derivations ('er', 'ly')
> prefixes and suffixes
> use of articles
> use of different sentence structures (passive, negative, interrogative, 'wh' questions)
> ambiguous sentences
> MLU
> the types of complex sentences (co-ordination, relative clauses 'subordination' embedded)
> the percentage of complex sentences attempted and the percentage correct
> the proportion of simple to complex sentences

(The last two areas can often be used as an index of improvement in children who are more fluent in the acute stage.)

Assessment tasks may include the use of visual stimuli (pictures of a cat and cats), sentence completion (e.g. She is teaching, She is a ...), production of sentences (e.g. Make up a sentence with the word 'farm', 'beneath', 'sadly') and the manipulation of given words to make sentences (e.g. 'is', 'hat', 'the', 'red'. Can the child make a statement and a question with the words?). The imitation of sentences of increasing complexity by the child (e.g. The boy hit the dog. The boy who was wearing a red cap hit the little dog.) may be useful to the clinician to evaluate the structures the child is able to imitate and possibly to produce spontaneously. Semantic understanding and short-term memory may influence the child's results. Short-term memory problems seen in the child with acquired aphasia are similar to those observed in the learning disabled child (Wiig and Semel, 1984). The literature discussing the learning disabled child reports in more detail the effects of short-term memory problems on imitation tasks and syntactic structures (Wiig and Semel, 1984; Wallach and Butler, 1984).

Semantics

As with acquired aphasia in adults, a deficit in the ability to produce language content is also a characteristic of acquired aphasia in childhood. This lack of content is similar to that heard in the expressive language of many learning-disabled children although the child with acquired aphasia may have a more pronounced problem, especially in the early stages of recovery. Spontaneous or elicited language samples give some indication of the deficits experienced by the child with semantic language problems. Semantic analyses (e.g. Bloom and Lahey, 1978; Prism-L/Prism-G analysis, Crystal, 1982) may be used to detail the presence of content categories or the usage of specific parts of speech.

Word-retrieval difficulties, dysfluency, semantic and literal paraphasias are common symptoms heard in the expressive language of a child with acquired aphasia. Word-retrieval problems and dysfluency characteristics need to be recorded when transcribing the sample. Qualitative analysis of a child's naming errors (Wiig and Semel, 1984) will give some indication of what types of semantic or literal paraphasias are used mostly by the child or whether many of his/her word retrieval problems are camouflaged by circumlocution. For example, when shown a picture of a boy writing and asked 'What is the boy doing?', one child replied, 'He's using a pencil. It's something to do with school'. When a phonetic cue was given the same child replied correctly, 'Writing'. The analysis of dysfluency characteristics may help the clinician decide whether the child has a comprehension difficulty and needs time to process the information, or whether there is a word-retrieval problem. The Double Administration Naming Technique (Fried-Oken, 1987) assists the clinician in determining whether the child has word-retrieval problems or expressive vocabulary limitations and further describes what cues (e.g. the object's function, its category, a description of the object or the sound at the beginning of the word) are best used for helping the child recall specific words.

Semantic and literal paraphasias should be noted and the percentage of occurrence in the sample calculated. The compilation of these percentages at intervals during recovery phases may be used as an objective measure of progress for, as recovery occurs, the percentage of paraphasias decreases.

Further assessment tasks should involve confrontation naming (e.g. body parts, colours, shapes, animals, common objects and actions), and automatic-sequential naming (e.g. the days of the week, the months of the year, counting). Expressive tasks similar to those proposed for assessing receptive skills may form part of the assessment, particularly with the older child when metalinguistic skills become important for classroom success. The child is asked to respond when given a verbal stimulus consisting of either a single word or short sentence. For example these expressive tasks may include:

antonyms ('up' – 'down')
synonyms ('happy' – 'glad' – 'elated')
homonyms ('meet – 'meat')
rhyming words ('cat' – 'hat' – 'fat')
definitions of words (What does 'jump' mean?)
categorization tasks (Tell me as many things as you can think of that we eat?)
figurative language (What does it mean if someone has a 'green thumb'?)
similarities and differences (How are wind-surfing and sailing alike and how are they different?)
convergent semantic tasks (Finish the sentence, 'I dig with a...')
divergent semantic tasks (If you can't use sugar in your tea to make it sweet, what (ingredients) could you use instead?)
sentence formulation using different parts of speech (Make me a sentence with the word 'emu' or 'beside' or 'except')
definition of mathematical terms ('divide', 'subtract', 'plus')

The choice of tests and tasks depends on the child's stage of recovery and their age and is greatly influenced by the clinician's knowledge of a child's normal language development. For example, metalinguistic tasks would neither be appropriate for the pre-school child nor the older child with severe expressive language difficulties.

Pragmatics
Behavioural changes in children who have sustained a brain lesion have been noted and reported in the literature. Parents frequently comment that their child's personality has changed (e.g. 'She is not a leader any more.'). However, as the child recovers, parents frequently report that the child is more like his/her previous personality.

It is commonly acknowledged that frontal lobe damage may contribute to disinhibited behaviour in adults. Similar behaviour has been observed in adolescents with known frontal lobe damage. Also, it seems that most children who sustain brain damage show some behavioural change. It is doubtful whether behavioural changes can be attributed solely to the brain lesion. Other influences such as the impact of the brain lesion on the child and his/her family must be considered. It would appear, in some cases, that the injury may exacerbate already existing problems. However, more research is needed in this area before conclusive statements can be made.

Regression of behaviour is known to be a coping mechanism that some children adopt when they have suffered any type of trauma. Also, while in hospital and particularly if their stay is lengthy, children's inappropriate behaviours are often reinforced by anxious parents and concerned hospital staff. This would seem a natural reaction on the part of the caregivers in these circumstances. The child was most probably dangerously ill and perhaps not expected to live. As the child recovers, the full extent of his/her injuries becomes apparent and parents and staff often 'spoil' the individual and accept behaviours which in normal circumstances would have been unacceptable to them.

When assessing the pragmatic behaviours of a child with acquired aphasia the clinician must be aware of the hospital and family situation before deciding whether some pragmatic behaviours are inappropriate and need specific treatment. As the child recovers and the family situation stabilizes the child's behaviour may also change without any direct treatment simply because normal expectations are placed on the child again.

There are acquired aphasic children, however, who continue to exhibit inappropriate behaviours and these behaviours persist even as their semantic and syntactic skills improve. Concomitant problems, particularly dysarthric symptoms such as disturbances in the rate of speech, prosody, volume and facial expression frequently influence pragmatic behaviours.

The children with persistent pragmatic problems appear to have significant difficulties in the social domain of pragmatics. They have difficulty in perceiving the social situation and in reading non-verbal cues. Consequently they fail to read that a person may be teasing, or is angry or in a hurry. They may address adults, persons in authority, strangers and friends in the same casual manner, they often invade personal space, make embarrassing personal comments, fail to turn-take or interrupt appropriately. For example, an 11-year-old girl with acquired aphasia used to tell strangers after only a few minutes conversation that she loved them and would often try to kiss or hold their hand. It transpired that in the hospital she had been making statements such as, 'If you come here, I'll punch you in the face'. Her mother had told her that she was not to say that even as a joke because she must love everyone because they were helping her. The girl then told everyone indiscriminately that she loved them. Reports from the school she attended before her injury did not indicate any previous problem with social skills.

Children with acquired aphasia usually have difficulties in the linguistic and cognitive domains of pragmatics. Their deficits in semantics and syntax decrease their ability to clarify or explain a statement, to use language imaginatively or to be specific. These disabilities impinge on their conversational skills and prevent them meeting the obligations of discourse. They often have difficulty with topic coherence, turn-taking, repair and revision and role adjustment.

Assessment of pragmatic skills is best done from observation or from a videotape of the child with another speaker (see Appendix 3). A spontaneous language sample will assist the clinician with the evaluation of discourse skills. The literature on the normal development of pragmatic skills is relevant to the assessment of the child with acquired aphasia. Several descriptions of pragmatic behaviours are to be found in tests on the normal development of language and in the literature describing the learning-disabled child (Miller, 1981; Prutting and Kirchner, 1983, 1987; Ripich and Spinelli, 1985; Simon, 1985; Wiig and Semel, 1984). Procedures such as the Pragmatic Protocol by Prutting and Kirchner (1987), the Clinical Discourse Analysis (Damico, 1985) and the Graphic Conversational Profile (Wilks and Monaghan, 1988) may be used.

Narratives
Narratives are mid-way between oral and literate language and require planning and the dynamic integration of content, form and use. In recent years a significant amount of research has accumulated on the difficulties experienced by learning disabled students on producing narratives and the implications this has on their education. Children with acquired aphasia appear to be similar in many respects to learning-disabled individuals (see Ch. 1) so that it is logical to assume that they too may encounter problems with narratives.

The literature on reading and writing skills of the child with acquired aphasia states that difficulties persist in these two areas of language. Specific help with narrative skills may then facilitate the recovery of reading and writing abilities. Therefore, in the latter stages of recovery when the child with acquired aphasia is using complex language, the narrative abilities of the individual should be assessed. Westby (1984) stated that the more traditional testing methods used with the learning-disabled child will not detect the language difficulties that become apparent on narrative analysis.

It has also been noted that children who have made a good recovery from acquired aphasia continue to have problems with academic learning although on traditional language tests, the same that are used with the learning-disabled students, their scores are within the normal range. Westby (1984) believed that this discrepancy arises because language tests are concerned with the components of language (i.e. vocabulary, morphology and syntax) rather than the integrative process. Narrative analysis, therefore, may be one way of tapping the higher abstract learning skills which are often difficult to assess in the child with acquired aphasia. Further research is needed to determine whether children with acquired aphasia and learning-disabled students do have similar difficulties with narrative tasks and whether specific intervention will improve their skills and facilitate reading and writing abilities.

Writing
In the early stage of recovery of a child with acquired aphasia concomitant problems such as visual perceptual deficits and hemiplegia or sensory deficits of the dominant hand may prevent the assessment of writing skills. The literature reports that writing

deficits tend to persist and are in most cases certainly slower at recovering than oral language abilities. The recovery of writing skills appears to follow similar stages to those of reading skills. The older child who already has some written language ability will regain his/her skills along with oral abilities but the young child who has never learned to spell may have difficulty acquiring these new skills. Word-retrieval difficulties may affect the child's ability to write words and sentences. As with reading the assessment of writing skills requires a team approach.

The child may be asked to copy letters or words, write letters and words from dictation, construct sentences and paragraphs. Phoneme to grapheme relationships may also be evaluated. Dysorthographic errors need to be noted and consideration given to how the child made them (e.g. Was the phoneme-grapheme relationship correct? Did the child sound out the word correctly?). As with adult aphasic clients the small abstract words such as 'was', 'saw' or 'the' appear to pose persistent problems. For example, we observed a 9-year-old girl who was making an excellent recovery in other language areas but her spelling of abstract words remained poor. When asked to spell 'this' she might write 'there' or 'that' and then comment that she knew it looked something like the word she had written. She did not appear to use any strategy to help her spell the words correctly.

Play

Observation of the play of children who have had a brain lesion may help in the assessment of their language abilities. Imaginative or pretend play, particularly when interacting with peers, requires a child to organize events, sequence the events, take roles and distance themselves from the 'here and now'. Researchers have suggested that pretend play and narratives are closely linked (Westby, 1984).

There is an interdependent relationship between language and play and gains in both areas are related to cognitive development. The three processes seem inextricably interwoven. Play appears to serve as preparation for children to live in society while language allows children to master their environment, which in turn contributes to their cognitive development (Irwin, 1975). Through play a child learns to use many pragmatic functions (regulatory, permission, imaginative). Assessment of the child with a brain lesion should involve some evaluation of the child's play skills. Observations (depending on the age of the child) may include: transcriptions of the complexity of language used (in play situations a child often uses more complex structures than when in 'formal' situations), a judgement on whether the child understands the group rules of the game, whether he/she contributes ideas, protests over the role allotted him/her, uses verbal reasoning skills for compromising or collaborating and whether the child seems to be part of the group or just an observer tolerated by the other children.

A child's ability to play is often compromised by concomitant problems and it is interesting to note what strategies the child may use to circumvent these difficulties, strategies which may be adapted for use in daily living situations. For example, one quadriplegic boy seen in our clinic had a talking tracheostomy tube (consequently the volume of his voice was soft and he required frequent breaths) and a loud whistle on his chair. When he wanted to contribute anything to the group discussion he whistled and the group would quieten and listen to him. His pragmatic skills were good (e.g. He waited for a break in the conversation before he whistled.). This whistle has now become his way of interrupting appropriately and he uses it with discretion, a soft whistle to let you know he is there or a loud, long whistle if the message is urgent.

Summary of Assessment Procedures

The assessment of a child with acquired aphasia is an ongoing process and continues as part of treatment activities. Ideally, the assessment should be comprehensive and include a selection of standardized and non-standardized tests and observations. The team approach to assessment of a child with a brain lesion is the only method which will provide all persons concerned with the child's welfare with an adequate understanding of the child's problems.

Formal tests used in assessing the child with acquired aphasia may include those shown in Table 2.1. The steps taken in assessing children with acquired aphasia are summarized in Figure 2.1.

Treatment of Acquired Childhood Aphasia

General Considerations

The clinician when formulating treatment goals for the child with acquired aphasia should be cognizant of the normal development of speech and language skills and the treatment procedures applicable to children with developmental language delays. As previously stated, many of the treatment techniques used with the learning-disabled child and those used with adult aphasic clients have relevance to the child with acquired aphasia.

Children with acquired aphasia although exhibiting similar difficulties to both learning-disabled children and adult aphasic clients do differ in a number of ways and the clinician must be aware of these differences. For example, while some children with a severe head injury may be unable to learn new material or strategies to compensate for their disability, others may learn rapidly. Such a range of learning ability is not seen in the learning-disabled population. Also, a child with acquired aphasia may have a wide scattering of abilities, some skills being severely depressed while others are near the norm for his/her age. This range of abilities within the one child is usually not so great in the child with a learning disability. Memory problems also may be far greater in the aphasic child than those exhibited by learning-disabled children. One major difference between adults with acquired aphasia and children with acquired aphasia that needs to be taken into account when developing treatment strategies is the fact that language skills are still developing in children.

When treatment goals are selected they should take into account the child's age, his/her interests, and the concomitant problems which may affect his/her performance (e.g. short-term memory deficits, visual perceptual problems or the presence of primitive reflex patterns such as the asymmetrical tonic neck reflex). Goals formulated by other health professionals should be reinforced in the speech and language sessions whenever possible (e.g. transferring from a wheelchair to a chair for the session, correct postural positioning and use of the affected arm when performing activities).

Treatment sessions with children with acquired aphasia, when they are in the period of spontaneous recovery, should be frequent and occur at the time of day when the child is alert. In most cases this occurs in the morning. The clinician must remain aware that children with a brain lesion fatigue easily and that this tiredness may continue for many months. The duration of time that fatigue continues to be an important consideration in therapy seems to be highly variable among children (e.g. Parents reported that their 13-year-old daughter was still going to bed at 7 p.m. or 7.30 p.m. 12 months after the injury and that by the weekend she was 'absolutely exhausted' and would sleep even longer.)

The length of treatment sessions may need to be kept short initially (15 minutes, twice a day) and then gradually lengthened when the child is able to cope better with increased demands. While the child continues to show good progress the frequency of therapy should be maintained (not less than three times per week in most instances). Clinicians in busy general clinics may need to decide which clients have priority and timetable accordingly. The child with a brain lesion is usually considered a priority particularly if the child is still improving his/her communication skills.

Other professionals who are concerned with the child's rehabilitation may also wish to treat the child when he/she is fresh and alert. Unfortunately, this may not be possible and in such a situation a cooperative team approach is vital. Priorities, agreed on by all persons concerned with the care of the child, should be established and taken into account by each professional when deciding daily treatment goals. For example, a demanding language task may not be advisable after the child has just finished a difficult physiotherapy session. Instead, at this time the child might be better placed in a language group where other children would share the workload. Perhaps if the physiotherapist wishes to have the child stand at various times during the day she/he can do so in the language session. A committed team approach is essential if the child is to gain maximum benefit from his/her rehabilitation programme.

Activities and materials used in the session should be functional and interesting to the child although making all activities into games is not usually necessary for school age children. Close liaison between the teacher and the clinician helps the clinician formulate language goals that are pertinent to the child and reinforces the communicative and academic skills required in the classroom. School reading texts, spelling lists and other general English activities may be incorporated into many treatment sessions (e.g. An activity that requires the child to rearrange words to make a satisfactory sentence may include words which the child is reading in school or those that he is learning to spell.).

A child's strengths and weaknesses should be considered when structuring tasks for treatment sessions. For example, if a child is helped by visual cues, either pictures or written words, when given a verbal task then these should be used and gradually faded as the child is better able to cope with the task. An hierarchy of steps may need to be devised so that only one variable is introduced at any one time. For example, short-term memory activities would use familiar materials initially. When the child is able to respond consistently at one level then the task is made more demanding by either adding another familiar item or keeping the same number of items but adding a word or object that has not been used previously. As the child progresses, steps may be missed (e.g. more items as well as unfamiliar ones may be added) but the clinician must always be ready to return to an easier step if the child is unable to cope.

The first sessions may need to have behavioural rather than linguistic goals. Children may be uncooperative (which is understandable considering the trauma that has occurred) in the new setting and try the limits. These goals may include, besides cooperation with activities, increased attention to a task and the completion of a set task in a given time. Often some activity which the child is capable of doing (e.g. a simple puzzle or matching of objects or pictures) may be used which will allow him/her to succeed and be positively reinforced. This same type of task may also be used to gain the child's cooperation. Operant conditioning principles may be used effectively in these situations. Children may respond best and be cooperative if they know exactly what is expected of them. For example, 'John, you have these (indicating the number of picture cards) to do then you may play a game' or using a cardboard clock face and showing the child how long he has before the activity changes, 'John, when the big hand reaches this point, then you may choose a game to play'. The clinician moves the hand of the clock after the completion of each activity. When a child is transferred to another rehabilitation facility these goals may need to be restated because the child may again try the limits of the new staff involved with his/her treatment. Also, contributing factors to uncooperative behaviour are the fact that emotional ties he/she has forged with the staff in the former facility have to be cut and that frequently the therapy and behavioural demands in the new setting have been increased to keep pace with his/her recovery.

In each treatment session the clinician must be alert to any situation in which pragmatic behaviours may be encouraged. For example, when the child first comes into the treatment room, he/she can be expected to give eye contact and greet the clinician appropriately (the expected behaviour would be dependent on the child's abilities) and then use appropriate leave-taking skills. If the clinician is working on some particular concept then a situation may be engineered in the session. Most children love actively participating in the session (e.g. taking the game from a box, choosing which colour token to have and which to give the clinician or going to the cupboard to collect the game). The clinician may tell the child, 'Get the game on top of the cupboard', 'Find the game in the cupboard on the bottom shelf'. The complexity of the oral directions may be increased or the concept chosen be more advanced each session in line with the child's abilities. The integration of form/content/use would be a goal in each treatment session.

Since children with acquired aphasia who appear to have recovered have been shown to have subtle problems, particularly in the areas of syntax and lexical retrieval (see Ch.1 and 3), it would appear that strategies to help the child in these areas need to be given to the parents before the child's discharge.

Treatment Goals

Treatment goals may be formulated when relevant information has been gathered and priorities formulated. The treatment of morphological, syntactical, semantic and pragmatic problems would be based on the interpretation of test results, information gleaned from non-standardized tests and from observation. Activities used in treatment sessions may include tasks similar to those previously employed to assess the child's communicative skills. These tasks should consist of both comprehension and expressive activities and should use the developmental order of acquisition of morphemes, sentence structures, content categories and pragmatic behaviours as guidelines when selecting treatment goals.

Syntax

Content/form/use interact and are inseparable, but when introducing new morphemes and sentence structures, content and use must be controlled. The semantics of the task need to be restricted (e.g. use words which are simple and familiar to the child) and initially only require the child to use the structure in one functional context (e.g. in a game format, 'Does your mystery person have . . . ?'). Immediate auditory memory problems may require consideration when more complex sentence structures are introduced and the sentence length restricted as much as possible.

Visual material, in most instances, assists the child with comprehension or expressive tasks. Children enjoy seeing photographs of themselves or friends so pictures of them doing various activities may be used for eliciting certain sentence structures. For example, subject-verb-object, 'I am eating a banana' or subject-verb-object-adverbial, 'I am eating my banana under the tree'. An activity such as cooking which the child may have done in her/his occupational therapy session can be photographed and used successfully in a language session to facilitate the use of 'after' or 'before' (e.g. After I put butter on my toast, I ate it.) The clinician, when playing games such as 'Fish' or 'Memory' may require the child to use certain grammatical question structures (e.g. 'Have you got the . . . ? Will you give me the . . . ?').

Children learn by doing. Activities which involve the child doing an action (provided the child's physical problems do not restrict her/him too much) may be used to help the child understand and express tenses. For example, the child walks around the room. The clinician asks, 'What are you doing?'. The expected reply is, 'Walking'. The child sits down. 'What did you do?' The reply, 'Walked'. Past, present and future tenses may be elicited in this manner as well as prepositions and adverbial phrases (e.g. 'climbing under the table').

Imaginative play situations, if the child is capable, may be enjoyable for the child and be designed to help facilitate more complex sentence structures. For example, she/he could pretend to be a fireman, going to a fire, fighting the fire and returning to the station. The child may use 'ing' endings while describing the activities she/he is playing and then past tense with complex sentence structures to tell what she/he did (e.g. After I put the ladder up I climbed to the top and hosed the fire.)

Other treatment activities may include judgement tasks which require the child to decide on whether some structure or morpheme is correct or incorrect and may involve tense, case and any part of speech. For example, the child is shown a picture of a man walking. The clinician says, 'The man is walking. She is walking. Is that right or wrong?' or 'Yesterday, I am walking. Correct or incorrect?' Activities comprising scrambled sentences, sentence completion, sentence formulation and sentence correction, may be designed for individual children. These activities should include morphemes and complex sentences of differing structures.

Semantics

Semantic tasks must be functional for the child with acquired aphasia, for example, the pre-school child may find attributes such as 'dirty' or 'sticky' more functional in her/his environment than the names of colours. The clinician needs to investigate what is meaningful for each child in the child's home and school environments and allow this information to direct the choice of materials and content in treatment sessions.

Simple comprehension activities may consist of asking the child to choose the correct object by name or function from a set number, maybe only a choice of two or three in the early stages of recovery. This activity may be varied using a variety of semantic categories (e.g. 'Show me the dirty car. Which dog is under the table?'). Categorization and association tasks may vary from the simple to the more complex as the child progresses. For example, the child may be required to place the pictures of animals and clothes in their correct piles or for a more difficult task, to distinguish between wild animals and farm animals or things made of plastic and those made of glass. Sorting by function or attribute (e.g. 'Put all the things you read together', or 'Find all the big objects'.) may be used and increased in complexity when necessary to make the task more demanding (e.g. 'Show me all the big blue things in this picture'.). A variation on a categorization or association that may ask the child to choose 'Which picture (or word) does not belong: apple, chair or orange?'. Comprehension and expressive tasks are often combined (e.g. the categorization task may involve confrontation naming or require the child to describe why pictures go together or why one object does not belong).

Judgement tasks involving the meaning of two sentences (e.g. Are these two sentences similar in meaning? 'Jim bought the table and chairs. Jim bought the fruit'.) are useful and children seem to enjoy them, particularly if some nonsense sentences are also added (e.g. 'I ate the cake and the icecream. I ate the furniture'.) Judgement of meaning can also involve antonyms, synonyms and homonyms (e.g. synonym – 'He yelled at the boys. He shouted at the boys. Same or different?').

Expressive tasks may require the child to explain the similarities and differences between two objects (e.g. 'glasses and a microscope'). Variations of the game of 'Twenty Questions' may be played where the clinician and the child take turns in giving short descriptions of some item in a designated category. For example, 'It is an animal. It has four legs. It lives on a farm. It gives us milk'. The child may choose from among four animal pictures in front of him/her: a horse, a cow, an elephant and a lion. A visual cue may not be needed as the child becomes more proficient in understanding and expressing language. The game of 'Twenty Questions' itself or an association game where the child has to guess what goes with some object (e.g. 'shoes and . . . ?') facilitates comprehension and expression.

The adult literature discusses convergent and divergent semantic tasks and their place in aphasia therapy to aid problem solving and pragmatic tasks such as getting and giving information (Chapey, 1981). These tasks are similar to examples of verbal elaboration (Wiig and Semel, 1984) used in therapy for learning-disabled children. Convergent tasks require the individual to give a specific commonly used response (e.g. You drink from a . . . 'cup' or 'glass' would be the usual response but not 'shoe' or 'hose'). Divergent production includes tasks which call for a variety of logical responses (e.g. 'Can you think of all the things which may be yellow?'). Many language stimulation activities used in the classroom with normal children to enhance their language abilities (e.g. Peabody Development Kits (Dunn and Smith, 1965)) contain similar suggestions to divergent semantic activities and may be adapted for use with children with acquired aphasia. Adaptation primarily is by controlling the semantic and syntactic aspects of the tasks.

The use of riddles and jokes may be employed to assist the child with multi-word meanings and phonological plays on words. For example, 'Why did the tomato blush? Because it saw the salad dressing.' What word has a double meaning and what are those two meanings? 'When do astronauts eat? At launch time.' What word was changed to make the joke? Selections from children's commercial joke and riddle books are a valuable and enjoyable resource for treatment activities. Also, the clinician may make use of children's favourite television programmes. The child is asked to identify what was funny about a situation, particularly if irony is involved. Homework, which includes watching a favourite television programme, is usually willingly done. This task may also involve narrative skills or the clinician may only choose to ask specific questions about the programme ('Why was it funny when . . .?'). These types of activities are particularly useful with the older child who has a good understanding of oral language.

The older child may also be given activities which require him/her to define words, formulate sentences which show that he/she understands the meaning of the words (e.g. 'steak', 'stake') or explain figurative language. For example, explain these sayings: 'Her skin was as white as snow, Too many cooks spoil the broth, I am pulling your leg'. Care should be taken when giving instructions to children that figurative language is not used with a child who has problems understanding colloquial and multi-meaning words (e.g. A child may seem to be uncooperative because he/she does not comply when asked, 'Hop up on the table'. He cannot 'hop' that far!).

Many children with acquired aphasia have significant word retrieval problems. The strategies used to facilitate word recall may be brought to the child's awareness during confrontation naming and rapid automatic naming tasks so that he/she may trigger the specific word himself/herself. These strategies may include:

> sentence completion – I cut with a . . .
> opposite cues – old and . . .
> association cues – It goes with shoes. Shoes and . . .
> descriptions of object – It's found in the bathroom. You wash your hands in it
> category cues – It's an animal
> syllable or sound cues – 'pot' for potato, /f/ for fire
> rhyming cue – It sounds like 'rain' for train.
> pantomime cue – Pretending to bounce the ball for ball

Teaching strategies may involve taking the child through the 'thinking' process. For example, picture the object in your mind. What do you do with it? Make a sentence in your mind about the function (e.g. I cut with the....). Can you think of what sound it starts with? Some children, as they recover their language skills, may become proficient in using synonyms although this is not a common occurrence and these children have usually had excellent vocabularies before their brain lesion.

Reading and writing

Treatment in these areas may mostly involve the clinician in a supportive role to the teacher. Many of the activities used in the treatment of auditory comprehension and expressive skills may be adapted to the written mode (e.g. sentence correction and sentence formulation). Liaison with the teacher about the child's difficulties in oral language will help the teacher decide on her/his expectations for the child in reading, spelling, sentence formulation and essays. Reading and spelling may be used as visual cues in oral language tasks and this in turn also reinforces written skills. In a group situation in the classroom the teacher may also be able to reinforce narrative and metalinguistic treatment goals.

Pragmatics

Pragmatic problems may be best treated in a group situation. With older children (10 years and over), specific pragmatic or social skills groups can be successful particularly if video recording equipment is available. Younger children seem to respond best in situations where pragmatic situations occur naturally and the clinician can facilitate the appropriate behaviour. This approach is discussed further in the section on group therapy.

Individual work on pragmatic skills in the linguistic domain may be done in language sessions when they occur naturally in context (e.g. repair/revision skills may be facilitated if the child is explaining). Work on a child's narrative skills also provides an opportunity for teaching pragmatic abilities (e.g. requesting and giving specific information).

In recent years, clinicians in many disciplines have addressed the issue of social skills and how they can be taught (Foxx, 1985). An awareness of group dynamics and how to structure the group is an important consideration before deciding to work directly on social skills. In a pragmatic or social skills group, ideally involving another team member such as the occupational therapist, the teacher, the social worker or the psychologist, a target behaviour (e.g. a greeting) is selected and task analyzed by the group members. It is useful if the team members involved role play the appropriate speech act before any discussion takes place. Each group member is then given the chance to role play the situation while it is video recorded. The group can then discuss whether the behaviour was appropriate or inappropriate and decide if a breakdown occurred and if so how to correct it (e.g. 'Did the child fail to make eye contact? Did the child call out when the person was too far away to hear? Did the child fail to say the person's name or use an appropriate greeting?') Besides analyzing various speech acts it is also useful to discuss non-verbal behaviour and what facial expressions or various tones of voice mean, as well as to assist the children to read social situations, start or finish conversations, decide on what the main topic of conversation was and what they could contribute to the discourse. Once the child has become proficient in the group then the behaviour needs to be transferred into other situations.

In groups such as this it is the responsibility of the speech and language clinician to decide on what is appropriate linguistically for each individual. For example, eye contact, a smile and 'Hello, Chris' may be all that a child with dysarthria can manage whereas a child with good language skills may have the same non-verbal goals but say, 'Hello, Chris, how are you today?'.

Group Treatment

Backus and Beasley (1951) advocated that group instruction form the core of speech and language treatment. They believed that it was the forces operating in the interpersonal relationships between the child and the clinician and among children as a group that brought about the appropriate changes in their speech and language behaviour. Since 1951 these forces have been identified and analyzed and the importance of these pragmatic aspects of language realized. Language allows us to master and manipulate our environment to our advantage and competence in communicating is important for social, educational and personal development.

Children with acquired aphasia benefit from group treatment. It allows these children to put into practice the language behaviours that they have learned in their individual sessions (e.g. Asking permission using a particular syntactic structure, 'Can I have the glue, please?'), and gives them the opportunity for interacting naturally in a controlled learning situation.

Group treatment sessions with the child with acquired aphasia may take many forms and include both homogeneous and heterogeneous populations. Language groups directed by the speech and language clinician may involve engineered tasks. For example, in a group addressing mostly pragmatic behaviours, something may be placed in the doorway so that a child in a wheelchair is unable to enter. The clinician can remain close and prompt the child, if necessary, to ask for specific help (e.g. 'Helena, would you move the chair please?'). Different tasks are devised for each child so as the child learns the appropriate behaviour, the prompts decrease in the language group situation. Generalization of this behaviour is helped by engineering similar situations in different contexts (e.g. going with the physiotherapist to another room and something is placed in the child's way). Other team members are aware of the behavioural goals and can prompt if necessary.

In other language groups the emphasis of the activities may be on semantics and syntax. Divergent semantic tasks are particularly successful in group situations because an idea given by one child may stimulate further ideas from other children (e.g. 'Think of all the things you could do with a box.' 'What would happen if we did not have water?'). Their ideas may be written or drawn on the board so that revision may take place. Turn-taking and repair/revision skills may also be reinforced. Barrier games facilitate specific word usage and aid organizational skills. For example, the children have a number of objects in front of them and arrange them in some way. The clinician has the same objects behind a barrier and the children must tell her how to arrange the objects. It is helpful to have two team members involved, one behind the barrier and the other to facilitate specific instructions.

Interdisciplinary or transdisciplinary groups, where the emphasis is not primarily on communcation skills, provide numerous pragmatic situations and facilitate the generalization of skills learned in individual language sessions. A fine motor control group directed by the occupational therapist may involve cutting and pasting skills. It also provides the children with an opportunity for learning requesting behaviours (e.g. 'Chris, may I have the scissors please?' or 'Chris, scissors please.'). Care must be taken in such groups that the language demands do not overshadow the other activities. It is best to focus on only one communication skill (e.g. The goal for each child might be to give eye contact and say the name of the person they are addressing.). Other team members ensure that this occurs while the speech and language clinician may help individual children to frame their present request in the most appropriate language depending on their language abilities.

Creative dramatics is a group activity which is closely linked to the dramatic play of children and is a technique that, when adapted, offers the clinician another treatment procedure. It is an informal spontaneous drama situation which allows a leader to structure and give form to the imaginative play of children. Because of the nature of the activities it provides numerous pragmatic opportunities for the children involved as well as stimulating divergent semantic behaviour.

The guided activities used in creative dramatics give children a chance to examine life in a more concrete form through the development of replica-of-life situations. This allows them to gain insight into their own and others' feelings and learn to understand and adapt to a variety of situations because they can experience present and future events and re-examine past ones.

There are several aspects to creative dramatics and each step may be successfully adapted for use with children with acquired aphasia. Simple activities such as 'Simon says', action songs, finger plays or a simple 'Guess what I am doing' activity may serve to introduce children to the imaginative situation. As they become more confident sensory awareness activities incorporating all senses may be suggested (e.g. concentrate on a real or imaginary object and discuss everything about it or listen to all the sounds in the room and name them. Pretend you are bush walking. What sounds can you hear?).

Movement activities (e.g. pretend to be raking leaves, reading a book, picking apples from a tree) follow sensory awareness tasks. Because the situations are imaginary it does not matter whether the children can actually do the physical actions well. Some severely disabled children use only small arm or finger movements yet enjoy the activity and make suggestions for further activities. Characterization and improvization are more demanding imaginary tasks but often facilitate the use of spontaneous language. Before beginning characterization or improvization activities, discussion takes place. For example, How would you know whether someone was a fireman or a policewoman? What do they do? How do you know someone is old? Improvization involves dialogue. Again discussion centres on what a person would say if they were: buying an ice-cream, calling a puppy, or selling tickets on a wheel of fortune; situations which some children would find difficult, such as asking for help or information, may be included in the imaginative situation. Children never play themselves in creative dramatics and so the demands to produce language correctly are lessened.

The final stage in creative dramatics is the dramatization of a chosen theme or story and this is excellent for improving children's narrative and sequencing skills. Stories chosen for dramatization may be those which are the children's current favourites or the 'classics' such as 'The Three Billy Goats Gruff' or 'The Ginger Bread Man'. For younger children stories with repetition are excellent because the more able child may serve as a model for another child. Discussion plays an important role in deciding what and how the actions are to be played. Children need to have a firm idea of the sequence of the story, what is to happen in each scene, where and why it happens, what characters are involved and how they react. A scene or the story is played and an evaluation of the playing takes place immediately (e.g. The character or action is discussed but the children's names are never used. 'Was the king angry enough when . . . ' not 'Was Alex angry enough when . . . '). The story, with improvements, may be played again with a further evaluation.

Initially, older children may be inhibited but these barriers gradually disappear as they become more secure in the group situation and with the activities. Older children particularly enjoy problem-solving situations. For example, they are members of a company and because of a strike by the pilots they cannot send their goods by air. What will they do? They play out the situation and the solutions. Many children with a brain lesion may not be able to cope with the final stage of creative dramatics but find enjoyment and benefit in short improvization situations and other earlier stages. The speech and language clinician may direct creative dramatic activities but if the school the children attend has access to a drama specialist then her/his expertise is extremely valuable and the sessions may be jointly planned with all team members involved and goals for each child established. For clinicians who wish to learn more of creative dramatics a reading list has been provided in Appendix 4.

The assessment and treatment of the pre-school child with a brain lesion presents a challenge to the rehabilitation team. Many pre-school children may appear to be developing normally and their subtle problems taken for immaturity rather than as symptoms of a brain lesion. Frequently, comments such as 'She'll be fine when she gets to school. She'll settle down there, or He seems to mix quite well with the other children', are heard and a referral is not made to the rehabilitation team. Subtle problems such as a poor attention span, impulsive behaviour, word retrieval difficulties and a difficulty learning new concepts may be observed in these children. If their problems are missed at this early age and go untreated then their difficulties may manifest in the early school years as they try to cope with the increased linguistic and cognitive demands in the schoolroom.

Treatment techniques successfully used with the pre-school child with a brain lesion are similar to those used with the language-delayed child, although the clinician must remain aware of the difficulties these children may have with cognitive tasks (e.g. problem solving, sustained representational or imaginative play). Treatment in a interdisciplinary or transdisciplinary group seems to be a particularly valuable treatment approach.

Problem Solving

Problem solving and organizational deficits have not been specifically addressed in this text but they are problems shown by many children with acquired aphasia. Problem solving, sequencing and organization should be inherent in treatment methodology. For example, if the clinician chooses to play a game with the child to facilitate specific semantic and syntactical structures then the problem-solving strategies used by the clinician when playing the game should be demonstrated to the child by thinking aloud (e.g. If one of your two mystery people has yellow hair and the other has black, then that means I can take out all the people that have brown or white or red hair.). Many commercial board games and some computer software can provide excellent therapy material. In the treatment of reading and written expression organization and problem-solving strategies may be discussed. For example, if a child is writing a short essay then there must be a beginning, a middle and an end. Discussion on what information needs to be given first, to let the reader know what the situation involves, what information should be in the middle section and how to end the story appropriately, may be a treatment goal.

Use of Computers in the Assessment and Treatment of Acquired Childhood Aphasia

The computer can be a valuable clinical tool. Besides using it for administrative tasks it may be used in assessment and therapy. A number of analysis and assessment programs have been developed including the Language Assessment and Screening Procedure (LARSP) (Bishop, 1984), Computerized Profiling (Long, 1986), Systematic Analysis of Language Transcripts (SALT) (Miller and Chapman, 1983), Lingquest I: Computer Assisted Language Sample Analysis (Mordecai *et al.*, 1982), and Lingquest II: Computer Assisted Phonological Analysis (Palin and Mordecai, 1982). The amount of qualitative and quantitative information generated by many of these programs is often far greater than the amount that can be analyzed 'manually'. Also, the computer is usually faster completing this analysis thus saving clinical time, particularly if a detailed linguistic analysis is necessary. For example, the microanalysis on the LARSP can yield printed information on how many times the child used the past tense and what regular and irregular verbs were selected or how often the child used a subject-verb-object construction and the specific sentences that were generated. With this information the clinician may note that the child used the verb 'made' 15 of the 20 times he used the past tense. Therapy goals or further assessment probes can then be formulated to address this deficit. Many of the assessment programs are expensive but in the long-term the cost effectiveness of such a program can be justified.

The computer has a wide application as a therapy tool. Most children appear to be highly motivated when given the opportunity of using the computer in therapy. There are few programs available, within an acceptable price range, that have been designed primarily for the language-disordered child. With a little ingenuity, however, many educational software programs can be adapted for both comprehension and expressive tasks.

Graded reading games have proved useful for both verbal and written comprehension activities. Initially, the child with acquired aphasia may be unable to read or even recognize letters. At this stage, the clinician may read the passage and the answers, with adjustment of language if necessary, and assist the child to choose the correct response. The choice of answers may also be reduced. As the child recovers his reading abilities he can be encouraged to read larger amounts of information with gradually decreasing assistance from the clinician. The semantic content and syntactic complexity in the programs is increased as the grade levels become higher.

Many families have computers and it may be possible to lend programs to the family for use at home, particularly if the parent has been instructed on how to adapt the program. Matching and association games are available as well as numerous programs requiring word, sentence and sequencing skills.

Expressive tasks may involve the same reading games (e.g. the clinician reads the passage and asks the child to retell the story). Spelling may be helped with programs which include games such as 'Hangman' or cross-word puzzles. Strategies to help the child with spelling can be brought to the child's awareness. For example, in 'Hangman', the first letter may be 't' and the third a vowel. It is not possible for the second letter to be an 'f' or a 'q'. It has to be a consonant that is found in a 't' cluster, such as 'w' or 'r'. If the clinician thinks aloud and the child can hear the reasoning process then it is possible that this technique may help the child develop or enhance his/her own logical thinking skills which, in children with acquired aphasia, are frequently depressed.

Software which allows children to draw or use graphics to make their own pictures can be used to facilitate children's knowledge of concepts, generate simple or complex sentences as descriptions of the picture they have drawn or used as stimuli for a narrative. Older children may enjoy using the word processor for writing sentences or short essays.

Mystery games or those programs where a child can choose a number of responses, some of which will allow different actions to occur and give the child the ability to decide the outcome of the story, may help facilitate problem solving skills, narrative and sequencing abilities. When these programs are used in small group situations they promote group discussion and cooperative problem solving.

There are some useful options available with many computer programs which enhance their value as clinical tools. Many commercial programs allow the user to store pertinent written information on the program disk or on a student disk. Sentence completion tasks or spelling lists from the child's school work can be incorporated into the format of the commercial game (e.g. 'Hangman'). This option is particularly useful for clinicians dealing with children with acquired aphasia whose linguistic deficits are usually widely variable. With this option, each game may be individually tailored for each client.

Some of the problem-solving programs will take a few treatment sessions to complete so that a save option which allows the clinician to save a half-completed game, as well as a number of games on a disk, is valuable. Good graphics are also important. Children seem to lose interest if the graphics are only line drawing or if the pictures are difficult to recognize.

It needs to be remembered that the computer is only one of a number of clinical tools. Although some children with acquired brain damage may find working through a program on their own useful, the most satisfactory treatment results seem to be obtained when the clinician assists the child with the program and facilitates the correct response.

Summary

Both the reports of practising clinicians and the descriptions of children with acquired aphasia documented in the literature seem to suggest that children with a brain lesion may present with communicative difficulties similar to those problems experienced by learning-disabled children and the adult aphasic population. Assessment and treatment procedures may be successfully adapted for the child with acquired aphasia from techniques used with both learning disabled and adult aphasic clients. Although the populations have some symptoms in common there are differences and it is hoped that future clinical research will provide more definitive descriptions of language assessment and intervention in acquired aphasia in children. Steps to be taken during the treatment of acquired childhood aphasia are summarized in Figure 2.2.

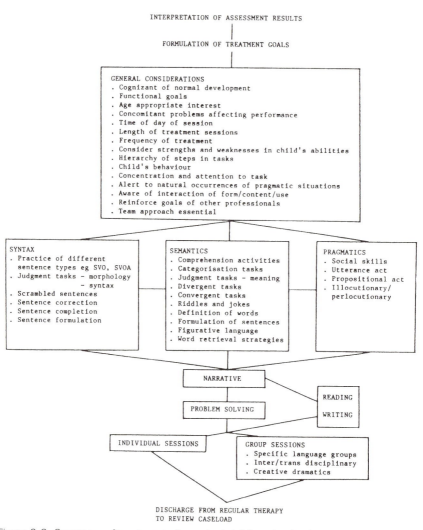

Figure 2.2 Summary of treatment of acquired childhood aphasia

Case Reports

To illustrate the major features of the assessment and treatment of children with acquired aphasia outlined above and to place them in a clinical context, two case reports are presented.

Case One

The client, Sandra, a 4½-year-old girl of part-Aboriginal descent was referred to a neurologist when she was 8 months old with a 5-month history of left-sided weakness.

Neurological examination

An initial CT scan at 8 months of age revealed a right cerebral hemisphere infarct secondary to occlusion of the right middle cerebral artery with subsequent porencephaly developing in the cerebral cortex and associated with atrophy of the right cerebral hemisphere. A subsequent EEG revealed prominent right posterior abnormalities suggestive of epileptic activity.

Speech and language assessment

At 3 years of age she was accepted at a special pre-school and referred for further occupational therapy and physiotherapy. The referring letter reported that she had good speech development and would not require speech therapy. Most people, including her mother, felt that Sandra had no difficulty with speech and language skills.

After a few months in pre-school, however, it was noted that Sandra had some difficulty understanding age-appropriate concepts as well as a marked difficulty with word retrieval and a lack of specificity in her language. Her attention to task was poor and she flitted from one activity to another. Her concentration span was not comparable to that of her peers.

At 3½ years of age on the TACL-R she performed between the 42nd and 56th percentile on all subtests except Grammatical Morphemes which was at the 27th percentile. A LARSP analysis confirmed her difficulty with morphemes on an expressive as well as receptive level. On the PPVT her score was at the 37th percentile. On a Bloom and Lahey Content/Form analysis (Bloom and Lahey, 1978) she was using and combining the early content categories with no apparent difficulty. The language samples, however, did show evidence of verbal and literal paraphasias (e.g. 'table' for 'chair', 'dog thing' for 'bone' and 'keffle' which seemed to be a combination of 'kettle' and 'coffee'). Essentially, though, Sandra's speech and language skills were within normal developmental limits. Yet both the speech and language clinician and the pre-school teacher believed that she had some language difficulties. The formal language tests available, however, did not appear sensitive enough to reveal her problems.

Extension testing confirmed that when more than two semantic elements were contained in a verbal command and no visual or situational cues were used then Sandra could not respond appropriately. Two elements presented no difficulty. She also had problems with 'wh' questions particularly when a 'what' or a 'where' question could be asked. For example, in response to a picture of a man eating an apple in the kitchen and being asked, 'What is the man eating?' Sandra would often answer with an adverbial phrase rather than the name of the object (e.g. 'in the kitchen' instead of 'an apple'). It was also noted that if Sandra could not retrieve the word she used circumlocution. Tangential ideas were also triggered by her circumlocution. For example, when shown a picture of a sheet Sandra replied, 'It's used on the bed. You pull it up. My Mum went mad on my brother'. When then asked some searching questions, it appeared that her brother had either ripped the sheet or used it to make a cubby house and was in trouble with his mother.

The Double Administration Naming Technique (DANT) (Fried-Oken, 1987) was administered and confirmed that Sandra had problems retrieving words. No reliable cue was found to help her retrieve the appropriate word. It was difficult to determine whether Sandra had word-finding problems or whether she had a reduced expressive lexicon from which to retrieve the names. It would appear from observation that Sandra had difficulties in both areas.

Pragmatically, Sandra appeared age-appropriate in the cognitive and social domain. As a result of her expressive difficulties her skills in the linguistic domain were not comparable with her peers (e.g. her inability to answer specifically or to give well sequenced simple explanations).

Current status including concomitant problems

Sandra attends a special pre-school twice a week where she receives speech and language therapy as well as occupational and physiotherapy. She also attends another pre-school three times a week which was especially established for aboriginal and Torres Strait Islander children. This latter pre-school is in a low socio-economic area. When her language difficulties were discussed with her mother, her mother commented that Sandra's brother had similar problems (i.e. non-specific language).

Sandra has a left-sided hemiparesis but can walk and run independently with the aid of a left leg calliper. Her main physical problem seems to be with fine motor control in her left hand. There is associated tone of effort in her left upper limb during right hand activity and she is unable to effect a pincer grasp. However, although she is reluctant to use her left limb, she can use it sometimes as a stabilizer or when performing bilateral activities. Initially, the neurologist reported that her attention span was short and that there was some associated behavioural problems. Sandra's impulsive behaviour often causes problems in pre-school (e.g. she falls over objects because she is walking and not looking where she is going or turns quickly and knocks a cup or a toy from the table). Although she had never had any seizure activity it was thought that she might require some anti-convulsant therapy in the future. To date this has not happened.

A language sample at 4 years of age showed that her syntactical structure had increased in complexity and the content had become more specific over the previous 6-month period. Pragmatically, she maintained topic and answered questions appropriately. Generally, her concentration had improved, she is now less impulsive and will attend to task.

At $4\frac{1}{2}$ years of age, testing on the Boehm Test of Basic Concepts-Revised (Boehm, 1986) placed her on the 10th percentile of the lower socio-economic group. However, visual perceptual difficulties appear to have influenced Sandra's score (e.g. she missed 'behind' yet she uses it appropriately in expressive situations and can carry out a command requiring her to go or put an object behind something). It should be noted that situational cues are at a minimum in this test.

The pre-school teacher from the Aboriginal pre-school reported that Sandra was a leader and had no problems when compared with her peer group. A summary of the speech and language tests used for the assessment of case 1 is outlined in Table 2.2.

Therapy

Because Sandra only attends the rehabilitation pre-school twice a week and because of the clinician's other caseload commitments she is not seen for regular individual therapy. Consequently, most of her therapy needs have to be met in the group situation. Occasionally she receives some individual treatment when resources permit. She is involved in a number of inter-disciplinary groups which include at least two team

Table 2.2 Case 1. Summary of assessments used

Age	Assessments	Comments
3½ yrs	Observation	• Difficulty understanding age-appropriate concepts • Word-retrieval problems • Lack of specificity in language • Poor attention to task
	TACL-R (Carrow-Woolfolk, 1985)	• Word classes and relations — 42nd percentile • Grammatical morphemes — 27th percentile • Elaborated sentences — 56th percentile
	Language samples LARSP (Crystal *et al.*, 1982)	• Confirmed morpheme difficulty
	Content/form (Bloom and Lahey, 1978)	• Early content categories → locative action: present • Neologisms • Literal and verbal paraphasias • Circumlocutions • Lack of specificity
	Extension testing (Non-standardized)	• Difficulty when instructions 3 + elements • Difficulty understanding 'Wh' questions
	DANT (Fried-Oken, 1987)	• Confirmed word-retrieval problems • No reliable cue to assist word retrieval
4 yrs	Language sample LARSP Content/form	• Greater variety and complexity of structures • Improvement with morphological endings • Coordination and causality category used
	Observation	• Improved attention to task • Greater specificity • Fewer paraphasias
4½ yrs	Boehm Test of Basic Concepts-Revised (Boehm, 1986)	• 10th percentile. Lower socio-economic group

Patient not yet discharged — therapy continuing.

members from the following: the speech pathologist, the teacher, the physiotherapist or the occupational therapist. Two groups where her language skills are specifically targeted are one involving gross and fine motor skills and another involving language and imaginative play. The staff present in each group are aware of her language goals and how to facilitate her language skills. For example, they require specific language from Sandra (e.g. She must ask 'Can I ride on the horse?' not 'Can I go on that?' and point).

In the language group, requesting behaviour has been particularly targeted primarily because most children in the group are physically disabled and often needed to ask for help. Imaginative play situations (which the children loved and would often suggest) were devised where the children had to request help and learn to be specific in their requests (e.g. pretending to shop in a supermarket). Some items which they were asked to buy were too high for them to reach or they were asked to get too many items and they could not carry them all. A team member was always near and the children were encouraged to request help. Sandra had been observed in numerous situations to cry and say 'I can't do it' when she needed help. However, she would not look to anyone for assistance and just kept repeating her utterance until someone observed her difficulty and responded.

Before each imaginative play activity discussion and demonstrations of the linguistic skills required took place. Even after a short demonstration of the specific task Sandra had to be cued into the situation. For example, 'Do you need some help, Sandra?' 'Yes', she would answer. 'What do you do when you need help?' 'Ask', she would say. 'Yes. What do you say?' 'Kathy (teacher), will you get the milk, please'. Her response was usually correct. Practice of these skills would then occur in other groups particularly in the fine motor group where Sandra often needed assistance.

In the fine motor group, led by an occupational therapist, Sandra had to be specific when asking for what she wanted. When she requested help she was expected to give eye contact and use the name of the helper (e.g. 'Kathy, can I have the glue please?' instead of 'I want that' addressed to no one in particular). If she had difficulty retrieving the name of a specific item a team member would first try a sentence completion task (e.g. 'It's sticky. It's called . . . .'). If Sandra was able to name the object correctly she was then expected to frame the request as stated. If she seemed to be having problems with encoding then the team member would frame the request for her. She was encouraged to repeat but not expected to imitate the utterance. If she was unable to retrieve the word then a phonemic cue was given. If this failed then the name of the item was given and a few minutes later in the session a team member would ask her to name the item.

In the movement group, commands were kept short when new concepts were introduced (e.g. 'Sandra, go through the tunnel', 'through' being a new concept). Repetition was used as a learning strategy and after an obstacle course was completed the children were asked what they had done using the course as the visual cue to help recall the sequence of actions and the concepts employed (e.g. 'over', 'under', 'up', and 'down'). Concepts such as 'first', 'last', and 'next' were also stressed. At all times during group activities appropriate greeting behaviours, eye contact as well as turn-taking were expected from Sandra.

Individual sessions, when possible, stressed classification and association tasks using a variety of activities (e.g. a simple guessing game similar to 'Twenty Questions'). Activities based on Bloom and Lahey's Content/Form categories (Bloom and Lahey, 1978) were also part of a therapy programme (e.g. coordination of locative action and attribution in an appropriate syntactical utterance with three constituents or learning to express causality using 'because'). A behaviour modification programme was initiated to improve Sandra's attention to task. For example, she was given a stick or a stamp or promised a game after she had completed a set of number of items in a task regardless of whether they were correct or incorrect.

Although Sandra's brain lesion is in the right hemisphere she still appears to have some language problems, particularly with word retrieval. She has similar problems, as reported in the literature, to other children with acquired brain damage in the right hemisphere, being impulsive and having visual perceptual problems. It is difficult to conclude, however, whether her language problems can be attributed solely to her brain lesion or whether an heredity/environmental factor also plays a major role.

Case Two

The patient, Narelle, was a 9½-year-old, right-handed girl who had been hit on the head by a falling tree branch. She remained unconscious after the injury, and while being transported to hospital first the left and then the right pupil dilated. Prior to a CT scan examination she underwent an urgent craniotomy. She remained in intensive care for 3 weeks during which time she underwent surgery for removal of the extensive fragmented fracture and the repair of her dura. Two weeks after admission extubation was attempted but was unsuccessful because her vocal cords had developed extensive granulation tissue. A tracheostomy had to be performed.

Neurological examination

A month after her injury Narelle's neurological status was assessed. Although she was conscious and alert the examining neurologist reported severe expressive dysphasia and a moderate receptive dysphasia. Visual acuity in both eyes was poor, with the left eye in particular being virtually blind. Also present was a complete left third cranial nerve palsy and a temporal hemianopia in the right eye. All other cranial nerves appeared normal although her tongue deviated to the right. She had a dense right hemiparesis but was able to walk with assistance.

Neuroradiological examination

The CT scan performed after the craniotomy showed extensive left temporoparietal fracture complex with extensive contusion of the underlying left temporal lobe. The following day a further CT scan showed haemorrhagic contusion in the left temporal region with considerable blood and some dilation of the lateral ventricles. A month later a CT scan showed significantly advanced ventricular dilation and a ventricular peritoneal shunt was inserted. The CT scan taken 4 months after the injury showed that the catheter was in a good position and there was some reduction in the size of the lateral, third and fourth ventricles. The left cerebellar-pontine subdural collection was no longer apparent.

Concomitant problems

Narelle made a good recovery of movement and strength in her right side. Although the initial dense hemiparesis in her right upper limb resolved to near normal motor functioning, she exhibited marked sensory deficits particularly on the palmar surface. These deficits hampered her functional ability but she continued to be right hand dominant in most activities except writing. Her visual acuity improved but the visual field deficit persisted and caused some minor motor incoordination of the eye- and figure-ground difficulties but she compensated by good visual scanning. Perceptually, she scored within the average range.

Speech and language recovery

A month after her admission she had no meaningful vocalization and her responses to 'yes/no' questions were inconsistent. Oral feeds were commenced and she tolerated a soft diet. Two weeks later her responses to 'yes/no' questions were consistent and she had some automatic expressive language such as 'no' and 'bye'. She was able to imitate some vowels and consonants with effort. Feeding was no problem. Seven weeks after the accident, Narelle was able to understand some complex sentences (e.g. 'The boy is running and the girl is jumping' but not 'Show me all of the red lines except the last one') and responded to social language appropriately. Her expressive skills were grammatically correct at this time but lacked content words.

Eight weeks after injury, when her irritability had decreased, an informal but systematic speech and language assessment was attempted. Receptively she could identify objects by name, colour, function, size and position, and could follow simple instructions. When sentences were semantically and syntactically complex she failed to comprehend. Her reading abilities were also severely affected. She could match letters and some letters to phonemes. She was also able to recognize some simple words (e.g. 'dog', 'cat').

Severe difficulties in using semantically important words in utterances and verbal and literal paraphasias characterized her expressive language. Her sentences were grammatically correct but with few content words. She usually required a sentence completion or a phonemic cue before she could produce a content word. Articulation was characterized by problems sequencing phonemes in complex words and exacerbated by literal paraphasias.

Written expression was complicated by fine motor deficits. She was able to write from dictation some letters of the alphabet, her name and some simple sentences which she initiated (e.g. 'The cat is black'.).

Language evaluation

Narelle was discharged from speech therapy 14 months after injury because her family were moving to another state. During the period before her discharge, Narelle made significant gains in the comprehension and expression of oral language. Three months after her accident the Clinical Evaluation of Language Functions (CELF) (Semel and Wiig, 1980) was attempted. The production subtests of the CELF were not administered because Narelle could not cope with these subtests and became distressed. She only managed to produce one name for each category on the Word Associations subtest and then only when prompted (e.g. At breakfast we eat bacon and . . . .). Literal paraphasias were numerous during the Word Series subtest and she refused to continue because she was aware of her failures. Her Processing Score was below the 5th percentile with a language age of 5 years 5 months (chronological age = 8 years 9 months). All subtests were below criterion level. Significant problems were noted on the Processing Spoken Paragraphs subtest. She was unable to answer any of the questions correctly. On the Peabody Picture Vocabulary Test (PPVT) (Dunn, 1965) she scored at the 30th percentile. Visual field deficits negatively influenced her PPVT score.

Seven months after her injury her Processing Score on the CELF was at the 5th percentile with a language age of 6 years 9 months (chronological age = 9 years 1 month). Linguistic Concepts, Relationships and Ambiguities subtests were above the criterion level and her performance on the Word Classes subtest was borderline. She was still having significant problems with expressive tasks and most of the production subtests of the CELF were not attempted. However, she was willing to attempt Word Associations and the Formulated Sentences subtests. Her sentences were simple when given the stimulus word (e.g. 'car' : 'I can see a car.' or 'children': 'I like children.') but sentences requiring conjunctions or adverbs were incorrect (e.g. 'because' : 'because I said so' and 'slowly' : 'My friend is slow at running.'). Her word associations tended to consist of broad categories (i.e. 'fruit', 'vegetables', or 'meat') and the animals named were mostly farm animals. Word-retrieval problems had decreased since her previous assessment. On the PPVT she scored at the 50th percentile, compensating well for her visual field deficit.

Twelve months after the accident her Processing Score on the CELF was at the 30th percentile and her Production Score at the 10th percentile yielding language ages of 9 years for processing and 7 years 3 months for Production (chronological age = 9 years 7 months). The subtest giving her the greatest problems was Processing Spoken Paragraphs. Her score on the PPVT at this time was at the 90th percentile.

Spontaneous speech

Narelle's spontaneous speech recovered quickly. Within 7 weeks of injury her communication progressed from no meaningful vocalization to grammatically correct sentences lacking content words. She had severe word-retrieval difficulties. When she was asked specific questions she would often pantomime her reply (e.g. getting on the floor and doing exercises to denote physiotherapy). Her language was circumlocutory with numerous literal paraphasias and some verbal paraphasias. Because her communication lacked content her listeners often did not understand her message.

There was gradual decrease in paraphasias and circumlocution over the 14-month period of speech and language therapy. Literal and verbal paraphasias disappeared first from her spontaneous speech. Content words specific to the 'here and now' seemed to be the easiest for Narelle to recall, followed by recall of the immediate past (e.g. the activities she had just completed at school before coming to therapy). Word retrieval was particularly difficult when she was required to explain or clarify her meaning. Memory did not appear to play a significant part in these problems. On discharge, 14 months after her injury, Narelle had few problems if the linguistic demands of conversational speech were minimal. Literal and verbal paraphasias were rarely heard and word-retrieval problems were few. Difficulties with word retrieval still persisted, however, when she was required to clarify or explain her meaning she gave her listeners enough content (often a context clue, e.g. 'beach' or 'holidays') for them to understand her message. Two years after the injury, when speaking with Narelle on the phone, the clinician noted that Narelle had no apparent problems in conversation and could explain logically what had happened at school and in her family life since her discharge.

Humour

Initially Narelle could only understand humour when it was concrete (i.e. 'slap-stick comedy'). If a joke or riddle was dependent on a word having two or more meanings, Narelle could neither understand the joke nor retell it (e.g. 'How do you stop a herd of rhinoceroses from charging?' Answer, 'Take away their credit cards.'). Further, she could not answer riddles even when presented with options from which to choose (e.g. 'What goes up but never comes down?' Answer, 'Smoke'). Narelle also had problems in accepting good-natured teasing from her peers. She failed to read their non-verbals or understand the incongruities in their language. This would often lead to frustration and arguments. However, as her language comprehension improved so did her ability to cope in these situations.

Narrative

Narelle's written stories before the accident were well above average for her age. After the injury, as her written language recovered her narrative was a series of short simple sentences in a sequence (e.g. The family is at the beach. The boy is swimming. The girl is making a sand castle.). As her recovery continued her narratives appeared to progress through the normal developmental stages even though therapy did not stress these steps. Her main difficulty in the latter stages of recovery was the lack of specificity and organization. Verbal difficulties were mirrored in her written work, for example, her stories contained a predominance of simple sentences or complex sentences with 'and then' as the conjunction rather than coordinators such as 'before', 'after', 'but', 'when' or 'because' which she had used before her injury. Nine months after her injury, a narrative, the story of Cinderella which she knew well, was analyzed. It was cohesive, sequenced correctly and used a variety of conjunctions and syntactical structures. Word-retrieval problems, however, were still in evidence and seemed to be the cause of pauses, often two to three seconds in duration, and false starts and repetitions. However, the organizational framework (i.e. a beginning, middle and end with specific descriptions of the characters and their relationship to one another), was apparent.

Play

From observation Narelle was able to play imaginatively as soon as she was physically able. However, her play involved much pantomime and action with little verbal reasoning skills required (e.g. pop-stars singing on stage or mothers and fathers). When her class was involved in drama sessions with a visiting drama specialist Narelle initially was unable to cope because her comprehension and verbal reasoning skills were inadequate; she became extremely frustrated during these sessions.

In one imaginative situation the children in her class pretended to be a group of scientists who were concerned about pollution on Earth. The scenario was as follows. The scientists had decided to escape from Earth and had discovered another planet which was similar to their world. Unfortunately, it was inhabited by a few survivors of a superior race who did not want the Earth people to settle there. The aliens were scared that the scientists would bring pollution to their planet. The same things that were happening to Earth had happened on their planet aeons ago and virtually destroyed their civilization. The alien planet had few trees, flowers, birds or animals and over the centuries fewer and fewer children were being born so that now the survivors were unable to have children.

These drama sessions continued for 1½ hours for 10 weeks during which time the children had to decide what action they could take. Following their decision the children then had to negotiate with rather hostile aliens (played by the speech pathologists). As part of this negotiation the children had to convince the aliens that they had skills and resources that would help the planet.

Towards the end of the 10 weeks Narelle was able to contribute ideas and understand the reasoning process. Both her mother and previous teacher reported that Narelle would have had no difficulty participating in such an activity before the accident. By observing her difficulties in these sessions further therapy goals were formulated. This situation provided an excellent opportunity to sample a number of Narelle's linguistic and pragmatic skills and to observe her progress. The standardized tests used with Narelle failed to identify this verbal reasoning difficulty. However, extrapolation of her standardized test results would seem to suggest the probability of problems in this area. Also, a normal language sample may not have provided the same information because most samples do not place the child in such a demanding linguistic situation. This imaginative scenario required a high level of cognitive, comprehensive and expressive abilities. As yet, there is little information in the literature about verbal reasoning skills in acquired childhood aphasia.

Reading

Before her accident, Narelle had been an excellent reader and read for recreation. Her reading skills improved almost daily after the injury, progressing from matching letters and words to choosing the correct sentence for a picture. Her written difficulties mirrored her verbal difficulties but were slower recovering. It was the amount of information that she was required to process rather than specific syntactic or semantic elements that gave her problems; for example, breaking the passage she was to read into short sections facilitated her comprehension. As she recovered, the amount of written information that she could process accurately increased, although at the time of discharge, 14 months after the injury, she still had not started to read for pleasure again. She complained, at this time, that she did not understand the story.

Writing

Like her reading, her written language improved quickly, although sensory problems in her right hand and her need to use her left non-dominant hand interfered with activities involving handwriting skills. Narelle suffered fatigue easily while writing so a typewriter or computer was often used. It was the spelling of the small abstract words such as 'the', 'as' etc. which gave her the greatest difficulty. She would omit them or interchange them indiscriminately (e.g. use 'was' for 'the' without seeing that it was incorrect).

A letter received by one of us from Narelle some 2 years after her injury had no spelling mistakes and her syntax was correct. A note added by her mother said that Narelle had written most of the letter herself without help.

Behaviour

When admitted to a school for handicapped children Narelle was unhappy with her class placement. She wanted to return to her former school and found it difficult to settle into the educational situation with other disabled children, many in wheelchairs. Throughout the duration of her rehabilitation Narelle was anxious that all staff involved in her treatment be aware of her previous school achievements. She would constantly remind staff that she had come first in her class and that most of the activities done in therapy she used to be able to do easily. She would also keep her work books from her former school with her and often bring them to therapy. She was determined to succeed and return to her former school. Consequently, she worked hard at school, in therapy and at home in a very supportive family environment. However, she was often frustrated by her inability to do some activity. A summary of the speech and language tests used for the assessment of case 2 is outlined in Table 2.3.

Therapy

Close liaison was maintained with Narelle's teacher and having a school on the same premises as the therapy departments was a distinct advantage for language treatment. Language tasks, whether they were verbal or written, mostly involved work that she would be using in class or had difficulty completing at school. School and therapy staff worked closely together, for example, when the occupational therapist planned a cooking session with Narelle she would take photos of the sequence of steps and these would be used later in Narelle's language session for both verbal and written tasks. Likewise, her family would send photos of special occasions or of recent outings and these would also be incorporated into language treatment sessions.

Treatment was daily and covered many areas. The main focus of therapy, however, was on Narelle's word-retrieval difficulties and her problems processing varying amounts of verbal and written language. Word-retrieval strategies included: sentence completion using all parts of speech, associations and categorization tasks, questions about Narelle's home and school environments, description of objects in a 'Twenty Questions' format, rhyming words, and antonyms, synonyms and homonyms. Initially, word retrieval was significantly helped by visual cues. When she played various card games with matching cards or association cards Narelle could, herself, facilitate the retrieval of the word required, for example, 'I want something that goes with the cage'. At this stage she would be holding the picture of the cage. This

Table 2.3 *Case 2. Summary of assessments used*

Post Injury	Assessments	Comments
4 weeks	Observation	• No meaningful vocalization • Inconsistent responses to 'yes/no' questions • Soft diet tolerated
6 weeks	Observation/Informal	• Imitation of some vowel and consonant sounds • Spontaneous 'no' and 'bye' • Consistent responses to 'yes/no' questions • No feeding problems
7 weeks	Informal/observation	• Responses to social language appropriate • Grammatically correct sentences lacking content words • Pantomime used for clarification • Severe word-retrieval problems • Understood complex sentences up to four semantic elements
8 weeks	Non-standardized systematic speech and language assessment	• Severe word-retrieval problems • Verbal and literal paraphasias • Sentences (SVOA) grammatically correct • Receptively could identify common objects by name, function, colour, size and position • Followed simple directions • Failed to understand semantically and syntactically complex sentences • Could not understand verbal humour • Verbal reasoning skills poor • Could match all letters of the alphabet • Write some letters to dictation — inconsistent responses • Write some self-generated simple sentences: 'The cat is black.' • Pragmatic skills appropriate except in linguistic domain • Some problems with understanding when peers were teasing • Play — imaginative but verbal reasoning skills poor

Table 2.3 Continued

Post Injury	Assessments	Comments
12 weeks	CELF (Semel & Wiig, 1980)	• Processing score below 5th percentile • Major difficulty processing paragraphs • Production subtests not completed because patient too distressed • Literal paraphasias predominate
	PPVT-R (Dunn & Dunn, 1981)	• 30th percentile
	Observation	• Verbal reasoning skills in play improving
28 weeks	CELF	• Processing score 5th percentile • Production subtests attempted but not all completed. Confrontation naming caused distress • Word-retrieval problems decreasing in conversational speech and in language treatment sessions • Reading and comprehending short paragraphs — approximately three sentences • Writing — problems spelling small abstract words 'was', 'that'
	Narrative	• Sequences
	PPVT-R	• 50th percentile
	Observation	• Play — contributes to argument in discussion
12 months	CELF	• Processing score 30th percentile • Production score 10th percentile
	PPVT-R	• 90th percentile
	Reading	• Volume of written information retained — increasing
	Writing	• Persistent spelling problems — sentences simple but grammatically correct

Table 2.3 Continued

Post Injury	Assessments	Comments
	Narrative	• Primitive narrative — conjunction mainly 'and then' • Lack of specificity — some word-retrieval problems, circumlocutionary language
14 months	Observation	• Word-retrieval problems few — present when tasks linguistically demanding
	Reading	• Not yet reading for pleasure — complains cannot understand the story
	Writing	• Complexity of sentences increasing
	(Discharged — moving to another state)	
2 years	Observations of phone conversation	• No apparent word-retrieval problems
	Writing	• Letter from patient — no spelling mistakes. Grammatically correct • Progressing well in a small class at school
3 years 3 months	A report from parent	• Doing well at school (two years behind peers) • Mother felt speech and language still improving • Above average in class, especially mathematics • Some difficulty with comprehension of 'mathematical' language • Good problem-solving skills • Persistent spelling problems — uses dictionary + • Reading for pleasure

would then facilitate the sentence, 'I want the bird'. Strategies which Narelle used to retrieve words were brought to her awareness and she was encouraged to use them in all situations, for example, thinking of what letter started the word or what was the object's function such as 'It flies. It is a bird'.

When helping Narelle with processing verbal and written information, stories from school reading programs were used, photocopied and cut into workable units starting with two sentences and increasing gradually until Narelle was able to do the complete card without any modification. The computer proved a highly motivating therapy tool. Computer reading programs were used for both verbal and reading exercises because the content was easy to modify. For example, the story could be read by the clinician and Narelle was asked to read silently the three answers given and choose the correct one. The game of 'Hangman' on the computer helped her with spelling. Verbal reasoning was facilitated with problem-solving computer games (e.g. 'Who done it' type mysteries). Fourteen months after the injury Narelle was discharged. She had achieved her pre-injury grade level in mathematics (still a year below her age-appropriate level) and a further grade below this level in English. Her language recovery had not plateaued and she was referred for further language therapy.

Concluding note

In recent contact with the family, 3 years and 3 months after the injury, her mother reported that Narelle was doing extremely well in all areas. In sport she had won her age championship for the best all-round performance, winning the 100 and 200 metres sprint and coming third in the 800 metres run. She also had entered for the long jump and the high jump. She was learning the clarinet and coping well although she still had some sensory deficits in her right hand. She remained left-handed for writing because, as Narelle herself commented, she could write much faster with it, but she did practice with her right hand occasionally.

In the speech and language area, her mother felt that she was still improving. Narelle was placed in a normal classroom situation where she was 12–18 months older than most of her peers. Her report card showed that she was above average in her academic marks, particularly in mathematics, and the teacher commented that she coped far better with mathematical processes than with language. In the areas of language, mathematics and science her teacher also reported that Narelle had excellent problem-solving skills and thought of the solution to many of the problems herself. She was also able to predict the outcome of science experiments. From further comments on her school report she appears to have difficulty understanding some abstract terms such as 'parallel' and in music has problems understanding rhythmic patterns. Generally, her report card showed marked improvement in all areas of language.

Narelle's written narrative was cohesive although some sentence structures were incorrect and obscured the meaning (e.g. 'There he was stolen up in the hills called The Fox View,' meaning the horse was stolen and hidden in the hills.). Her mother reported that she was reading for pleasure again. Her main difficulty in the language area appeared to be with spelling. When tested with a new list of words at the beginning of the school week Narelle only got two or three correct out of 15 but after learning them she would usually achieve 12 or 13 correct, which she then remembered. She appeared to have a problem transferring from the oral to the written form. Her mother reported that she would spell the word correctly orally but then write it incorrectly transposing letters. Narelle believed that she had no problems with word finding and during the phone conversation there was no indication of any difficulty. Her mother commented that Narelle was almost back to her previous personality. Her confidence had improved with her recent achievements and she had assumed a leadership role again among her peers. She was determined to do well in all areas.

Comment

Although Narelle has made a good recovery, some aphasic symptoms still persist in the higher level language areas. However, it seems probable that Narelle may overcome many of her difficulties because she has good problem-solving skills and uses strategies to help her achieve in academic areas.

References

BACKUS, O. and BEASLEY, J. (1951) *Speech Therapy with Children*, Boston, Houghton Mifflin Company.

BISHOP, D. (1984) *Language Assessment, Remediation and Screening Procedure (LARSP)*, Newcastle, University of Newcastle upon Tyne.

BLANK, M., ROSE, S. A. and BERLIN, L. J. (1978) *Preschool Language Assessment Instrument*, Orlando, Harcourt Brace Jovanovich.

BOEHM, A. E. (1986), *Boehm Test of Basic Concepts-Revised*, New York, Psychological Corporation.

BLOOM, L. and LAHEY, M. (1978) *Language Development and Language Disorders*, New York, John Wiley and Sons.

CARROW–WOOLFOLK, E. (1985) *Test of Auditory Comprehension of Language-Revised*, Allen, DLM Teaching Resources.

CHAPEY, R. (1981) 'The assessment of language disorders in adults', in Chapey, R. (Ed.) *Language Intervention Strategies in Adult Aphasia*, Baltimore, London, Williams and Wilkins.

CHAPEY, R. (1986) 'The assessment of language disorders in adults', in Chapey, R. (Ed.) *Language Intervention Strategies in Adult Aphasia*, 2nd ed., Baltimore, Williams and Wilkins.

CRYSTAL, D. (1982) *Profiling Linguistic Disability*, London, Edward Arnold.

CRYSTAL, D., FLETCHER, P. and GARMON, M. (1982) *The Grammatical Analysis of Language Disability*, London, Edward Arnold.

DAMICO, J. S. (1985) 'Clinical discourse analysis. A functional language assessment technique', in Simon, C. S. (Ed.) *Communication Skills and Classroom Success: Assessment of Language-Learning Disabled Students*, San Diego, College Hill Press.

DI SIMONE, F. (1978) *The Token Test for Children*, Hingham, MA, Teaching Resources.

DUNN, L. M. (1965) *Peabody Picture Vocabulary Test*, Circle Pines, MN, American Guidance Service.

DUNN, L. M. and DUNN, L. M. (1981) *Peabody Picture Vocabulary Test-Revised*, Minnesota, American Guidance Service.

DUNN, L. M. and SMITH, J. O. (1965) *Peabody Language Development Kits*, Circle Pines, American Guidance Service.

FOXX, R. M. (1985) 'Social skills training: The current status of the field', *Australian and New Zealand Journal of Developmental Disabilities*, **10**, pp. 237–43.

FRIED-OKEN, M. (1987) 'Qualitative examination of children's naming skills through test adaptations', *Language, Speech and Hearing Services in Schools*, **18**, pp. 206–16.

GADDES, W. H. and CROCKETT, D. J. (1975) 'The Spreen–Benton aphasia tests, normative data as a measure of normal language development', *Brain and Language*, **2**, pp. 257–80.

GUILFORD, A. M. and NAWOJCZYK, D. C. (1988) 'Standardization of the Boston Naming Test at the kindergarten and elementary school levels', *Language, Speech and Hearing Services in Schools*, **19**, pp. 395–400.

HAMMILL, D. D., BROWN, V. L., LARSEN, S. C. and WIEDERHOLT, J. L. (1987) *Test of Adolescent Language*, Austin, Pro-Ed.

HAMMILL, D. D. and NEWCOMER, P. L. (1988) *Test of Language Development-2 Intermediate*, Austin, Pro-Ed.

HOLLAND, A. L. (1980) *Communicative Abilities in Daily Living*, Baltimore, University Park Press.

IRWIN, E. C. (1975) 'Facilitating children's language development through play', *The Speech Teacher*, **24**, pp. 10–12.

JORGENSEN, C., BARRETT, M., HUISINGH, R. and ZACHMAN, L. (1981) *The Word Test: A Test of Expressive Vocabulary and Semantics*, Illinois, Lingui Systems Inc.

KAPLAN, E., GOODGLASS, H. and WEINTRAUB, S. (1983) *The Boston Naming Test*, Philadelphia, Lea and Febiger.

LONG, S. H. (1986) *Computerized Profiling*, Arcata, Cal., Computerized Profiling.

MILLER, J. F. (1981) *Assessing Language Production in Children*, Baltimore, University Park Press.

MILLER, J. F. and CHAPMAN, R. S. (1983) *SALT – Systematic Analysis of Language Transcripts*, Wisconsin, University of Wisconsin–Madison.

MORDECAI, D., PALIN, M. and PALMER, C. (1982) *Lingquest I: Language Sample Analysis*, Napa, Cal., Lingquest Software.

NEWCOMER, P. L. and HAMMILL, D. D. (1988) *Test of Language Development-2 Primary*, Austin, Pro-Ed.

PALIN, M. and MORDECAI, D. (1982) *Lingquest II: Phonological Analysis*, Napa, Cal., Lingquest Software.

PORCH, B. F. (1974) *Porch Index of Communicative Ability in Children*, Palo Alto, Consulting Psychologists Press.

PRESSLEY, M. and BRAINERD, C. J. (1985) *Cognitive Learning and Memory in Children*, Berlin, Springer-Verlag.

PRUTTING, C. A. and KIRCHNER, D. M. (1983) 'Applied Pragmatics', in Gallagher, T. M. and Prutting, C. A. (Eds) *Pragmatic Assessment and Intervention Issues in Language*, San Diego, College Hill Press, Inc.

PRUTTING, C. A. and KIRCHNER, D.M. (1987) 'A clinical appraisal of the pragmatic aspects of language', *Journal of Speech and Hearing Disorders*, **52**, pp. 105–19.

REYNELL, J. (1977) *Reynell Developmental Language Scales-Revised*, Oxford, NFER Publishing Company Ltd.

RIPICH, D. N. and SPINELLI, F. M. (1985) *School Discourse Problem*, London, Taylor and Francis.

SEMEL, E. and WIIG, E. H. (1980) *Clinical Evaluation of Language Functions*, Columbus, Charles E. Merrill Publishing Company.

SEMEL, E., WIIG, E.H. and SECORD, W. (1987) *Clinical Evaluations of Language Fundamentals-Revised*, Orlando, Harcourt Brace Jovanovich Inc.

SHULTZ, T.R. (1976) 'A cognitive-developmental analysis of humour', in Chapman, A.J. and Foot, H.C. (Eds) *Humour and Laughter: Theory, Research and Applications*, London, John Wiley and Sons.

SIMON, C.S. (1985) *Communcation Skills and Classroom Success: Therapy Methodologies for Language-Learning Disabled Students*, London, Taylor and Francis.

SPREEN, O. and BENTON, A.L. (1969) *Neurosensory Centre Comprehensive Examination for Aphasia: Manual of Directions*, Victoria B.C., University of Victoria.

WALLACH, G.P. and BUTLER, K.G. (1984) *Language Learning Disabilities in School Age Children*, Baltimore, Williams and Wilkins.

WESTBY, C.E. (1984) 'Development of narrative language abilities', in Wallach, G.P. and Butler, K.G. (Eds) *Language Learning Disabilities in School Age Children*, Baltimore, Williams and Wilkins.

WIIG, E.H. (1982) *Let's Talk Inventory for Adolescents*, Ohio, Charles E. Merrill Publishing Company.

WIIG, E.H. and SEMEL, E. (1984) *Language Assessment and Intervention for the Learning Disabled*, Ohio, Charles E. Merrill Publishing Company.

WILKS, V. and MONAGHAN, R. (1988) 'The graphic conversational profile: A possible intervention tool for people with communication deficits following closed head injuries', paper presented at the Annual Conference of the Australian Association of Speech and Hearing, Brisbane.

YLVISAKER, M. (1985) *Head Injury Rehabilitations: Children and Adolescents*, San Diego, College-Hill Press.

Chapter 2 — Appendix 1 Informal assessment of acquired childhood aphasia

Name:

Aetiology: Date of Onset

Items	✓	x	Comments/Observations
Yes/No Questions (1) Is your name . . . ? (2) Are your a boy/girl? (3) Do you got to . . . school (4) Are you in school now?			
Body Parts (1) Show me your nose (2) Show me your leg (3) Show me your arm (4) Show me your eyes (5) Show me your ears			
Two Stage Commands (1) Touch your nose and your leg (2) Touch your ear and your arm (3) Close your eyes, and then open your mouth (4) Move your arm, nod your head			
Three Stage Commands (1) Touch your nose, leg and arm (2) Touch your eye, leg and nose (3) Close your eyes, open your mouth, move your arm			
Matching *Object to Object* chair, bed, bath *Object to Photo* bed, car, table *Photo to Photo* bath, table, chair *Photo to Picture* bed, chair bath			
Function (1) Which one do you sleep in? (2) Which one do you wash in? (3) Which one do you drive in? (4) Which one do you sit in?			

Chapter 2 — Appendix 1   Continued

Items	✓	x	Comments/observations
Size			
(1) Show me the big chair			
(2) Point to the small bed			
(3) Give me the little person			
(4) Which is the biggest boy?			
Semantic Relations			
(1) Are you older than your Dad?			
(2) Are you heavier than a car?			
(3) Is a plane faster than a motorbike?			
(4) Do you have lunch before breakfast?			
(5) Does Christmas come after Easter?			
(6) The ball was in the cupboard. The cupboard was in the house. Was the ball in the house?			
(7) Bill came behind John. Who was in front?			
(8) Mary stood next to June. Was June beside Mary?			
(9) The lion was chased by the hunter. Who was chased?			
(10) Daniel was hurt by Tim. Was Tim hurt?			
Concepts			
(1) Put the girl on the table.			
(2) Put the man under the bed.			
(3) Put the boy in the box.			
(4) Who's under something?			
(5) Who's in something?			
(6) Who's on something?			
Naming			
What's this?			
bed, chair, bath, table, man, car, box, boy.			
Semantic cue			
Sentence completion cue			
Phonemic cue			
Function			
What do you do with this?			
bed, chair, bath, table, car, box			

Chapter 2 — Appendix 1 Continued

Items	✔	x	Comments/observations
Behaviour			
(1) Alert to situation			
(2) Greeting behaviours			
(3) Eye contact			
(4) Appropriate social interaction			
(5) Turn-taking			
(6) Cooperation			
(7) Attention to task			

Materials Required:-

Toys — Two of everything matching: kitchen table and chair, lounge chair, bed, bath, car (large enough for a toy person to sit in), box.

Photography — Two sets of photographs of the above toys.

Pictures — One set of pictures (e.g., from a language test), similar but not the same, of the above toys.

Chapter 2 — Appendix 2   Observational checklist

Language Behaviours	Number	Examples/Comment
Syntax In, on, under Plural 's' ing Possessive-s Articles Regular past-tense Contractible copula 'be' Irregular past Regular 3rd person singular-s Irregular 3rd person singular-s Uncontractible copula 'be' Contractible auxillary 'be' Uncontractible auxillary 'be'		
Semantics Existence Non-existence Recurrence Rejection Denial Attribution Possession Action Locative action Locative state Other:-		

Pragmatics	Appropriate	Inappropriate	Comment
Intelligibility Fluency Prosody Facial Expression Eye gaze Lexical/Specificity/Accuracy Work order Ability to take speaker and listener roles Maintain topic Turn-taking Repair/Revision/Contingency Pause time			
(1) Was the message received by the listener?			

General impressions (Comment)

Appendix 3

Analysis of a Video Tape Recording — Example

Observation by the speech and language clinician confirmed reports from other team members that Joseph, 8 years, was having problems with requesting. A video tape recording was made of an occupational therapy group session in which seven children were making mobiles. Activities included cutting and pasting, sprinkling, and manipulating pipe cleaners. All activities were difficult for the children and most required some help. Three adults were involved in the session.

Before analyzing the recording, the speech and language clinician, decided on which verbal and non-verbal behaviours constituted a request.

Requesting

1 Stopping work and glancing around the table with a look of expectation.
2 Choosing the appropriate person to ask. To do this successfully the individual would need to perceive the situation. He/she must look for the nearest person to them, or the nearest person to the object he/she might want. Then, he/she would need to decide whether that person was free to help or should someone else be asked.
3 Making eye contact and holding his/her gaze steady with the person to be asked.
4 Saying 'Excuse me' and identifying the person by name.

(Three and four may be reversed. It would depend on whether the child made eye contact and when they looked around the table.)

5 Saying 'Will you help me . . . please.' Language should be specific e.g. cut the paper, or glue the picture.

The team then watched the video and noted all Joseph's requests and decided whether they were appropriate or not and if they were inappropriate just where did the breakdown occur.

1 Did the child look up, or stop work, or give some indication non-verbally that he was seeking help?
2 Did the child choose the nearest appropriate person or just the nearest person regardless of what that person was doing. Did the child always request the same person e.g. the teacher, regardless of what the teacher might be doing?
3 Was eye contact made and maintained for the appropriate length of time?
4 What did the child say to initiate the request? Was it appropriate? Did the child use the person's name?
5 Was the child's language specific or did the child indicate non-verbally what the request was? Was this acceptable?

A record was kept of all request interactions in the sample. The team then decided whether it was a skill that Joseph was learning or whether direct intervention was necessary. In this instance, Joseph's requesting behaviour broke down most often at step 1. He tended to keep requesting 'I can't do it', but made no attempt to look around and seek help. Direct intervention by the speech and language clinician was necessary and treatment goals were reinforced by other team members.

Video tape recording may be used to identify very specific behaviours such as requesting, greetings etc. or be used for spontaneous language sampling when the child's use of semantics, syntax and pragmatic behaviours is documented.

Appendix 4

Reading List for Creative Dramatics

BORDEN, S. D. (1970) *Plays as Teaching Tools in Elementary School*. New York: Parker Publishing Co., Inc.

BURGESS, L. and GAURY, P. (1985) *Time for Drama: A Handbook for Teachers*. Cheshire: Longman.

HEINIG, R. B. and STILLWELL, L. (1974) *Creative Dramatics for the Classroom Teacher*. New Jersey: Prentice-Hall, Inc.

JENNINGS, S. (1974) *Remedial Drama — A Handbook for Teachers and Therapists*. New York: Theatre Arts Books.

SIKS, G. B. (1958) *Creative Dramatics: An Art For Children*. New York: Harper.

SLADE, P. (1954) *Child Drama*. London: University of London Press Ltd.

WARD, W. (1957) *Playmaking with Children*. New York: Appleton-Century-Crofts.

WAY, B. (1967) *Development through Drama*. Atlantiac Highlands, N.J.: Humanities Press.

Chapter 3

Speech and Language Disorders Following Childhood Closed Head Injury

Faye M. Jordan

Introduction

Loss of the ability to communicate effectively is a frequent finding secondary to severe head trauma. In the last decade the importance of the recovery of speech and language skills to the long-term quality of life subsequent to closed head injury has been recognized, particularly in the paediatric population. The significance of speech and language deficits after head trauma has been minimized in the past. The reasons for this lack of recognition include: a failure of researchers in this area to agree on an accepted set of terminology that accurately describes the communication deficits, a lack of empirical data relative to the treatment of communication disorders resulting from head trauma, and a failure of researchers and clinicians to recognize that communication deficits secondary to head injury deserve special attention because they represent a unique speech and language symptomatology. With reports in recent years that persistent speech and language deficits may occur subsequent to closed head injury and the recognition of their important consequences for the long-term quality of life of the head-injured patient, there has been a corresponding surge in research into the communicative abilities of head-injured persons. The present chapter will address issues arising from research into the recovery of linguistic skills secondary to closed head injury in the paediatric population.

Mechanisms of Injury

Holbourne (1943) deduced that the effects of head injury on the adult brain were determined by the physical properties of the brain and skull — in particular the contrast beween the rigid skull and the less rigid but incompressible brain. A head injury produces relative movement between the brain and the skull with resultant rotation of the brain and contact with the inside of the skull. The resultant forces are maximal between the soft frontal and temporal lobes and the bony sphenoid prominences (Jellinger, 1983).

Bruce *et al*. (1978) suggested that the pathophysiology and symptomatology of head injury are different in children when compared with adults. Similarly Levin *et al*. (1983b) referred to the greater capacity of young children to survive severe closed head injury as compared with adults and attributed this increased survival to anatomical and physical features of head injury in the paediatric population that differ from the adult population. According to Jellinger (1983), the morphology of cranial injuries in infancy and childhood is somewhat different from that in adults. This is because the anatomical structures have different proportions and the physical events taking place at the moment of trauma are different. For instance, a newborn infant's brain weight is about one-quarter of that of the adult, although its body weight is only 5 per cent of the adult. By the end of the second year of life brain weight is 75 per cent of the adult weight and reaches over 90 per cent of the adult weight by the end of the 6th year (Jellinger, 1983). Friede (1975) reported that the brain weight comprises 15 per cent of the body weight at term and 3 per cent in the adult.

The skull of an infant and young child is characteristically pliable and the existence of unfused sutures and open fontanelles means that it is more susceptible to external forces than in later years. The floors of the middle cranial fossa and the orbital roofs continue to be relatively smooth and offer little resistance to the shifting brain. These basic anatomical differences and the deformability of the young skull mean the pattern of brain lesions in the infant resulting from closed head injury differ from those observed in older age groups (Lindenberg and Freytag, 1969). Some researchers suggest, however, that the greater flexibility of bones in childhood may enhance the capacity of the skull to absorb traumatic forces rather than making it more vulnerable to injury (Craft, 1972; Gurdjian and Webster, 1958). Despite these identified differences Jellinger (1983) noted that infants comprise only a small proportion of the paediatric head injury population and that lesions found in children over 1 or 2 years of age do not differ in principle from those seen in adults.

Biomechanics of Head Injury

Head injuries generally result from some form of short mechanical impact to the skull. Two broad categories of head injury exist: those occurring subsequent to penetrating injuries or open head injury, and those resulting from an impact transmitted to the brain with or without skull fracture but failing to perforate the dura or closed head injury. In that during peacetime the most frequent type of head injury is closed head injury, the present review will be confined to an examination of the literature relating to speech and language disorders following closed head injuries.

Head injury may be defined in terms of the physical forces that occur at the time of impact. There are two types of injury using this classification system — compression or impression injury due to an impact to the fixed head and acceleration/deceleration injury due to an impact to the freely movable head. Acceleration trauma may be translational or rotational or a combination of these forces (Pang, 1985).

Impression injury is caused by a blow to the resting head and results in local indentation and a depressed fracture of the skull with brain damage occurring directly beneath the site of impact (Pang, 1985). Acceleration injury produces acceleration and deceleration forces which affect the movable head. The rotation and shearing stresses that result cause damage at sites distant to the place of impact and throughout the brain. Translational acceleration results when the resultant vector of a force applied to the head runs through or near the centre of the head. In this instance all individual particles within the brain will travel at the same acceleration and in the same direction and therefore will sustain no intermolecular stress (Pang, 1985). In contrast, angular acceleration results if the resultant force vector does not pass through the centre of the head. In this instance the head will assume an angular acceleration and will rotate around its own centre of gravity. Most frequently acceleration injuries are neither purely translational nor angular, but result from a combination of these forces. Such combined forces produce complex traumatic damage to the brain, skull and spinal cord (Jellinger, 1983)

Types of Brain Damage Subsequent to Head Injury

Brain damage subsequent to closed head injury can be divided into two distinct classes — primary damage, which occurs at the time of injury, is the result of distinct mechanical factors and is seldom aided by treatment, and secondary damage which is the consequence of some form of complication and is therefore potentially preventable or reversible with treatment. Teasdale and Mendelow (1984) suggested that there are many mechanisms that can cause brain damage after head injury; the type, severity and location of damage determine the effects on the patient in both the acute and long-term stages.

Primary brain damage

Immediate or impact brain damage results in two types of lesions, contusions and diffuse axonal injuries. Research by Adams *et al.* (1980) indicated that, regardless of the site of impact, the maximal location for contusions was the frontal region. Haemorrhagic contusions are reported to occur on the crests of the gyri of the cerebral cortex (Teasdale and Mendelow, 1984). Haemorrhage may vary in extent from a superficial layer of blood to one which involves the whole depth of the cortex and several adjacent gyri. It has in the past been commonly believed that contusions remote from the site of impact are produced by a *contra-coup* mechanism, with the force of the blow transmitted to the opposite side of the brain from impact. Ommaya *et al.* (1971), after carrying out experimental studies on monkeys, found that contusions were maximal in the frontotemporal region, regardless of whether or not the skull was struck in the frontal or occipital region. This finding was confirmed by Adams *et al.* (1980). Gurdjian and Gurdjian (1976) stated that *contra-coup* contusions result from relative movement of the brain during impact. They suggested that frontotemporal contusions secondary to frontal or occipital impact are *contra-coup* because these result from movement of the brain against the bony irregularities at the base of the skull, however, this is again consistent with the findings of Ommaya *et al.* (1971).

It has been frequently reported that diffuse cerebral injury produced at the moment of impact is the primary mechanism of brain damage in closed head injury (Adams *et al.*, 1977; Levin *et al.*, 1982a). In addition, the severity of diffuse brain injury is an important determinant in the quality of recovery. According to Bruce (1983), however, cerebral laceration and contusion are uncommon in children, occurring in only 2–3 per cent of children sustaining head trauma.

The most important mechanism of primary traumatic brain injury is diffuse axonal injury in the white matter (Adams *et al.*, 1977; Levin *et al.*, 1982a). A shearing mechanism serves to explain diffuse axonal injury, in this instance produced by the movement between different components of the brain itself. The forces required to produce this shearing strain result from rotational acceleration. Numerous researchers have reported that in the case of rotational acceleration more severe lesions occur in the cerebral hemispheres than in the brainstem (Adams *et al.*, 1982; Holbourne, 1943; Ommaya and Gennarelli, 1974). Bruce *et al.* (1981) placed major significance on this diffuse axonal injury, particularly in children, and in fact suggested that the degree of recovery is probably dependent on the degree of axonal injury. These conclusions were based on the outcome of a study by Bruce *et al.* (1981) that examined a series of children with closed head injury in relation to traumatic brain swelling and subsequent recovery. The findings of this study indicated that children suffering brain swelling subsequent to closed head injury, but in the absence of concomitant primary diffuse impact injury to the white matter, made a rapid recovery with little residual neurological damage. In contrast, children suffering a significant amount of primary impact damage to the white matter, in addition to cerebral swelling, demonstrated a more complicated neurological recovery with persistent and significant neurological deficits.

Secondary brain damage

Secondary brain damage, which occurs as the result of a complication relating to the primary damage, is an important consideration in the management of closed head injury in children. Bruce (1983) suggested that children may be at greater risk of secondary injury than adults. There are two main groups of factors responsible for secondary brain damage: intracranial and extracranial. Intracranial factors include intracranial haematomas, brain swelling, infection, subarachnoid haemorrhage and hydrocephalus. Extracranial factors include respiratory failure and associated hypoxia, and hypotension.

Intracranial factors

Bleeding inside the skull following head injury results in the development of a clot and subsequent compression of the brain. An extradural haematoma (a clot between the skull and meninges) or an intradural haematoma (a clot deep to the dura mater) may form following head trauma. An extradural haematoma is classically a complication of a skull fracture that has damaged the middle meningeal artery. More frequently occurring are the intradural haematomas which may be either subdural or intracerebral or in some cases a mixture of both. Acute subdural haematomas which carry the highest mortality of all acute cerebral traumatic lesions in adults, however, are uncommon in children and adolescents, occurring in only 5 per cent of childhood head injury cases (Bruce, 1983).

Another intracranial factor which may influence the outcome of a closed head injury is brain swelling. This may be due to either an increase in cerebral volume (engorgement) or an increase in the amount of intra- or extracellular fluid (oedema) and may affect the whole or only part of the brain. A generalized increase in brain volume within 24 hours of a head injury is reported to be common in young patients (Levin *et al.*, 1982a), with a computed tomographic (CT) pattern of generalized brain swelling being a frequent finding subsequent to head trauma in children (Zimmerman *et al.*, 1978). Although focal hemispheric swelling has been documented in adults, symmetrical diffuse swelling of the brain is seen particularly in children and adolescents (Bruce, 1983). Such diffuse cerebral swelling is reported to result from hyperaemia or cerebral blood flow in excess of the metabolic needs of the brain. In this condition the ventricles and cisterns appear compressed. Bruce *et al.* (1978) reported that the brain swelling in their series of head-injured children appeared to be due to cerebrovascular dilatation and increased cerebral blood volume, not the decrease that would be present if the swelling were due to oedema.

Factors such as the development of brain swelling or a haematoma may lead to an increase in intracranial pressure and can also produce a resultant brain shift or herniation. Elevated intracranial pressure has been reported to occur in more than 75 per cent of patients with severe closed head injury (Miller *et al.*, 1977). According to Bakay and Glasauer (1980) uncontrolled intracranial pressure is likely to account for almost 50 per cent of the mortality rate after closed head injury. Such an uncontrolled increase in intracranial pressure results in diffuse ischaemic brain damage.

Brain shift typically occurs in a number of identifiable patterns. Tentorial herniation (also referred to as transtentorial or uncal herniation) results in the compression of the oculomotor nerve and is characterized by ptosis, dilation of the pupil and loss of eye movements. Distortion of the brainstem and the blood supply lead to dysfunction of the midbrain and characteristically decerebrate rigidity. Lesions in the brainstem that result from such herniation may also cause loss of consciousness (Levin *et al.*, 1982a). Martin (1974) suggested that the stretching of reticular structures that occurs subsequent to herniation is, in fact, the major cause of loss of consciousness following a closed head injury. Tonsillar herniation results in displacement of brain structures from the posterior fossa into the spinal canal through the foramen magnum and leads to compression of the medulla oblongata, thereby causing vasomotor and respiratory disturbances.

Secondary brain damage may also take the form of infection which may manifest as either a brain abscess or meningitis. The predisposing factors that allow the invasion of microorganisms are compound depressed fractures of the vault of the skull or fractures of the skull base or nasal sinuses. Brain abscess may produce brain shift or increased intracranial pressure or both. Meningitis may produce increased intracranial pressure or communicating hydrocephalus.

Other intracranial mechanisms that cause secondary brain damage include subarachnoid haemorrhage and hydrocephalus. Subarachnoid haemorrhage occurs in a high proportion of head injuries and may lead to vasospasm with reduced cerebral blood flow and ischaemic brain damage (Macpherson and Graham, 1978). The hydrocephalus that occurs early after a head injury is due to the failure of cerebrospinal fluid absorption in the arachnoid villi which become blocked with blood cells.

Extracranial factors

An accident that results in a head injury often results in injuries to other parts of the body which may in turn damage the brain by causing either hypoxia or hypotension. Both intracranial and extracranial abnormalities can cause hypoxic brain damage. For instance, deficient respiratory function causes brain damage even if the cerebral circulation is normal. In contrast to this, brain damage occurs with a normal arterial oxygen content when there is a failure of cerebral circulation and ischaemia, either generalized or local. This may result from systemic hypotension or from raised intracranial pressure, both of which lead to a fall in cerebral perfusion pressure. There are two major patterns of damage resulting from hypoxia, one corresponding to the territory of one of the major intracranial arteries, usually as a consequence of the artery being occluded during an episode of transtentorial herniation and the other typically occurring in areas such as the basal ganglia and hippocampus (Graham *et al.*, 1978).

Characteristics of Speech and Language Disturbances Subsequent to Closed Head Injury in Children

The traditional view of childhood recovery subsequent to closed head injury has held that recovery is rapid and complete, particularly when compared with similarly injured adults. Much of the current literature, however, suggests the presence of a subclinical aphasia characterized by subtle high level language deficits subsequent to closed head injury in both adults and children (Ewing-Cobbs *et al.*, 1987; Jordan *et al.*, 1988; Levin *et al.*, 1976; Sarno and Levin, 1985). One of the difficulties that arises when examining research data in this area is the great variability in the methodological approaches which have been employed. An attempt will be made, however, to provide an historical perspective and then to establish the current status of research on the recovery of linguistic skills in children subsequent to closed head injury.

It is suggested that aphasia is probably the earliest recorded neuropsychological sequelae of closed head injury (Levin *et al.*, 1982a) with historical documents dating its existence back to AD 30. Aphasic disturbance in children tends to be non-fluent (Ewing-Cobbs *et al.*, 1985; Levin *et al.*, 1983a). Ewing-Cobbs *et al.* (1985) suggested that children with traumatic injuries characteristically exhibit expressive deficits and generally have a good prognosis when compared with children suffering vascular lesions which are reported to produce more persistent language disorders.

Alajouanine and Lhermitte (1965) reported findings in a group of 32 children who they described as suffering acquired aphasia. This group included 13 children whose cerebral damage was the result of traumatic contusion, with the remaining subjects suffering a variety of other causes including vascular malformation, aneurysm or angioma, occlusion of the middle cerebral artery and 'no precise   diagnosis — meningoencephalitis?, phlebitis?' Alajouanine and Lhermitte (1965) reported that the most striking characteristic of the aphasic disorder identified in their subjects was the reduction in 'expressive activities', with each child demonstrating a reduction in oral and written language and a reduction in the use of gestures. Some subjects also presented with dysarthria. These findings suggested the persistence of a linguistic disorder subsequent to traumatic head injury. It must be noted, however, that despite the detailed description of the linguistic skills of the subjects provided by Alajouanine and Lhermitte (1965), there were methodological flaws in their study which limit the usefulness of the reported information. For instance, it is difficult to determine the relevance of the general conclusions of their study to any one group of children in particular, for example head-injured children, because of the wide range of causes in the subject group. Any form of generalization of the results must, therefore, be necessarily guarded. In addition the subject group was described as having injury to the left hemisphere only. Such a neurological presentation would be atypical for a group of head-injured children who generally present with diffuse bilateral damage. The speech and language abilities of a series of 52 patients who had sustained head injuries and were comatose for more than a week were described by Brink *et al.* (1970). The re-learning of intelligible speech by this group is reported to have paralleled the recovery of motor function, with only one member of the group unable to communicate basic needs. The remainder of the group demonstrated varying degrees of recovery with 16 attaining 'normal speech', 20 presenting with articulation deficits and six with some degree of aphasia. Again, the results of this study indicated the presence of a persisting linguistic disorder subsequent to a childhood closed head injury; however, the recovery interval was not reported making interpretation of the findings difficult.

Hécaen (1976) reported the language features of 26 cases of acquired childhood aphasia. The aetiology of the group was mixed, but included 16 cases of head trauma. Hécaen described acquired childhood aphasia as being characterized by a period of mutism followed by the recovery of language, marked by decreased initiation of speech, naming disorders, dyscalculia and dysgraphia. Receptive disorders were less frequent, occurring in one third of his children with acquired aphasia.

The Neurosensory Center Comprehensive Examination for Aphasia (NCCEA) (Spreen and Benton, 1969) was used by Levin and Eisenberg (1979a) to examine the language recovery of a group of children and adolescents with closed head injury. Linguistic deficits characterized by dysnomia for objects presented visually or tactually to the left hand were identified in about 12 per cent of the group studied. Deficits in auditory comprehension were identified in 11 per cent of the group and verbal repetition was impaired in only 4 per cent. In a similar study, Levin and Eisenberg (1979b) reported that one-third of a series of 45 children and adolescents with closed head injury presented with significant linguistic deficits.

Further evidence for the presence of continuing linguistic deficit subsequent to closed head injury was provided by Gaidolfi and Vignolo (1980) who examined the language performance of a group of young adults who had suffered closed head injury while schoolchildren. Language was examined by tests of oral expression, auditory verbal comprehension, writing and reading comprehension. Although a poor performance was noted on the oral expression test, this was reported to be due to an overall reduction of spontaneous speech rather than specific aphasic errors.

A prospective study of children suffering head injury was carried out by Chadwick *et al.* (1981a) over a period of 27 months post-onset. These researchers reported that head injury was more likely to lead to visuospatial deficits than verbal impairment. This finding was based on interpretation of the verbal and performance IQ scores on the WISC. In a companion paper Chadwick *et al.* (1981b) described the specific cognitive deficits they identified in the same group of head-injured children and reported that these children demonstrated deficits in speed of naming objects. Although these researchers dismissed the existence of a significant verbal impairment following paediatric closed head injury, the presence of a deficit in the speed of naming objects is indicative of a high-level language disorder.

Winogran *et al.* (1984) carried out a retrospective study of three groups of children who had sustained head injuries of different degrees of severity. Psychological outcome was assessed by a comprehensive neuropsychological test battery in compliance with the Knights–Norwood Neuropsychological Test Administration Manual (Knights and Norwood, 1979). The subject groups consisted of 17 children sustaining a severe head injury, 17 sustaining a moderate injury and 17 sustaining a mild injury. Significant group differences were reported for performance on the verbal fluency test, the severely head-injured group demonstrating a decreased verbal fluency relative to the moderately and mildly head-injured groups. These researchers suggested that the test performances most affected by head injury are those dependent on the child's ability to respond quickly. This finding is consistent with the earlier findings of Chadwick *et al.* (1981b) who, as indicated above, identified a deficit in the speed of naming objects.

A study by Ewing-Cobbs *et al.* (1985) employed the NCCEA to determine the presence of linguistic impairment in children and adolescents with closed head injury. Their results indicated that during the early stages of recovery (less than 6 months after the trauma) a significant percentage of the subject group achieved scores which indicated the presence of a linguistic impairment. Naming disorders, dysgraphia and reduced verbal productivity were identified as the most significant linguistic impairments. Ewing-Cobbs *et al.* (1985) concluded that the language disturbance identified was evidence of a subclinical aphasia rather than a frank aphasic disturbance. Comparison of recovery related to the severity of injury indicated that children with moderate–severe closed head injury were more likely to demonstrate poorer performance on the naming and graphic subtests when compared with their mildly head-injured counterparts. These workers also reported that the severity of acute linguistic disturbance was comparable in children and adolescents, however, written language was more affected in children than adolescents. According to Gibson and Levin (1975) written language skills develop most rapidly between 6 and 8 years of age. The finding that graphic skills were disproportionately affected in children was therefore considered by Ewing-Cobbs *et al.* (1985) to indicate that skills that are in a rapid stage of development may be more affected by cerebral injury than well-consolidated skills. This suggestion is consistent with the hypotheses proposed by Hebb (1942) and Rutter (1981) that brain injury may predominantly affect the acquisition of new skills or may produce deficits which reflect the degree to which the skill had been acquired, skills in a rapid stage of acquisition being more vulnerable to injury.

A further study by Ewing-Cobbs *et al.* (1987) examined the linguistic performance of 23 children and 33 adolescents who had sustained a closed head injury. The NCCEA was administered to all subjects less than 15 years of age. Subjects older than 15 years were administered the Multilingual Aphasia Examination (Benton and Hamsher, 1978). Results of this study indicated that a large proportion of the sample demonstrated 'clinically significant language impairment', with expressive and graphic functions most affected. The conclusions of this study indicated that age at injury and severity of injury are significantly related to language performance. Again written language was significantly more affected in children than adolescents.

The most recent evidence for the existence of long-term linguistic deficits secondary to paediatric closed head injury was provided by Jordan *et al.* (1988) who examined the speech and language functioning of a group of 20 children 8–16 years of age who had sustained a closed head injury at least 12 months previously. The subjects were administered a battery of speech and language assessments including an articulation/phonological assessment, oromotor assessment, overall measure of language performance and specific language skills assessments. The performance of the head-injured group was compared with that of a group of non-neurologically impaired accident victims matched for sex, age, and socio-economic status. The findings of this study indicated that the head-injured children achieved lower scores on tests of overall language performance and naming skills when compared with the control group. There were no deficits identified in articulation skills. A follow-up study on the same group of subjects was carried out by Jordan and Murdoch (1990); the results provided support for the earlier findings. A persisting problem in verbal fluency was also documented. The conclusions of the two studies suggested that the language abilities of children who have sustained a closed head injury are mildly impaired when compared with those of an age- and sex-matched control group. The identified language impairment was characterized by a mild dysnomia and reduction in verbal fluency. A more detailed examination of the naming errors produced by the group with a closed head injury in the above study was carried out by Jordan *et al.* (1990). The results indicated that although the closed head injury group produced more errors on a test of naming ability than did the controls, the error pattern mimicked that of the controls.

In summary, research over the last two decades has confirmed the existence of language deficits subsequent to closed head injury in children. This is contrary to the traditional view which holds that children make a rapid and full recovery from brain trauma, particularly when compared with similarly injured adults. Frank aphasia is evident in only a very small proportion of children suffering a closed head injury, if at all. Language impairment subsequent to closed head injury is characterized initially by reduced verbal output or in its most severe form, mutism, which is followed in the long-term by subtle high-level language deficits. Subclinical language disturbance, as reflected in impoverished verbal fluency, dysnomia and decreased word-finding ability, is consistently reported in the literature. These findings are not unlike those reported in the literature on adult closed head injury. A number of studies have also reported the presence of dysarthria and articulation problems in children with closed head injury; however, these are much less consistent findings.

Comparison of Child and Adult Language After Head Injury

Several researchers have characterized the long-term linguistic outcome of closed head injury in adults over the past two decades. Thomsen (1975) reported that aphasia subsequent to closed head injury was typically characterized by residual deficits in higher-level language skills, such as verbal description and the use of antonyms, synonyms and metaphors. These findings were supported by Levin *et al.* (1976) who described anomia and verbal associative difficulty as prominent sequelae to closed head injury in adults.

Similarly, Sarno (1980) described a subclinical aphasia following closed head injury that was characterized by decreased verbal fluency. Sarno (1980) also noted the presence of dysarthria in a number of subjects. Levin *et al.* (1981) described the long-term outcome of acute aphasia in a group of adults with closed head injury and found that 43 per cent demonstrated a 'full' recovery of language with the remaining cases demonstrating a residual anomia or a marked global impairment of language concomitant with a cognitive impairment. Further research by Sarno (1984) and Sarno *et al.* (1986) again demonstrated that adults who had suffered severe closed head injury demonstrated persistent linguistic deficits.

Clearly, the presentation of the adult with closed head injury is not dissimilar to that of the child with closed head injury. Both children and adults have been found to present with persistent and frequently high-level language deficits subsequent to closed head injury. This conclusion is contrary to the previously popular belief that children make a rapid and full recovery after closed head injury compared with a slower and less complete recovery in the adult population.

Other Neurological and Neuropsychological Sequelae of Paediatric Closed Head Injury

The most frequent consequence of head injury is an altered level of consciousness or cerebral concussion (Jellinger, 1983). According to Teasdale and Mendalow (1984) different durations of unconsciousness indicate differing degrees of diffuse axonal injury. In the case of deep and persistent coma, axonal damage is likely to be severe and widespread. In contrast to this, if the ability to verbalize returns soon after a head injury, severe primary damage cannot have been sustained. Teasdale and Mendalow suggest, however, that even with brief loss of consciousness as observed in concussion, the basis for altered consciousness is a degree of diffuse axonal injury in which most fibres escape permanent structural damage. Evidence of persisting but subtle deficits subsequent to even minor head injury provide support for this theory (Gronwall and Sampson, 1974). Ewing-Cobbs *et al.* (1985) suggested that cognitive impairment frequently persists after severe closed head injury in children despite the resolution of focal motor and sensory deficits and the resumption of daily activities.

Brink *et al.* (1970) studied 52 head-injured children and reported that the majority of subjects showed impairment in academic performance, with intellectual deficits more pronounced in the younger age group than in the adolescents. Klonoff *et al.* (1977) reported the findings of a 5-year follow-up of head-injured children and adolescents. The neuropsychological findings of their study indicated that, after 5 years, 23.7 per cent of their sample continued to show impaired neuropsychological performance. Levin and Eisenberg (1979a, b) evaluated intellectual recovery in a group of children and adolescents with closed head injury. The findings indicated that neuropsychological impairment was present in more than a third of the subjects and that the degree of neuropsychological impairment was directly related to the duration of coma.

Chadwick *et al.* (1981b) examined the intellectual recovery in a group of 25 children subsequent to severe head injury and found them to be impaired on measures of IQ when compared with a control group of orthopaedically-injured children. Chadwick and co-workers also reported that performance measures were more affected than verbal measures. In addition, infants and toddlers have been identified as being more vulnerable to long-term cognitive impairment than their older counterparts (Levin *et al.*, 1982a). Levin *et al.* (1982b), in a study of children and adolescents who had suffered severe closed head injury, reported that global intellectual deficit was confined to patients who were younger than 13 years of age when injured, and it was a frequent concomitant of impaired memory storage.

The neuropsychological recovery of three groups of children including a severely, moderately and mildly head-injured group was examined by Winogran *et al.* (1984). The outcome of this study indicated that scores on the performance component of the IQ test were significantly related to the severity of injury with the more severely injured subjects achieving a poorer score. Costeff *et al.* (1988) carried out neuropsychological testing on a group of head-injured children 3–10 years after injury. Their findings indicated that subjects who were initially identified with more severe injuries continued to demonstrate inferior performance on IQ tests than the less severely injured group.

According to Ewing-Cobbs *et al.* (1985) school achievement is frequently significantly affected by moderate or severe head injury. Reading skills is one area that has been identified as being vulnerable to head injury (Chadwick *et al.*, 1981c; Shaffer *et al.*, 1980). Numerous studies have reported the need for special school placement subsequent to severe head injury (Brink *et al.*, 1970; Fuld and Fisher, 1977; Klonoff *et al.*, 1977).

In addition to the generalized cognitive impairment that has been identified, memory impairment has frequently been reported as a common deficit subsequent to head injury in children. Richardson (1963) examined memory in ten patients with closed head injury, 5–18 years of age, and concluded that all patients showed memory deficits despite improvement in fine motor skills and in adjustment to daily living. Similarly, Fuld and Fisher (1977) reported that the head-injured patients in their study demonstrated reduced recovery of long-term memory compared with motor skills. Support for the existence of a memory deficit subsequent to closed head injury in children has also been supplied by Levin and Eisenberg (1979b). Levin *et al.* (1982b) studied the recovery of memory function (verbal and visual) in a group of children and adolescents with closed head injury at least 6 months after the injury. Subjects who had sustained severe head injuries as determined by the Glasgow Coma Scale (Teasdale and Jennet, 1974) (severe less than 8) demonstrated a persistent impairment in the retrieval of information from long-term storage. In addition, children, but not adolescents, with severe head injuries showed residual deficits in recognition memory as compared with age-matched patients with milder head injuries.

In summary, there appears to be clear evidence of a persisting cognitive deficit subsequent to severe closed head injury in children. Memory has been identified as being particularly vulnerable. The presence of such a global cognitive impairment will clearly affect the prognosis for the recovery of speech and language skills.

Mechanisms of Recovery

Robinson (1981) stated that a widely-held view with regard to recovery following brain trauma is that the young brain, as a result of its greater neuronal plasticity, recovers better from such events than the mature brain. Cotard (1896, cited in Levin *et al.*, 1982a) did much to advance the theory of brain plasticity when he reported that early or congenital left hemisphere damage did not lead to aphasia. This theory of brain plasticity was supported by the findings of Kennard (1938). Kennard reported an absence of severe motor deficit subsequent to ablation of the motor cortex in infant monkeys. Similar lesions in adult monkeys, however, were observed to produce severe motor impairment. Kennard did observe, however, that as the operated infants matured they showed motor incoordination and spasticity. According to Levin *et al.* (1983b) the clinical literature supporting neuronal plasticity in children consists of studies of recovery from focal lesions. There is no substantial evidence, however, to indicate that immaturity offers any advantage in withstanding the effects of diffuse cerebral trauma (Levin *et al.*, 1982a). Levin *et al.* (1983b) identified the issues that complicate comparison of recovery from brain injury at different ages: differences in the pathophysiology of brain injury, the chronicity of brain injury in the infant population compared with adults, and the variety of insults producing both focal and diffuse injury.

Studies of outcome after closed head injury have shown a lower mortality rate for children as compared with adults (Levin *et al.*, 1983a). Similarly, brain lesions in childhood have been reported to have different effects from those sustained in adulthood (Bishop, 1981). The effects of age on the quality of recovery from closed head injury is less well documented.

Satz and Bullard-Bates (1981) reviewed the literature relating to acquired childhood aphasia including those works which examined the speech and language recovery of children subsequent to traumatic brain injury. They concluded that, although spontaneous recovery of speech and language skills occurs in a large majority of children with acquired aphasia, it is not invariable, with several instances of persisting speech and language deficits being reported.

The general pattern of findings, then, seems too suggest that contrary to the previously expounded theory that children make a rapid and full recovery from closed head injury, cognitive impairment frequently persists despite the resolution of gross signs of impairment, such as focal motor or sensory deficits.

Recovery of Function

Early recovery of function following closed head injury is most likely to be the result of the cessation of some disorder of neuronal function which is reversible, for example, resolution of brain swelling (Teasdale and Mendelow, 1984). Late recovery, in contrast, is largely dependent on the extent of primary irreversible brain injury. Bruce *et al.* (1981) contend that the degree of recovery following closed head injury is determined by the degree of initial axonal injury.

Teasdale and Mendelow (1984) provided two theories to explain late recovery subsequent to head injury. The first theory hypothesized that the recovery of function reflects the use of neuronal pathways other than those initially damaged. They suggested that these pathways may be alternative pathways or may be previously re-dundant connections. The use of other pathways is considered a learning phenomen-on. This first theory proposed by Teasdale and Mendelow (1984) has gained some support following studies by Soh *et al.* (1977) who demonstrated that attempts to speak by dysphasic patients did not show the expected increase in blood flow in the speech areas of the brain but instead showed an increase in flow in the adjacent subfrontal and parietal regions of the cortex. Teasdale and Mendelow (1984: 29) suggested that it is 'not surprising that children are most rapid in relearning whereas elderly people recover more slowly and less completely'. This theory was also considered by Bishop (1981) who suggested that the degree of functional plasticity of the brain may depend on the availability of synaptic sites for the development of new compensatory pathways. Bishop (1981) proposed that the recovery observed in children following brain damage is therefore different rather than better when compared with adults. If Bishop's theory relating to the availability of synaptic sites is correct, it could be expected that head-injured children would present with more generalized brain impairment than head-injured adults. According to Bishop's theory, in children neurons mediating both verbal and non-verbal abilities compete for a limited number of synaptic sites, thereby reducing the potential synaptic connections for both types of function. In contrast, brain-damaged adults present with specific rather than general skill deficits as their neuronal sites have already been committed to other functions and it is only the specific skill area that is competing for synaptic connections. Robinson (1981) failed to support Bishop's hypothesis and suggested that there does not seem to be an excess of synaptic sites formed at birth. In addition, synaptic density reaches adult levels during the second year of life, hence, it cannot provide an explanation for the enhanced recoverability in children proposed by Bishop (1981).

The alternative theory of late recovery involves the transfer of functions subsequent to structural changes in the traumatized brain to non-damaged areas of the brain. Teasdale and Mendelow (1984) proposed that diffuse axonal injuries typical of head injury may result in axonal damage with intact glial sheaths, so that the opportunity for regeneration may be significant. Other researchers (Daniel and Pritchard, 1975; Maxwell and Krugner, 1964) have reported the regeneration of nerve fibres in animal subjects subsequent to traumatic brain damage. Generalization of this concept of structural neuronal regeneration to recovery in the human population must obviously, however, remain guarded.

Assessment and Treatment of Speech/Language Disorders Following Closed Head Injury

Assessment of Speech/Language Disorders Subsequent to Closed Head Injury

The speech and language evaluation of a child with a closed head injury involves the careful review of relevant medical and biographical information, the formation of a differential diagnosis and the determination of a prognosis for the recovery of communicative function. The assessment should incorporate analysis of motor speech skills, receptive and expressive language abilities, cognitive ability and the child's general physical and emotional recovery processes. In light of the high-level language deficits identified in the literature, assessment of the linguistic performance of children with closed head injury needs to include sensitive measures of higher level language functions.

Assessment of the motor speech skills of the child with closed head injury should involve evaluation of muscle strength and coordination during both speech and non-speech activities and evaluation of the adequacy of respiration, phonation, resonance, prosody and articulation. A review of the literature would indicate that although speech disorders occur in the closed head injury paediatric population, the majority of children with closed head injury will not present with significant speech disorders subsequent to the injury.

Language evaluation needs to include a wide range of formal and informal procedures to ensure detection of subtle high-level language deficits typical of the closed head injury population. Adult aphasia examinations such as the NCCEA or the Western Aphasia Battery (WAB) (Kertesz, 1982) have frequently been used by a number of researchers to determine the existence of a language deficit. These evaluations, however, were not designed for use with children, hence there are obvious limitations in their use and interpretation. For example, a reading item in the NCCEA is 'screwdriver' which is not a familiar word to many young children. Adult aphasia tests do serve, however, to examine skills not necessarily included in developmental assessments of language such as verbal fluency, and memory-based tasks which, in the light of the available research, are areas which obviously require close attention. Assessment of speech and language skills subsequent to childhood closed head injury should also include a developmental test as well as tests of specific skill areas, such as a visual naming test to determine the presence of a dysnomia which is a frequently-documented sequelae to closed head injury in children. A language evaluation would not be complete without the inclusion of a language sample which can be analyzed in terms of syntax, semantics and pragmatics. It may only be in careful examination of such samples that subtle deficits may become evident.

Implications of Neuropsychological Deficits for Language Assessment

It is obvious that children suffering a closed head injury frequently present with a linguistic deficit concomitant with neuropsychological impairment. This is of particular concern to the speech pathologist who must determine the extent of linguistic disorder and differentially diagnose a cognitively-based language deficit due to a global reduction in skills, a memory-based language deficit and a specific linguistic impairment. Many speech and language impairments shown by head-injured patients are secondary manifestations of cognitive disorganization (Smith, 1974). The neuropsychological recovery of the child with a closed head injury must, therefore, be considered in the speech/language management of the child.

Treatment of Communication Disorders Subsequent to a Closed Head Injury

The speech pathologist should be an integral member of the rehabilitation team working with a head-injured child. Once a differential diagnosis has been established the speech pathologist can proceed to design a rehabilitation programme which caters for the specific needs of the patient. Children who have suffered a closed head injury may present with a wide range of deficits dependent on cause, site and size of lesion, age at time of injury and premorbid skills. Obviously each programme must be designed to meet the specific needs of the child in question. Communication management may require the use of augmentative communication systems in the cases of mutism or severely impaired motor speech skills or may involve the use of facilitative techniques which enable a child to manage their communication deficits more effectively. There is no prescriptive or standard approach to therapy with these children and intervention must be sensitive to the needs of each individual child.

Case Report

In order to place the preceding information in a clinical context, a typical course of treatment and recovery is described in a child with a closed head injury.

Case Description

The patient, a 9-year-old female, was admitted to hospital following a horse-riding accident. The child had fallen from the horse, hitting her head. She had not suffered any loss of consciousness immediately following the accident; however, she was unresponsive to commands. On admission to hospital the child was described as irritable and thrashing about and her eyes were deviated to the left. Her Glasgow Coma scale (Teasdale and Jennet, 1974) score was 7 and she showed focal fitting. A computerized tomographic (CT) scan performed shortly after admission was normal with the exception of a fracture of the skull in the region of the left occiput.

At 1 day after the trauma the child appeared to recognize her mother, but made no atttempt to communicate. During the following 24 hours rapid deterioration occurred to a state of deep coma. A repeat CT scan at this stage demonstrated right cerebral oedema, with compressed ventricles and some midline shift. The child was electively ventilated and paralyzed until 1 week after the trauma, at which time she was weened-off the ventilator and medication. Focal seizures continued but by 9 days after the accident the patient was able to open her eyes and follow simple commands. By 2 weeks after the accident the child was bright and enjoyed watching television, however, she did not initiate communication and failed to respond socially. Response to 'yes/no' questions was demonstrated by the use of eye closing. Four weeks after the trauma, the child showed socially appropriate but simplified language. Her speech was described as laboured. She was discharged from hospital with regular medical and paramedical follow-up.

Speech/Language Evaluation

Initial standardized evaluation of the child's speech and language skills was carried out 4 weeks after the accident. The following test battery was administered: the NCCEA, the Test of Language Development-Intermediate (TOLD-I) (Hammill and Newcomer, 1982), the Boston Naming Test (BNT) (Kaplan *et al.*, 1983), selected subtests of the Clinical Evaluation of Language Functions (CELF) (Semel-Mintz and Wiig, 1982) and the Frenchay Dysarthria Assessment (Enderby, 1983). In addition to these standardized tests a conversation sample was also collected and analyzed.

NCCEA
The child did not show any significant deficit areas according to the NCCEA with the exception of the word fluency subtests where responses were slow, but appropriate.

TOLD-I
The child achieved a Spoken Language Quotient of 83 which falls more than one standard deviation (S.D.) outside the mean score for the average population as provided by test norms ($\times$ = 100, S.D. = 15). Other quotient scores appear in Table 3.1. These results indicated that the child was performing just outside the normal range according to the test norms.

BNT
A raw score of 38 was achieved on the BNT which corresponds to the test norms for a child of 7 ; 6 years to 8 ; 6 years. The child's chronological age at the time of testing was 9 years, hence performance of the BNT was slightly poorer than would be expected according to the test norms. In addition the child's performance on the BNT was marked by numerous semantic errors such as 'dice' for 'dominoes', 'penguin' for 'pelican', 'escalope' for 'stethoscope'. These errors were indicative of a word-finding difficulty.

CELF Confrontation Naming Subtest.
The child's accuracy score for the confrontation naming subtest was well within normal limits, however, speed of performance was markedly reduced.

CELF Word Association Subtest
Performance on the word association subtest which requires the naming of animals and food within a prescribed period was within normal limits.

Frenchay Dysarthria Assessment
The child had some difficulty with the coordination of respiration and vocalization which frequently resulted in inappropriate pitch and loudness. Speech was slow but intelligible. All other oral motor skills were considered within normal limits.

Conversation Sample
The conversational interaction was evaluated using the pragmatic protocol developed by Prutting and Kirchner (1987). All communicative acts identified in this protocol were found to be appropriate in the

Table 3.1 Quotient scores achieved on the test of language development — intermediate (Hammill and Newcomer, 1982)

	Assessment	
	1 month after injury	12 months after injury
Spoken Language Quotient	83	107
Listening Quotient	91	106
Speaking Quotient	81	106
Semantic Quotient	82	97
Syntax Quotient	87	113

child's sample. It was noted, however, that the child's conversational fluency was often interrupted by repetitions and circumlocutionary behaviour as she appeared to search for the appropriate word. It was also apparent from the conversation sample that the child had difficulty interpreting jokes in any more than a literal sense and also demonstrated some difficulty understanding complex instructions, with frequent repetitions required.

On the basis of the test results and observation and analysis of the child's conversational skills it was concluded that the child presented with a high-level language deficit affecting both verbal fluency and word retrieval and higher-level comprehension skills. Speed of response was also significantly impaired. These areas were considered appropriate for remediation as they were affecting the child's communicative competence.

Concomitant problems

Evaluation of the child's motor skills by the occupational and physiotherapists identified difficulties in strength, balance and endurance with particular difficulties in upper limb coordination, speed and dexterity. A strong intention tremor was noted in both hands and this significantly affected the child's fine motor performance. The child attended both physiotherapy and occupational therapy in order to help her overcome these difficulties.

Speech/Language Treatment

The child was seen by the hospital speech pathologist for the following 6-month period. During this time intervention aimed to provide the child with strategies to overcome word-finding difficulties and to increase language comprehension skills, with particular emphasis on figurative and imaginative language and the processing of complex oral commands. Therapy activities included convergent thinking tasks which required the child to identify the salient features of objects, the giving of directions, story construction, and the interpretation and explanation of jokes and ambiguous sentences. The child made significant progress in all areas of speech and language during the 6-month period and then was placed on a 6-monthly review programme.

Re-evaluation 12 months after the accident indicated the resolution of most deficits with the exception of the persistence of some subtle word-finding difficulties most evident in conversational interactions with the child. Quotients obtained on the TOLD-I at this time appear in Table 3.1. The child's progress will continue to be monitored in order to determine the long-term outcome of closed head injury on linguistic skills.

As is typical of the majority of children with a closed head injury, the present case recovered basic communicative competency within a very short period after the injury. Despite the rapid recovery of speech and language skills observed in the present case, she continued to show subtle high level language deficits, a feature typical of the majority of children with closed head injury. Such subtle deficits are particularly significant in terms of the child's long-term integration into school and social environments, and must be considered relevant in her long-term management.

Summary

Considerable heterogeneity exists in the speech/language recovery patterns of children subsequent to closed head injury. Mutism is common in patients during the early stages of recovery but this is rapidly succeeded by a return of basic communicative functions in most instances. Frank aphasic symptoms are evident in only a limited number of children after head injury. Language impairment is more frequently characterized by a persistent subclinical aphasia which has as its most predominant feature dysnomia and decreased verbal fluency. Children with a closed head injury often show concomitant neuropsychological deficits including memory impairment. The speech pathologist has a significant role to play in the assessment and long-term rehabilitation of the child with closed head injury. It must be recognized that the optimal recovery of speech and language skills must be achieved in order to facilitate successful integration of the child back into a society which makes demands for highly developed communication skills. This goal will only be achieved if the speech pathologist is included as a vital participant in the rehabilitation process of the child with a closed head injury.

References

ADAMS, J. H., GRAHAM, D. I., MURRAY, L. S. and SCOTT, G. (1982) 'Diffuse axonal injury due to non-missle injury in humans: an analysis of 45 cases', *Annals of Neurology*, **12**, pp. 557–63.

ADAMS, J. H., MITCHELL, D. E., GRAHAM, D. I. and DOYLE, D. (1977) 'Diffuse brain damage of immediate impact type', *Brain*, **100**, pp. 489–502.

ADAMS, J. H., SCOTT, G., PARKER, L. S. GRAHAM, D. I. and DOYLE, D. (1980) 'The contusion index: a quantitive approach to cerebral contusions in head injury', *Neuropathological Applications of Neurobiology*, **6**, pp. 319–24.

ALAJOUANINE, T. and LHERMITTE, F. (1965), 'Acquired aphasia in children', *Brain*, **88**, pp. 653–62.

BAKAY. L. and GLASAUER, F. E. (1980) *Head Injury*, Boston, Little, Brown and Company.

BENTON, A. L. and HAMSHER, K. (1978) *Multilingual Aphasia Examination*, Iowa City, Benton Laboratory of Neuropsychology.

BISHOP, D. V. (1981) 'Plasticity and specificity of language localisation in the developing brain', *Developmental Medicine and Child Neurology*, **23**, pp. 251–5.

BRINK, J. D., GARRETT, A. L., HALE, W. R., WOO-SAM, J. and NICKEL, V. L. (1970) 'Recovery of motor and intellectual function in children sustaining severe head injuries', *Developmental Medicine and Child Neurology*, **12**, pp. 565–71.

BRUCE, D. A. (1983) 'Clinical care of the severely head injured child', in Shapiro, K. (Ed.) *Pediatric Head Trauma*, New York, Futura Publishing Company.

BRUCE, D. A., ALAVI, A., BILANIUK, L., COLINSKAS, C., OBRIST, W. and UZZELL, B. (1981). 'Diffuse cerebral swelling following head injuries in children – the syndrome of malignant brain edema', *Journal of Neurosurgery*, **54**, pp. 170–8.

BRUCE, D. A., SCHUT, L., BRUNO, L. A., WOOD, J. H. and SUTTON, L. N. (1978) 'Outcome following severe head injury in children', *Child's Brain*, **5**, 174–91.

CHADWICK, O., RUTTER, M., BROWN, G., SHAFFER, D. and TRAUB, M. (1981a) 'A prospective study of children with head injuries: II Cognitive sequelae', *Psychological Medicine*, **11**, pp. 49–61.

CHADWICK, O., RUTTER, M., SHAFFER. D. and SHROUT, P. E. (1981b) 'A prospective study of children with head injuries: IV Specific cognitive deficits', *Journal of Clinical Neuropsychology*, **3**, pp. 101–20.

CHADWICK, O., RUTTER, M., THOMPSON, J. and SHAFFER, D. (1981c) 'Intellectual performance and reading skills after localised head injury in childhood', *Journal of Child Psychology and Psychiatry*, **22**, pp. 117–39.

COSTEFF, H., ABRAHAM, E., BRENNER, T., HOROWITZ, I., APTER, N., SADAN, N. and NAJENSON, T. (1988) 'Late neuropsychologic status after childhood head trauma', *Brain and Development*, **10**, pp. 371–4.

CRAFT, A. W. (1972). 'Head injury in children', in Vinken, P. J. and Bruyn, G. W. (Eds) *Handbook of Clinical Neurology, Vol: 23*, New York, Elsevier North-Holland.

DANIEL, P. M. and PRITCHARD, M. M. L. (1975) 'Studies of the hypothalamus and the pituitary gland: with special reference to the effects of transection of the pituitary stalk', *Acta Endocrinology*, **80**, pp. 201–16.

ENDERBY, P. (1983) *Frenchay Dysarthria Assessment*, San Diego, College-Hill Press.

EWING-COBBS L., FLETCHER, J. M. and LEVIN, H. S. (1985) 'Neuropsychological sequelae following paediatric head injury.' in Ylvisaker, M. (Ed.) *Head Injury Rehabilitation: Children and Adolescents*, London, Taylor & Francis.

EWING-COBBS, L., FLETCHER, J. M., LEVIN, H. S. and EISENBERG, H. M. (1987) 'Language functions following closed head injury in children and adolescents,' *Journal of Clinical Experimental Neuropsychology*, **5**, pp. 575–92.

FULD, P. and FISHER, P. (1977) 'Recovery of intellectual ability after closed head injury', *Developmental Medicine and Child Neurology*, **19**, pp. 495–502.

FRIEDE, R. L. (1975) *Developmental Neuropathology*, Wien, New York, Springer.

GAIDOLFI, E. and VIGNOLO, L. A. (1980) 'Closed head injury of school aged children: neuropsychological sequelae in early adulthood,' *Italian Journal of Neurological Sciences*, **1**, pp. 65–73.

GIBSON, E. J. and LEVIN, H. (1975) *The Psychology of Reading*, Cambridge, MIT Press.

GRAHAM, D. I., ADAMS, J. H. and Doyle, D. (1978) 'Ischaemic brain damage in fatal non missile head injuries,' *Journal of Neurological Science*, **39**, pp. 213–34.

GRONWALL, D. and SAMPSON, H. (1974) *The Psychological Effects of Concussion*, Auckland, Auckland University Press.

GURDJIAN, E. S. and GURDJIAN, E. S. (1976) 'Cerebral contusions: reevaluation of the mechanism of their development,' *Journal of Trauma*, **16**, pp. 35–51.

GURDJIAN, E. S. and WEBSTER, J. E. (1958) *Head Injuries: Mechanisms, Diagnosis and Management*, Boston, Little, Brown and Company.

HAMMILL, D. D. and NEWCOMER, P. L. (1982) *Test of Language Development — Intermediate*, Texas, Pro-Ed.

HÉCAEN, H. (1976) 'Acquired aphasia in children and the ontogenesis of hemispheric functional specialisation,' *Brain and Language*, **3**, pp. 114–34.

HEBB, D. O. (1942) 'The effect of early and late brain injury on test scores, and the nature of normal adult intelligence,' *Proceedings of the American Philosophical Society*, **85**, pp. 274–92.

HOLBOURNE, A. H. S. (1943) 'Mechanics of head injuries,' *Lancet*, **ii**, pp. 438–41.

JELLINGER, K. (1983) 'The neuropathology of pediatric head injuries,' in Shapiro, K. (Ed.) *Pediatric Head Trauma*, New York, Futura Publishing Company.

JORDAN, F. M. and MURDOCH, B. E. (1990) 'Linguistic status following closed head injury in children: a follow-up study,' *Brain Injury*, **4**, pp. 101–8.

JORDAN, F. M., OZANNE, A. E. and MURDOCH, B. E. (1988) 'Long term speech and language disorders subsequent to closed head injury in children,' *Brain Injury*, **2**, pp. 179–85.

JORDAN, F. M., OZANNE, A. E. and MURDOCH, B. E. (1990) 'Performance of closed head injury children on a naming task,' *Brain Injury*, **4**, pp. 27–32.

KENNARD, M. A. (1938) 'Reorganisation of motor functions in the cerebral cortex of monkeys deprived of motor and premotor areas in infancy,' *Journal of Neurophysiology*, **1**, pp. 477–97.

KAPLAN, E., GOODGLASS, H. and WEINTRAUB, S. (1983) *Boston Naming Test*, Philadelphia, Lea & Febiger.

KERTESZ, A. (1982) *Western Aphasia Battery*, Ontario, Grune & Stratton.

KLONOFF, H., LOW, M. and CLARK, C. (1977) 'Head injuries in children with a prospective four year follow up,' *Journal of Neurology, Neurosurgery and Psychiatry*, **40**, pp. 1211–19.

KNIGHTS, R. M. and NORWOOD, J. A. (1979) *A Neuropsychological Test Battery for Children: Examiners Manual*, Ottawa, Psychological Consultants.

LINDENBERG, R. and FREYTAG, E. (1969) 'Morphology of brain lesions from blunt trauma in early infancy,' *Archives of Pathology (Chicago)*, **87**, pp. 298–305.

LEVIN, H., BENTON, A and GROSSMAN, R. (1982a) *Neurobehavioural Consequences of Closed Head Injury*, Oxford, Oxford University Press.

LEVIN, H. and EISENBERG, H. (1979a) 'Neuropsychological impairment after closed head injury in children and adolescents,' *Journal of Paediatric Psychology*, **4**, pp. 389–402.

LEVIN, H. and EISENBERG, H. (1979b) 'Neuropsychological outcome of closed head injury in children and adolescents,' *Child's Brain*, **5**, pp. 281–92.

LEVIN, H., EISENBERG, H. M. and MINER, M. E. (1983a) 'Neuropsychological findings in head injured children', in Shapiro, K. (Ed.) *Pediatric Head Trauma*, New York, Futura Publishing Company.

LEVIN, H., EISENBERG, H. M., WIGG, N. R. and KOBAYASHI, K. (1982b) 'Memory and intellectual ability after head injury in children and adolescents,' *Neurosurgery*, **11**, pp. 668–73.

LEVIN, H., EWING-COBBS, L. and BENTON, A. L. (1983b) 'Age and recovery from brain damage,' in Scheff, S. W. (Ed.) *Aging and the Recovery of Function in the Central Nervous System*, New York, Plenum Publishing Corporation.

LEVIN, H., GROSSMAN, R. G. and KELLY, P. J. (1976) 'Aphasic disorder in patients with closed head injury,' *Journal of Neurology, Neurosurgery and Psychiatry*, **39**, pp. 1062–70.

LEVIN, H., GROSSMAN, R. G., SARWAR, M. and MEYERS, C. A. (1981) 'Linguistic recovery after closed head injury,' *Brain and Language*, **12**, pp. 360–74.

MACPHERSON, P. and GRAHAM, D. I. (1978) 'Correlations of angiographic findings and the ischaemia of head injury,' *Journal of Neurology, Neurosurgery and Psychiatry*, **41**, pp. 122–7.

MARTIN, G. (1974) *A Manual of Head Injuries in General Surgery*, London, Heinemann Medical Books.

MAXWELL, D. S. and KRUGNER, L. (1964) 'Electron microscopy of radiation induced laminar lesions in the cerebral cortex of the rat' in Hale, T. J. and Snider, S. J. (Eds) *Response of the Nervous System to Ionising Radiation*, Boston, Little Brown.

MILLER, J. D., BECKER, D. P., WARD, J. D., SULLIVAN, H. G., ADAMS, W. E. and ROSER, M. J. (1977) 'Significance of intracranial hypertension in severe head injury,' *Journal of Neurosurgery*, **47**, pp. 503–16.

OMMAYA, A. K. and GENNARELLI, T. I. (1974) 'Cerebral concussion and traumatic unconsciousness: correlations of experimental and clinical observations on blunt head injuries,' *Brain*, **97**, pp. 633–54.

OMMAYA, A. K., GRUBB, R. L. and NAUMANN, R. A. (1971) 'Coup and contracoup injury: observations on the mechanics of visible brain injuries in the rhesus monkey,' *Journal of Neurosurgery*, **35**, pp. 503–16.

PANG, D. (1985) 'Pathophysiologic correlates of neurobehavioural syndromes following closed head injury,' in Ylvisaker, M. (Ed.) *Head Injury Rehabilitation: Children and Adolescents*, London, Taylor & Francis.

PRUTTING, C. A. and KIRCHNER, D. M. (1987) 'A clinical appraisal of the pragmatic aspects of language,' *Journal of Speech and Hearing Disorders*, **52**, pp. 105–19.

RICHARDSON, F. (1963) 'Some effects of severe head injury. A follow up study of children and adolescents after protracted coma,' *Developmental Medicine and Child Neurology*, **5**, pp. 471–82.

ROBINSON, R. (1981) 'Equal recovery in child and adult brain?' *Developmental Medicine and Child Neurology*, **23**, pp. 379–83.

RUTTER, M. (1981) 'Psychological sequelae of brain damage in children,' *American Journal of Psychiatry*, **138**, pp. 1533–44.

SARNO, M. T. (1980) 'The nature of verbal impairment after closed head injury,' *Journal of Mental and Nervous Disease*, **168**, pp. 685–92.

SARNO, M. T. (1984) 'Verbal impairment after closed head injury: Report of a replication study,' *Journal of Nervous and Mental Disease*, **172**, pp. 475–9.

SARNO, M. T., BUONAGURO, A. and LEVITA, E. (1986) 'Characteristics of verbal impairment in closed head injured patients,' *Archives of Physical and Medical Rehabilitation*, **67**, pp. 400–5.

SARNO, M. T. and LEVIN, H. S. (1985) 'Speech and language disorders after closed head injury,' in Darby, J. K. (Ed.) *Speech Evaluation in Neurology*, New York, Grune & Stratton.

SATZ, P. and BULLARD-BATES, C. (1981) 'Acquired aphasia in children', in Sarno, M. T. (Ed.) *Acquired Aphasia*, New York, Academic Press.

SHAFFER, D., BIJUR, P., CHADWICK, O. and RUTTER, M. (1980) 'Head injury and later reading disability,' *Journal of the American Academy of Child Psychiatry*, **19**, pp. 592–610.

SEMEL-MINTZ, E. and WIIG, E.H. (1982) *Clinical Evaluation of Language Functions*, Columbus, Charles E. Merrill.

SMITH, E. (1974) 'Influence of site of impact upon cognitive performance persisting long after closed head injury,' *Journal of Neurology, Neurosurgery and Psychiatry*, **37**, pp. 719–26.

SOH, K., LARSEN, B., SKINHOJ, E. and LASSEN, N.A. (1977) 'rCBF in aphasia', *Acta Neurologica Scandinavia*, **56**, pp. 270–1.

SPREEN, O. and BENTON, A.L. (1969) *Neurosensory Centre Comprehensive Examination for Aphasia*, Victoria B.C., University of Victoria.

TEASDALE, G. and JENNET, B. (1974) 'Assessment of coma and impaired consciousness: A practical scale,' *Lancet*, **ii**, pp. 81–4.

TEASDALE, G. and MENDELOW, D. (1984) 'Pathophysiology of head injuries', in Brooks, N. (Ed.) *Closed Head Injury — Psychological, Social and Family Consequences*, Oxford, Oxford University Press.

THOMSEN, I.V. (1975) 'Evaluation and outcome of aphasia in patients with severe closed head trauma', *Journal of Neurology, Neurosurgery and Psychiatry*, **38**, pp. 713–18.

WINOGRAN, H.W., KNIGHTS, R.M. and BAWDEN, H.N. (1984) 'Neuropsychological deficits following head injury in children', *Journal of Clinical Neuropsychology*, **6**, pp. 269–86.

ZIMMERMAN, R.A., BILANIUK, L.T., BRUCE, D., DOLINSKAS, C., OBRIST, W., and KUHL, D. (1978) 'Computed tomography of paediatric head trauma: Acute general cerebral swelling,' *Radiology*, **126**, pp. 403–8.

Chapter 4

Communicative Disorders in Childhood Infectious Diseases

**Veronica Smyth, Anne E. Ozanne and
Lynn M. Woodhouse**

Introduction

Infectious diseases of the central nervous system (CNS) include diseases caused by viral, bacterial, spirochetal and other less common microorganisms and are classified according to the major site of involvement and type of infecting organism. Infection of the meninges (usually the leptomeninges) is called meningitis while inflammation of the brain is referred to as encephalitis. In some cases both the meninges and brain may be infected, a condition called meningoencephalitis. There are three major types of meningitis, including pyogenic meningitis caused by pus-forming bacteria (e.g. meningococci, pneumococci and the influenza bacillus), tuberculous meningitis caused by the tubercle bacillus, and viral meningitis caused by a variety of different viruses (e.g. polio, mumps etc.). Encephalitis is caused by either pyogenic bacteria or viruses. In addition, in some regions of the world encephalitis may also be caused by various other parasites acquired from animals. Childhood infectious diseases having the CNS as a primary site of infection are listed in Table 4.1.

Types of Infectious Disorders Affecting the Central Nervous System

Acquired Meningeal Infections

The CNS should be suspected as a site of infection in childhood illnesses whenever the patient's presenting signs and symptoms include fever, headache, altered states of consciousness ranging from drowsiness to coma, irritability, a high-pitched cry in infants, neck stiffness (especially inability to touch chin to chest), back stiffness (inability to sit normally), positive Kernig's sign (inability to extend knee when the leg is flexed anteriorly at the hip), positive Brudzinski's sign (flexion of the lower

Table 4.1   Primary central nervous system infections of childhood

VIRAL	BACTERIAL
Aseptic meningitis	*Neisseria meningitides*
Lymphocytic choriomeningitis	Meningococcal meningitis
Lassa fever (West Africa)	Diplococcal meningitis
Viral encephalitis	Pneumococcal meningitis
Bulbar polioencephalitis	Streptococcal meningitis
	Haemophilus influenzae
	(especially type B)
SPIROCHETAL	GRAM-NEGATIVE
Leptospirosis	*Escherichia coli*
Spirochetal jaundice	*Enterobacter aerogenes*
Syphilis	*Proteus morgani*
	Klebsiella pneumoniae
	Listeria monocytogenes
	Tuberculous meningitis
	RARE
	Salmonella
	Shigella
	Clostridium perfringens
	Neisseria gonorrhea

extremity with the head bent forward), projectile vomiting and shock. Other CNS signs may include bulging fontanelles, increased diplopia, increased cerebrospinal fluid (CSF) pressure, constriction of visual fields, papilloedema, slow pulse rate and irregular respiration. All the above signs and symptoms are regarded as meningeal and should be investigated clinically.

Clinically, pathological signs of meningeal infection depend on the underlying aetiology and may include petechial or purpuric rashes, conjunctivitis, arthritis, myocarditis, a history of upper respiratory tract infection or otitis, urinary tract or other localized infection, jaundice, albuminuria and oliguria. Laboratory findings are required to establish an accurate diagnosis of CNS infections, especially meningitis. Examination of the CSF will include cultures, glucose levels (decreased), lactic acid content (increased), protein (increased) and white blood count (increased). Results of these laboratory investigations provide the best indication of neurological damage and help to determine prognosis as well as final diagnosis. The most common CNS infection in childhood is undoubtedly meningitis, in particular bacterial meningitis, which may present with few or many of the signs and symptoms indicated above, depending upon the specific causative organism and the severity of the infection. The organisms which are most frequently responsible for bacterial meningitis include *Haemophilus influenzae* type B (HIB), *Neisseria meningitis* (meningococcus) and

Streptococcus pneumoniae (pneumococcus). The relative frequencies of various bacterial species in the aetiology of meningitis vary with age. In the neonatal period, gram-negative bacilli are the major cause of meningitis. Between 3 months and 5 years of age HIB is the most common causative bacteria of paediatric meningitis accounting for 75–80 per cent of paediatric cases of bacterial meningitis (Sell, 1987). Meningococcal meningitis occurs most frequently in children and young adults, although it may occur in all age groups. It is the only type of meningitis that may occur in large community-wide outbreaks. The incidence of pneumococcal meningitis is greatest in children and older adults.

The advent of antibiotics (e.g. penicillin and chloramphenicol) has greatly reduced the mortality rate of bacterial meningitis from about 90 per cent to less than 10 per cent (Dodge, 1986; Sell, 1987). Despite this reduction in the mortality rate, there is, however, a body of research to indicate that bacterial meningitis is associated with a high incidence of permanent neurological sequelae, including speech and language disorders, in those children who survive the disease. Therefore, as noted by Tejani *et al.* (1982), the reduction in mortality rate has not been matched with a decrease in morbidity. In addition to meningitis, other infections may also affect the CNS and these are noted later in this chapter.

Infectious Encephalitis and Para-infectious Encephalitis

Infectious encephalitis may result from either direct invasion of the brain tissue by arthropod-borne organisms or the enteroviruses (echo, coxsackie or polio), or indirectly by the mumps virus, herpes simplex virus or by other agents such as toxoplasmosis. Para-infectious encephalitis may follow infection with rubeola, rubella, varicella or infectious mononucleosis or follow vaccine inoculation.

The presenting signs of encephalitis are lethargy, coma, convulsions, headache, nausea, vomiting and cerebral oedema. Clinical findings may change depending on the extent of the oedema, with neck and back stiffness occurring. CSF findings contrast with meningitis in that glucose levels may be normal. Table 4.2 compares the pathological changes seen in the CSF in various CNS infectious diseases with the pattern seen in normal children.

Reye's Syndrome

This is an uncommon form of encephalopathy associated with influenza and varicella viruses. It is associated with hepatic failure. The prognosis is poor.

Table 4.2 Usual cerebrospinal fluid findings in central nervous system infections

Condition	Pressure mm H$_2$O	Appearance	White blood cells per cu mm	Sugar mg/100 ml	Protein mg/100 ml
1 Normal children	40–200	clear	0–5 (over 5 years)	40–80	15–40
2 Bacterial meningitis	300	turbid	500–15,000	low or absent	500
3 Tuberculous meningitis	300	clear or opalescent	30–500	0–45	300
4 Encephalomyelitis	normal	clear or opalescent	1000	normal	normal
5 Guillain-Barré syndrome	increased	clear	normal	normal	increased
6 Toxoplasma encephalitis	normal	clear or opalescent	30–2,000	normal	normal
7 Other encephalitides	normal	clear or opalescent	15–1,000	normal	60–200

Congenital and Perinatal Infectious Diseases Affecting the CNS

The capacity to cross the placental barrier has long been recognized as a characteristic of the TORCH (Pappas, 1985) group of infections: toxoplasmosis, rubella, cytomegalovirus (CMV), herpes simplex, hepatitis B, syphilis and others. Such maternal infections are well known causes of CNS disorders in the infant. Hearing loss is common in affected infants and mental retardation, blindness and less severe forms of CNS involvement are possible sequelae. The TORCH syndromes occur as a result of intra-uterine infection generally in the first trimester. However, the CMV appears to have the potential to affect the fetus beyond the first trimester. Other infections may also occur relatively late in pregnancy and affect the fetus. Table 4.3 lists infections known to affect the human fetus or neonates.

Clinical findings in CMV infection

Congenital CMV infection is accompanied by neonatal jaundice, hepatosplenomegaly, purpura, haematuria, encephalitis and abnormal blood findings including lymphocytosis, bilirubinaemia, erythroblastosis and thrombocytosis. Inguinal hernia, chorioretinitis and small size for gestational age are other signs that have been noted. (Note: acute acquired CMV infection may also occur. This resembles infectious mononucleosis in sequelae.)

Table 4.3 Infections able to produce disease in the human fetus or neonate (ranging from subclinical to severe mutli-facet CNS involvement)

Arboviruses
Coxsackie B virus
Cytomegalovirus
Herpes simplex
Varicella zoster
Influenza
Polioviruses
Rubella
Toxoplasmois (protozoal)
Syphilis
Echovirus
Coxsackie A virus
Measles
Streptococcus
Escherichia coli
Hepatitis B

Subclinical CMV infection is the most commonly occurring form of the disease. Children affected appear normal at birth but are at risk for late onset of a variety of CNS disorders including microcephaly, auditory pathway dysfunction, gross motor skill delays, behavioural problems, learning disabilities and intellectual retardation.

Long-Term Sequelae of CNS Infections in Childhood

In all types of CNS infection residual impairment of CNS function may range from nil to subtle to severe. Children may have peripheral hearing loss or central auditory processing dysfunction leading to varying degrees of learning disability. In some instances selective attention problems may occur and children may be hyperactive with significant behavioural problems. Pragmatic skills may be disordered or language development may be delayed. In the extreme instance intellectual retardation will result. Disturbances in equilibrium may lead to delays in motor skill development. The apparent severity of CNS infection does not correlate with residual functional disability and long-term monitoring is necessary. In many cases cause and effect relationships are difficult to ascribe with any degree of certainty or statistical reliability.

Hearing Disorders in Childhood Infectious Diseases of the CNS

Infectious diseases are found as significant aetiological features in many clinical histories associated with peripheral and central auditory disorders in children. Most infections in childhood which are recognized as having the potential to damage the hearing mechanism either transiently or irreversibly have been well documented. However, the causative relationship is not always certain or clear and the level of infection may not correlate directly with the degree or extent of auditory system involvement. Furthermore the cause of the auditory impairment may be the primary infection itself or a secondary association brought about by systemic reactions or by-products.

Causes and Course of Infection

Table 4.4 lists infections reported in children that have the potential to involve the CNS. Many of these infections have the capacity to cause hearing loss or related functional speech and language disorders.

W hether a primary or secondary focus, most infectious diseases affecting the CNS manifest peripheral sensorineural hearing loss as a complication in some children. The degree of hearing loss in the various infectious disorders is never predictable, although some sequelae are relatively constant. For example, a profound unilateral sensorineural

153

Table 4.4 Childhood infections which have the potential to involve the central nervous system

VIRAL	RICKETTISIAL
Echovirus	Typhus
Coxsackie virus	
Herpes simplex	FUNGUS
Epidemic parotitis (mumps)	Cryptococcosis
Infectious mononucleosis	
Rubeola (measles)	POST-VACCINAL
Varicella (rare)	e.g. smallpox
Influenza (rare)	
Herpes zoster	SEROUS OTITIS MEDIA
Epstein Barr virus	*Streptococcus pneumoniae*
Guillain-Barré syndrome	Group A streptococci
Reye's syndrome	*Haemophilis influenza*
Cat scratch disease	Gram-negative bacilli (neonates)
Brainstem encephalitis	
Progressive rubella panencephalitis	
Subacute sclerosing panencephalitis	

hearing loss is characteristic of hearing loss associated with mumps even though positive identification of the mumps virus may not be verified in the presence of such a hearing loss in every instance. Table 4.5 lists the infectious organisms known to cause deafness as a common complication in childhood, infancy, neonatal or fetal developmental periods.

Hearing Loss

Characteristics of the hearing losses reported in children with infectious disease states include: (1) variability in manifestation; (2) incidence and prevalence changes over time; (3) fluctuation in severity and outcome; and (4) substantially variable sequelae. This variability has, in the past, led to problems in detecting and defining hearing loss in children with CNS infections. In recent years developments and changes occurring in medical diagnostics and audiological management protocols have lead to more accurate identification of the organisms involved and more accurate monitoring of hearing status in children with CNS infections. Furthermore, the accuracy of neurological diagnosis is improving with the use of computed tomography (CT) to detect complicating hydrocephalus and brain abscess, and magnetic resonance imaging (MRI) which defines ischaemic disturbances of basal ganglia and the diencephalon as well as parenchymal signal abnormalities in the brainstem and adjacent temporal lobes (Schoeman *et al.*, 1988). Currently, treatment strategies available to cope with the infectious disorder at the time tend towards better accessibility and earlier diagnosis.

Table 4.5 Infectious organisms known to cause deafness as a common complication variously in childhood, infancy, the neonate or fetus

ORGANISM	AUDITORY SYSTEM INVOLVEMENT
Coxsackie virus encephalitis	Hearing loss
Echovirus 2 enteroviral encephalomyelitis	Hearing and vestibular dysfunction
Herpes simplex virus	Disturbance of memory — probably reflects bilateral temporal lobe involvement
Herpes simplex encephalitis	Extensive CNS involvement
Guillain-Barré syndrome	VIIth nerve involvement
Herpes zoster	VIIIth nerve is second most common sensory site
Ramsay Hunt syndrome	VIIth nerve involvement
Zoster encephalitis	Inflammation of the cochlea and maculae. (Geniculate ganglion inflammation)
Infectious mononucleosis and the EB virus	May involve any cranial nerve plus the brainstem
Epstein Barr (EB) virus	Implicated in nasopharyngeal carcinoma with posterior extension. May involve the VIIIth nerve
Cytomegalic inclusion disease	Hearing loss and impaired intellectual function, epilepsy, cerebral palsy (also cardiac and orthopaedic disorders)
Rubella. Progressive rubella panencephalitis (late onset > 8 years)	Hearing loss, mental retardation, growth retardation, microcephaly (also cardiac murmurs and cataract)
Bacterial meningitis	Hearing loss
Toxoplasmosis	Hearing loss
Syphilis	Hearing loss

At the same time diagnostic audiology has been undergoing change, for example in the decade 1970–79 the addition of impedance audiometry to the audiological test battery enabled more accurate diagnosis of middle ear dysfunction. During 1980–89 the increasing acceptance of auditory evoked response audiometry, especially the use of the auditory brainstem response (ABR) has provided the clinician with the means to detect hearing loss in otherwise difficult to test children without the need to defer assessment until behavioural responses could be obtained (Smyth, 1984).

Mechanism of Auditory System Involvement

The mechanism whereby infectious disease processes involve the auditory system is exemplified by the most common CNS causes of hearing loss. These are the bacterial meningitis strains: *Haemophilus influenzae* type B, meningococcus, *Neisseria meningitidis* and *Diplococcus pneumoniae*. Nadol (1978) cited these organisms as being responsible for 90 per cent of the hearing loss in bacterial meningitis. Inflammatory processes in the meninges lead to meningeal blood vessels becoming congested, with the formation of an exudate in the subarachnoid space. Keane *et al.* (1979) described the process as a diffuse, meningeal inflammation with purulent material concentrated within the basal cisternae and around the cerebellum, brainstem and internal auditory meatus. This purulent infiltration involved the arachnoid in the region of the internal auditory canal. Keane *et al.* (1979) speculated that this infiltration may produce a neuritis or perineuritis of the VIII nerve. However, the cochlear end organ may also be damaged significantly via either the cochlear aqueduct or the internal auditory canal leading to long-term fibrosis amd calcification. This is observed in some post-meningitis cochlear implant patients who in fact retain a scatter of residual VIII nerve activity, indicated by positive promontory stimulation obtained during pre-implant testing and successful psychophysical electrode array mapping post-implant.

As the subarachnoid space extends in a continuous manner to include the space around the brain, spinal cord and optic nerves and is connected either directly or by reflux through the basal foramens of Magendie and Luschke to the ventricles of the brain, meningitis is always cerebrospinal. The inflammatory reaction referred to by Keane *et al.* (1979) may impinge upon structures within the subarachnoid space (cranial and spinal nerve roots) or the ventricles (choroid plexuses) or reach adjacent structures: pial blood vessels, cerebellar and cerebral cortices, spinal cord white matter, peripheral optic nerve fibres, ependymal and subependymal tissues.

The pathogenesis of meningeal microorganisms is not always ascertained accurately. Predisposing factors for bloodstream entry include primary viral infections of the upper respiratory tract, lungs or meninges, trauma or circulating endotoxins. Other entries include middle ear disease, paranasal sinus infection, congenital defects, fractures or surgical sites or pre-existing disease states.

In young children, upper respiratory tract infection and middle ear infections commonly occur as antecedents, the onset of infection may be reported as being accompanied by seizures. Early identification and diagnosis is now an increasing likelihood. In a prospective study Smyth *et al.* (1988) reported that no apparent statistical relationship emerged between onset, hospitalization and auditory status outcome in a 12-month cohort of children admitted to a city hospital who had a confirmed diagnosis of bacterial meningitis. However, the average time between onset of signs and symptoms and admission to hospital was a mean of 3.2 days with a standard deviation of 2.2 days, with four children being admitted during day one of onset of their signs and symptoms. This indicates a trend towards better and earlier diagnosis and parental and caregiver awareness of the need to seek medical treatment.

Feigin and Dodge (1976) discussed host and environmental factors in children which predispose to bacterial meningitis. The host factors included:

1　Increased incidence in the very young
2　Increased severity in the very young
3　A male:female ratio of 1.7:1
4　Prematurity
5　At risk neonatal physiological factors leading to defects in the response of leucocytes to chemotactic factors
6　Deficiency in IgA and IgM which would protect normally against Gram-negative organisms
7　Congenital deficiency of immunoglobulins
8　Congenital functional defects
9　Pre-existing disease states
10　Specific antigen-antibody relationships.

Environmental factors included overcrowded living conditions or close contact between individuals. Contact with farm animals or wild animals is also a recognized infection route in the case of leptospirosis-related meningitis which occurs at sporadic intervals and should not be over-looked even in this decade.

Infectious Diseases and Prevalence of Hearing Disorders

The occurrence of hearing loss in children as a result of infectious diseases may be considered in relation to either the number of known clinical cases (incidence) or the rate of occurrence of clinical cases as a population ratio, for example, incidence per 1000 live births (prevalence). Prevalence estimates are generally considered a more realistic data base for the purpose of monitoring trends in the effects of diseases. Nevertheless, aetiological profiles differ when attempting to compare industrialized societies and developing Third World countries. Immunization and Public Health programmes in Western society have resulted in the control of diseases such as measles, rubella, whooping cough, meningitis and goitre to a large extent, thus time-series studies of prevalence data reveal differences in trends dependent upon the environment and disease being targeted. There is a paucity of scientifically-based studies available from developing countries.

Patterns and trends of prevalence can be illustrated best by studying representative examples of hearing loss in children caused by infectious disease. For example:

1　Rubella as a known cause of congenital deafness

2   Cytomegalovirus infection as an emerging cause of congenital deafness.
3   Meningitis as a known cause of acquired deafness
4   Unknown causes as an additional acquired deafness category

Because of the lack of scientifically-based studies available from developing countries, figures from industrialized countries only are considered here. Table 4.6 lists prevalence studies covering the period 1967 to the present for these four representative disease states. While a large proportion of the percentage of unknown causes may be attributable to autosomal recessive genetic causes, the apparent emergence of a new cause in CMV would suggest the possibility of unidentified viral infections also subsumed in the unknown category.

A study by Tomlin (1989) examined in fine detail the demographic characteristics of handicapping childhood hearing loss (for the state of Queensland, Australia), with handicapping defined as: requiring hearing aid fitting. Tomlin (1989) presented his data in the form of aggregate prevalence of each cause as a percentage of all known cases of hearing loss between 1950 and 1987. The acquisition of such data was possible since every child fitted with a hearing aid in Queensland was, and still is, listed in the records of the Australian Federal Government instrumentality (the National Acoustic Laboratories) which is responsible for the assessment and provision of free hearing aids for all children requiring them. The laboratories are recognized internationally as a unique entity. Because of the extended time-span, the sampling nature of the total cohort, its climatic setting which includes tropical, subtropical and temperate areas, mountainous country, flat lands, inland farming and grazing, large industrialized cities, and long stretches of coastal high-density population, the Tomlin study represents an important source of data for researchers concerned with aetiological trends in industrialized countries on a global basis.

Figures 4.1–4.5 depict the prevalence per 1000 live births for the infectious diseases under discussion for each year from 1950 to 1987, derived from Tomlin's data together with the overall prevalence. The overall number of hearing loss cases requiring hearing aids in that period was 3951 children, an aggregate incidence of 2.90 per 1000 live births. By excluding children under 7 years of age from the sampling window to avoid late onset/late detection contamination of data, the aggregate prevalence during 1950–81 becomes 3.32 per 1000 births for all causative factors. Table 4.7 lists the percentage of cases by our target infectious diseases from all cases of handicapping hearing loss in children born between 1950 and 1987. Tomlin's (1989) conclusions were as follows:

1   Rubella (congenital infection) see Figure 4.2
     The incidence of rubella-attributed congenital hearing loss between 1950 and 1987 was 550 cases. This indicates an aggregate prevalence for that period of 0.406 per 1000 live births. This was the highest aggregate of any known aetiological factor. The prevalence attributable to rubella reflects the 1964

Table 4.6 Hearing loss prevalence studies from industrialized countries 1967 onwards for representative aetiological factors

Authors	Study population	Rubella %	Cytomegalovirus %	Meningitis %	Unknown cause %
Martin *et al.* (1981) Martin (1982)	1969 birth year cohort (EEC) all 8 years old with 3 frequency. Average hearing levels > 50 dB.	16.0	—	6.0	42.0
Kankkunen (1982) Thiiringer *et al.* (1984)	Sweden n = 146 1970–79 birth years	5.0	1.0	5.0	12.0
Parving (1985)	Denmark n = 117 1970–80 birth years (every effort taken to identify unknown causes)	19.0	not stated	2.6	11.0
Feinmesser *et al.* (1986)	Israel n = 107 1967–78 birth years n = 62 000 children screened	6.5	not stated	3.7	28.1
Brown (1986)	USA n = 55 136 hearing impaired 1982–83 school year annual survey	16.3	not stated	7.3	39.5
Greville and Keith, (1978)	New Zealand	7.9	not stated	not stated	49.7

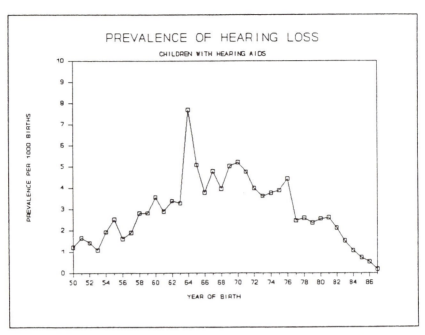

Figure 4.1   Prevalence of handicapping childhood hearing loss 1950–87

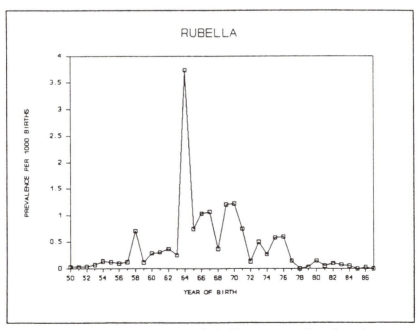

Figure 4.2   Prevalence of rubella during 1950–87 as a cause of handicapping childhood hearing loss

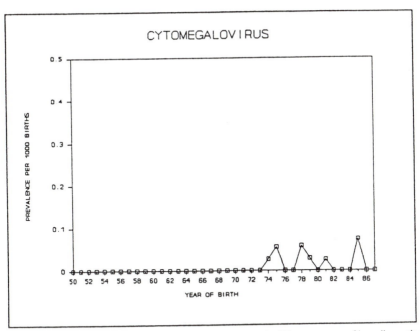

Figure 4.3 Prevalence of cytomegalovirus during 1950–87 as a cause of handicapping childhood hearing loss

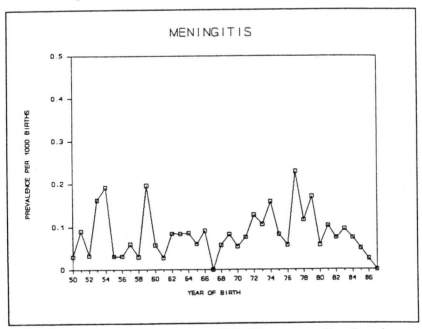

Figure 4.4 Prevalence of meningitis during 1950–87 as a cause of handicapping childhood hearing loss

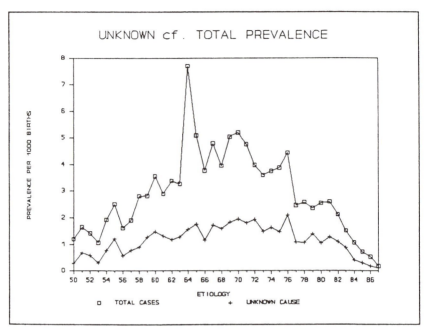

Figure 4.5 Prevalence of unknown factors during 1950–87 as a cause of handicapping childhood hearing loss

Australian rubella epidemic and presumably reflects the effects of aggressive immunization programmes in the smaller prevalence since 1977.

2   Cytomegalovirus, see Figure 4.3

The incidence of congenital hearing loss in Queensland attributed to cytomegalovirus between 1950 and 1987 was 10 cases. This indicates an aggregate prevalence for that period of 0.007 per 1000 live births. No child born before 1974 was identified as having a cytomegalovirus-caused hearing loss. The highest prevalence recorded was 0.07 per live births in 1985; however, this figure may be underestimated at this point since Tomlin (1989) found that although final incidence figures by 21 years of age, by 16 years and by 8 years are similar, a larger proportion may be unidentified before 8 years of age. This was supported by a regression analysis of relationships between total number of children fitted with hearing aid by ages 16 and 8 years which indicated that the number of children fitted with hearing aids by 8 years of age accounted for over 89 per cent of the overall incidence.

3   Meningitis, see Figure 4.4

The incidence of hearing loss in Queensland attributed to meningitis between 1950 and 1987 was 112 cases. This indicates an average prevalence for that period of 0.082 per 1000 live births. Despite atypical fluctuations, as in 1954

Table 4.7 Percentage of cases attributed to infectious diseases from all cases of handicapping hearing loss in children born between 1950 and 1988 for target factors (Queensland University study)

Authors	Study population	Rubella %	Cytomegalovirus %	Meningitis %	Unknown cause %
Tomlin (1989)	Queensland n = 3951 all children fitted with hearing aids 1950–88 (equivalent to all children in general population with handicapping hearing loss.)	14.0	0.2	2.8	38.8

and 1967 (see Figure 4.4), meningitis as an aetiological factor appears to have been increasing slightly in prevalence throughout the study period.

4   Unknown causes, see Figure 4.5.

The aetiology of hearing loss was unknown in 1561 cases during the period 1950–87, representing an aggregate prevalence of 1.128 per 1000 live births, a slight increase rising from below 4 per cent in the 1960s to around 50 per cent of cases in the 1980s.

The Aetiology of Hearing Loss During the Period 1950–88 — Queensland Data

The mean three frequency average hearing levels (3 FAHL) for the better hearing ear are indicated in Table 4.8. It can be seen that infectious diseases as causative factors each produced group mean hearing losses of 10dB (3 FAHL) or greater above the hearing handicapped population mean. Only mumps, of the infectious diseases recorded, produced a hearing loss below the overall mean. For the four representative factors considered here, the percentage of cases manifesting additional or associated handicaps are indicated in Table 4.9. The distribution of such associated handicaps is indicated in Table 4.10.

It can be seen from Tables 4.9 and 4.10 that the incidence of additional handicaps is seen to be highest in CMV both with reference to other causes and with respect to

Table 4.8 Mean three frequency average hearing levels (3 FAHL) for the better hearing ear according to aetiological factors

Aetiology	3 FAHL	SD
Rubella	82.0	26.0
Cytomegalovirus	85.0	23.0
Meningitis	78.0	32.0
Unknown	55.0	28.0
Study population mean	59.2	29.0

Table 4.9 Percentages according to aetiological factor associated with the handicap

Rubella	20.1%
Cytomegalovirus	40.0%
Meningitis	7.9%
Unknown	12.0%

Table 4.10 Distribution of handicaps according to aetiological factors

	Cerebral palsy and epilepsy %	Cardiac, orthopaedic or other physical handicaps %	Mental retardation alone or associated with other handicaps %	Visual impairment %
Rubella	1.0	3.0	7.5	4.5
Cytomegalovirus	10.0	1.5	>20.0	0.0
Meningitis	1.0	<1.0	6.0	0.0
Unknown	2.0	1.0	7.0	0.5

the overall incidence of such handicaps. However, studies such as those of Reynolds *et al.* (1974) have failed to find significant correlations between the degree of hearing loss and related handicaps such as intellectual retardation. A feature of cytomegalovirus infection is its chronic course and the persistence of active infection for many years during which period the child's auditory function may potentially undergo deterioration. Cytomegalovirus infection may be either symptomatic or asymptomatic and in either state hearing loss may occur (Conboy *et al.*, 1986). Other associated handicaps appear to centre around intellectual function, with learning disabilities and cognitive deficits cited most often. However, the Conboy *et al.* (1986) study concluded that children born with asymptomatic congenital cytomegalovirus infection and normal hearing are not likely to be at increased risk of mental impairment. Physical handicaps include cardiac disorders, epilepsy and cerebral palsy and orthopaedic problems. Unlike rubella, visual handicaps do not appear to be common with cytomegalovirus.

Prognosis for Hearing Disorders Associated with Infectious Diseases

The long-term recovery of children who have had significant infectious CNS diseases affecting their hearing is subject to much controversy. There appears to be no doubt that in some instances recovery (either complete or partial) of auditory function can occur following even profound hearing loss. Moreover, such recovery may occur over a prolonged time scale throughout childhood. There appears to be less conclusive evidence to support the hypothesis of hearing loss as a late-onset, late-occurring complication of infectious disease states, although deterioration in acuity levels to the point of total hearing loss is well documented especially in post-meningitic hearing loss.

Brookhouser *et al.* (1988) in one of the most recently published studies of patterns and stability of post-meningitic hearing loss in children, reported 31 per cent of a population of 280 children to have a sensorineural hearing loss. The losses were unilateral, bilateral, profound, anacusic, severe, moderate and mild. Configurations were varied and asymmetric. Thresholds changed over the $3\frac{1}{2}$-year mean course of the study, hearing was reported as improving, declining and fluctuating. Changes in benefit from amplification was also variable, suggesting the need for long-term surveillance. Clearly, the audiological management of the childhood infection involving the CNS needs to be carefully structured to fit the unique prevailing signs and symptoms of the individual patient.

Linguistic Disorders in Childhood Infectious Diseases of the CNS

Linguistic Deficits Associated with Childhood Encephalitis

No study to date has systematically evaluated the linguistic outcome of a group of children who had suffered encephalitis. Such cases, however, have often been included in studies of acquired childhood aphasia of mixed aetiology (Cooper and Flowers, 1987; Van Hout *et al.*, 1985). In such studies, however, the specific outcomes attributable to the encephalitis are usually lost in the group results. The few individual case studies reported in the literature in combination with the case descriptions included within group data do give however, some idea of the prognosis after encephalitis. In most reported cases the encephalitis associated with the occurrence of linguistic deficits has resulted from the herpes simplex virus.

From these case descriptions we can see the effects of encephalitis in the acute and recovery stages and then judge the outcome by assessing long-term deficits. For the sake of discussion we have taken the acute stage to represent the period while the child is still hospitalized. One deficit frequently described in the acute stages of encephalitis is impaired comprehension. This has been described as a severe comprehension deficit similar to that seen in global aphasia. Two cases described by Cooper and Flowers (1987) presented initially as mute. One with meningoencephalitis presented with global aphasia following this mutism, while the other case who only had suspected encephalitis presented with poor receptive language skills, paragrammaticism and naming difficulties when the mute period ended. Other aphasic symptoms described in the acute stage following an attack of encephalitis include paraphasias, poor repetition skills, stereotypes and perseveration (Cooper and Flowers, 1987; Van Hout *et al.*, 1985).

Van Hout and co-workers described two cases of acquired childhood aphasia resulting from infectious disease in terms of adult aphasic syndromes. The first case had an infection of unknown type and presented with an apparent conduction aphasia, as comprehension remained relatively intact in the presence of marked naming problems, slight paragrammaticism and phonemic paraphasias noted in spontaneous speech but more prominent on repetition tasks (Van Hout *et al.*, 1985). A second case with herpes simplex encephalitis was described in detail by Van Hout and Lyon (1986). They described their case, a 10-year-old boy, as presenting with a Wernicke's aphasia. His comprehension was severely affected and initially he presented in a perseverative state which lasted for 5 weeks. He then became anosognosic when he presented with logorrhea. Initially stereotypic behaviour which varied daily was also noted. As he became more fluent alliterative behaviour was evident in his spontaneous speech, his reading and on repetition tasks. Neologisms increased during this fluent period from 15 per cent on day 6 (after the perseverative period) to 65 per cent on day 16. Verbal paraphasias were absent on day 8 but up to 30 per cent on day 16, also showing an increase in the acute stage. In the recovery phase, however, there was a decrease in neologisms together with an increase in verbal paraphasias and circumlocutions. This change in the number of paraphasias, was observed between 2 and 8 months after the perseverative period. After 2 months the comprehension abilities of the case described by Van Hout and Lyon (1986) also showed some improvement.

The length of time children stayed in a paraphasic phase post-onset was used by Van Hout *et al.* (1985) to separate their 11 subjects with acquired childhood aphasia into three groups. It is of importance to note that four of the five children in whom paraphasias were evident months after onset had suffered from herpes simplex encephalitis. In this group phonemic paraphasias disappeared before the semantic ones and generally the overall number of paraphasias was greater than in the other two groups. This group had severe comprehension and aphasic symptoms and tended to have had longer coma periods, though the period of mutism did not differ from the other two groups. The second group, while comprised of only two cases, had paraphasias lasting weeks, moderate comprehension deficits but no history of mutism or coma. The aetiology for this group was also infectious in nature, one from measles and one from an infection of unknown origin.

The pattern of language deficits and strengths seen during this recovery phase, as measured on the Gaddes and Crockett (1975) norms of the Neurosensory Centre Comprehensive Examination of Aphasia (NCCEA), was similar for the two groups though generally more severe for those children who had had herpes simplex encephalitis. Generally the pattern was as follows: poor on visual and tactile naming tasks, sentence repetition, identification by sentence, good performance on naming by description of use, and moderate performance on digit repetition and word fluency. The greatest individual variation was on the tasks of sentence construction, identification by name and the number of words produced per minute.

During this recovery period (in this discussion taken to be up to 1 year post-onset) some individual cases were described as regaining functional communication skills within 1 month post-onset (Cooper and Flowers, 1987). One case had regained functional communication 4 months post-onset yet, at chronological age 12 years, her language skills were 6 to 7 years delayed. Specific deficits described in individual cases during this phase included: word finding and naming difficulties, difficulties associating and integrating verbal information, slow rate of speech and articulation difficulties, poor verbal memory, and difficulties with written language (Cooper and Flowers, 1987; Van Hout *et al.*, 1985).

One case of acquired childhood aphasia associated with encephalitis, described by Cooper and Flowers (1987) did not regain basic communication skills until 6 months post-onset. At that time he presented with impairments in both receptive and expressive language skills. This same case when assessed almost 4 years post-onset, presented with a delay in the language and academic areas tested. In addition, he was the only subject assessed by Cooper and Flowers (1987) who was intellectually handicapped and who had pragmatic deficits. Of all the cases of acquired childhood aphasia resulting from encephalitis reported in the literature, the prognosis for this latter case was the worst.

Another case of acquired aphasia occurring in a child following encephalitis was assessed by Cooper and Flowers (1987) as having a borderline intellectual handicap with poor performance on all language and academic skills assessed except reading ability. In the other cases described by these authors, intellectual functioning was within normal limits but specific language deficits were found on certain syntactic constructions and receptive vocabulary, and academic problems in the areas of arithmetic, reading and spelling. While Van Hout *et al.* (1985) did not give information on the intellectual functioning of their cases, they did describe long-term linguistic deficits. These included naming difficulties, poor verbal memory, written language problems and paralexia.

Therefore, it would appear from the few case descriptions outlined above that the prognosis is poor for linguistic and academic abilities of children who have suffered encephalitis. This particularly appears to be so when the outcome of these cases is compared with cases of acquired childhood aphasia from other causes (Cooper and Flowers, 1987; Van Dongen and Visch-Brink, 1988; Van Hout *et al.*, 1985). This generally poor prognosis may be due to bilateral brain damage, for while some cases of acquired childhood aphasia associated with encephalitis reported in the literature showed unilateral lesions, and indeed others presented with normal CT scans, it would seem that infections are likely to involve both cerebral hemispheres. In view of the severe comprehension deficits displayed by a number of the cases described and the presence of two cases where intellectual functioning has been affected, it is imperative that linguistic functioning is evaluated in the light of cognitive functioning. It is important that clinicians publish detailed longitudinal case studies of children with encephalitis.

Neurological Problems Associated with Childhood Meningitis

A number of researchers have reported neurological sequelae after an episode of meningitis. These sequelae include ataxia, paralysis, elevated muscle tone, clinically significant hearing deficits, seizures, visual disturbances, depressed IQ, behavioural changes (Feigin and Dodge, 1976), learning problems (Taylor *et al.*, 1984), social adjustment deficit (Sell, 1987), receptive and expressive language delays (Jadavji *et al.*, 1986) and 'soft' neurological signs.

Although some of these researchers have noted the presence of speech and language deficits among the sequelae of meningitis (Feldman *et al.*, 1982; Jadavji *et al.*, 1986; Taylor *et al.*, 1984) there is a paucity in the literature of detailed linguistic outcome subsequent to recovery from bacterial meningitis. In the following general review of the literature on the neurological sequelae of childhood meningitis emphasis is given to studies that have highlighted speech and language deficits as specific sequelae.

Bacterial meningitis

Bacterial meningitis in childhood may result in neurological sequelae of varying types and degree. Jadavji *et al.* (1986) looked at neurological sequelae in children (4 days to 18 years) after bacterial meningitis. These children were treated with ampicillin or chloramphenicol. The pathogens responsible for the meningitis in the study group included *H. influenzae* type B (HIB; 70 per cent), *Strep. pneumoniae* (20 per cent) and N. *meningitidis* (10 per cent). Of the 171 follow-up assessments performed on the subjects, 20 per cent had mild to severe handicaps. Children recovering from meningitis caused by *Strep. pneumoniae* had a 57 per cent frequency of handicap. HIB resulted in 14.5 per cent handicap and there were no subsequent handicaps noted in the children with *N. meningitidis* meningitis.

It is particularly important to note that 5 per cent of the group studied by Jadavji *et al.* (1986) had a disorder of language, i.e. 8 of the 171 subjects. Over 16 per cent of the children with *Strep. pneumoniae* meningitis had receptive and/or expressive language delay in comparison to 2.4 per cent of the children with HIB meningitis with language delays. An identifiable developmental delay was present in 5.3 per cent of the children. Jadavji *et al.*, (1986) did not specify the speech and language tests used in the analysis. Long-term assessment of the children was carried out by an infectious disease consultant, neurologist, audiologist, ophthalmologist and psychologist.

Haemophilus influenzae type B (HIB) meningitis

Many studies have detailed the incidence and type of sequelae due to HIB meningitis. The incidence of sequelae noted in subjects varies among researchers. Of the 75 subjects monitored by Sell *et al.* (1972a), 29 per cent had severe or significant handicaps and 14 per cent had possible neurological sequelae. Sproles *et al.* (1969) indicated that 55 per cent of the subject group of 45 children with influenza meningitis had permanent effects. Eight per cent of the subject group of a study by Feigin and Dodge (1976) had neurological or intellectual deficits.

Sell *et al.* (1972a) looked at the long-term sequelae of HIB meningitis. Significant handicaps included mild spastic hemiparesis, moderately/severe mixed type hearing loss, hyperactivity, slow learning, poor speech and left spastic hemiplegia. These authors highlighted that prevention of this disorder should be of a primary concern, because of the long-term neurological sequelae.

In another study Sell *et al.* (1972b) reported on two controlled studies of the psychological sequelae subsequent to bacterial meningitis. The first study considered the WISC scores for HIB survivors. The second study compared children's performances following meningitis with those of their classroom peers. The children were assessed on the Illinois Test of Psycholinguistic Abilities (ITPA) (McCarthy and Kirk, 1961), the Frostig Developmental Test of Visual Perception (Frostig, 1963) and the Peabody Picture Vocabulary Test (PPVT) (Dunn, 1965). The first study showed that the post-meningitis group had a mean IQ of 86, while the control group had an IQ of 97. The second group of children, who had had meningitis, were selected because it was considered that there were no apparent sequelae from their meningitis. The results of the PPVT indicated that the vocabulary quotient for the post-meningitis group was 90.96 per cent, with the control group at 12.60 per cent. This was significantly different at the 0.35 level. In both cases the subject group performed at a significantly lower intellectual level than the control group.

Feldman *et al.* (1982) attempted to ascertain if the concentrations of *H. influenzae* type B in the CSF before treatment had any relationship to later sequelae. The results of the study showed that patients who had 1×10^7 CFU (colony forming units) of *H. influenzae* type B per ml of CSF were significantly more likely to have abnormalities of speech and hearing and more severe neurological sequelae than those with a lower concentration at the acute stage. Forty-five subjects were evaluated in the study, with 12 subjects having a speech delay and three with expressive speech defects. Five subjects had a bilateral and sensorineural hearing loss, with three having a unilateral sensorineural hearing loss. The results of the study indicated that the concentration of HIB in the CSF prior to treatment was predictive of the sequelae. This study indicated that further research was needed to ascertain whether pre-treatment concentrations of *H. influenzae* is an indicator of intellectual ability.

Taylor *et al.* (1984) investigated the neurological sequelae of HIB meningitis in 24 children 6–8 years after recovery. They tested the children for intellectual, neuropsychological and achievement outcomes using a test battery which included among others the WISC-R (Wechsler, 1974), the Token Test for Children (Di Simoni, 1978), and the Expressive One Word Picture Vocabulary Test (Gardner, 1979). The performance of the HIB children was compared with an appropriately matched control group. The HIB subjects performed more poorly than the control subjects on tests that required verbal comprehension and memory, verbal list learning and visuomotor dexterity. Academic achievement, however, was not adversely affected in the HIB subjects. It was suggested by Taylor *et al.* (1984) that a further study should monitor the performances of the HIB children through the school years. While the morbidity of meningitis is measurable, Taylor *et al.* (1984) suggested other factors must be considered when predicting the long-term effects on the child.

Feldman and Michaels (1988) looked at academic achievement in children several years after an episode of HIB meningitis. Using specific academic tests, they showed that the children continued to perform well academically 10–12 years after recovery from the episode. The only test that showed any statistically significant difference was in reading accuracy (i.e. the fluency of reading paragraphs).

In contrast to the findings of the studies outlined above, Emmett *et al.* (1980) were unable to find any major neurological sequelae in children who had had HIB meningitis. Based on the findings of a range of psychological tests, which included the WISC and the Frostig and Bender Psychological tests, they concluded that children promptly diagnosed and treated for HIB have no detectable residual deficits. Emmett *et al.* (1980), however, did note that prolonged fever during the meningitis was associated with poorer results in psychological tests.

Streptococcal meningitis

Incidence figures vary on the neurological sequelae of Group B streptococcal meningitis. Chin and Fitzhardinge (1985) reported that 36–44 per cent of survivors of streptococcal meningitis in their study had long-term sequelae. Other authors, however, such as Baker and Edwards (1983), Barton *et al.* (1973) and Edwards *et al.* (1985) have found that up to 50 per cent of survivors of Group B streptococcal meningitis show long-term sequelae. In their study of 38 infants with bacteriologically-proven Group B streptococcal meningitis, Edwards *et al.* (1985) identified 29 per cent as having major sequelae and 21 per cent with mild to moderate deficits. In particular they noted that subtle deficits in cognitive abilities and language or learning deficits may not be manifest until later years.

Wald *et al.* (1986) also looked at the performance of children subsequent to Group B streptococcal meningitis. They found the mortality rate to be 27 per cent, with another 12 per cent of the subjects having major neurological sequelae. The study did, however, indicate that there was no significant difference between the subject group and a control group in communication behaviour, if the children with major neurological sequelae were excluded.

Aseptic meningitis

The term aseptic meningitis refers to a clinical syndrome characterized by signs of meningeal inflammation, fever and pleocytosis (presence of a greater than normal number of cells) of the CSF with bacteriological sterility of the CSF. Although most frequently associated with viral infections, other agents may also cause this disorder. Fee *et al.* (1970) evaluated the long-term effects of aseptic meningitis by following the neurological, behavioural and visuomotor perceptual development and electroencephalographic changes in a group of 18 children for a period up to 10 years after meningitis. Based on their findings, Fee *et al.* (1970) concluded that the majority of children with aseptic meningitis showed only mild abnormalities in the long-term, although no definite pattern of deficit was identified. It was noted, however, that behaviour and school performance of children following aseptic meningitis should be monitored, especially in those cases where seizures accompany the original illness.

Implications of Childhood Meningitis for Speech and Language Function

The information in the literature on speech and language deficits subsequent to meningitis is inconsistent. While some researchers have indicated a deficit in communicative abilities as one neurological sequela, others have not. One reason for this discrepancy may lie in the different types of research designs used by different authors to investigate the long-term outcomes of meningitis. Tejani *et al.* (1982) stressed the need to carefully evaluate the control group used in particular studies. The use of a sibling control group, for instance, may lend weight to the conclusion that a neurological deficit observed in the subject group is the result of the meningitis rather than the outcome of some environmental or educational factor. In addition, the failure of some specific linguistic test to indicate the presence of a linguistic deficit may not in itself signal that communication skills are appropriate. Further, when considering speech and language deficits it is important to note that these deficits may not fully manifest themselves until later years. Haslam *et al.* (1977) acknowledged that although they observed no significant differences in language testing of their subject group after recovery from meningitis, the children had not progressed to the 3rd and 4th grades where learning difficulties become evident. Similarly Edwards *et al.* (1985) indicated that it is difficult to identify neurodevelopmental disorders at an early age. They recommended a 3-year follow-up period to assess linguistic delay or mild/moderate mental retardation.

Although discrete speech and language tests may highlight specific deficits in the younger child, as the child matures and academic skills are monitored, further deficits may become obvious. High-level speech and language deficits which impinge on the child's abilities may also become evident and these deficits may then pervade other aspects of the child's learning. Swartz (1984) discussed the need for more information in order to define factors that may be responsible for neurological damage and to design strategies beyond prompt administration of appropriate medication to alleviate such factors after meningitis.

Overall, more information is needed on linguistic aspects of meningeal complications including (1) an examination of the onset time of the meningitis (pre- or post-linguistic) and its effect, and (2) the aetiology of the meningitis (viral or bacterial). Linguistic skills need to be analyzed thoroughly and patterns detailed if present. Ongoing monitoring, with assessment at critical academic stages, needs to be instituted. These issues need to be considered in relation to the implications for long-term management of speech/language pathology. They are also vital in considering long-term academic programming.

Summary

Communicative disorders following childhood infectious diseases represent a significant area in which available knowledge in the literature is sparse and fragmented. The CNS diseases occurring in children are variable in onset, manifestation and outcome. The incidence of handicapping sequelae documented in the literature and the severity of such sequelae suggests the need for clinical surveillance well beyond the normal medical regimen in order to detect residual deficits which range from hearing impairment to subtle cognitive dysfunction and possible speech/language disturbances.

References

BAKER, C. J. and EDWARDS, M. S. (1983) 'Group B streptococcal infections', in Remington, J. S. and Klein, J. O. (Eds) *Infectious Diseases of the Fetus and Newborn Infant*, Philadelphia, W. B. Saunders.

BARTON, L. L., FEIGIN, R. D. and LINS, R. (1973) 'Group B beta-hemolytic streptococcal maningitis in infants', *Journal of Pediatrics*, **82**, pp. 719.

BROOKHOUSER, P. E., AUSLANDER, M. C. and MESKAN, M. E. (1988) 'The pattern and stability of post-meningitic hearing loss in children', *Laryngoscope*, **98**, pp. 940–7.

BROWN, S. C. (1986) 'Etiological trends, characteristics and distributions', in Shildroth, A. N. and Karchmer, M. A. (Eds) *Deaf Children in America*, San Diego, College Press, pp. 33–54.

CHIN, K. C. and FITZHARDINGE, P. M. (1985) 'Sequelae of early-onset Group B haemolytic streptococcal neonatal meningitis', *Journal of Pediatrics*, **106**, pp. 820–3.

CONBOY, T. J., PASS, R. F., STAGNO, S., BRITT, W. J., ALFORD, C. A., McFARLAND, C. E. and BELL, T. J. (1986) 'Intellectual development in school-aged children with asymptomatic congenital cytomegalovirus infection', *Pediatrics*, **77**, pp. 801–6.

COOPER, J. A. and FLOWERS, C. R. (1987) 'Children with a history of acquired aphasia: Residual language and academic impairments', *Journal of Speech and Hearing Disorders*, **52** pp. 251–62.

DI SIMONI, F. G. (1978) *The Token Test for Children*, Boston, Teaching Resources.

DODGE, P. R. (1986) 'Sequelae of bacterial meningitis', *Pediatric Infectious Diseases*, **5**, pp. 618–20.

DUNN, L. M. (1965) *The Peabody Picture Vocabulary Tests*, Circle Pines, American Guidance Service, Inc.

EDWARDS, M. S., RENCH, M. A., HAFFAR A. A. M., MURPHY, M. A., DESMOND, M. M. and BAKER, C. J. (1985) 'Long-term sequelae of Group B streptococcal meningitis in infants', *Journal of Pediatrics*, **106**, pp. 717–22.

EMMETT M., JEFFERY, H., CHANDLER, D. and DUGDALE, A. (1980) 'Sequelae of *Haemophilus influenzae* Meningitis', *Australian Paediatric Journal*, **16**, pp. 90–3.

FEE, W., MARKS, M., KARDASH, S., REITE, M. and SEITZ, C. (1970) 'The long-term prognosis of aseptic meningitis in childhood', *Developmental Medicine and Child Neurology*, **12**, pp. 321–9.

FEIGIN, R. D. and DODGE, P. R. (1976) 'Bacterial meningitis: newer concepts of pathophysiology and neurologic sequelae', Symposium on Pediatric Neurology, *Pediatric Clinics of North America*, **23**, pp. 541–56.

FEINMESSER, M., TELL L. and LEVI, H. (1986) 'Etiology of childhood deafness with reference to the group of unkown cause', *Audiology*, **25**, pp. 65–9.

FELDMAN, H. and MICHAELS, R. (1988) 'Academic achievement in children 10–12 years after haemophilus influenzae meningitis', *Paediatrics*, **81**, pp. 339–44.

FELDMAN, W. E., GINSBERG, C. M., MCCRACKEN, G. H., ALLEN, D., AHMANN, P., GRAHAM, J. and GRAHAM, H. (1982) 'Relation of concentration of *Haemophilus influenzae* type B in cerebrospinal fluid to late sequelae of patients with meningitis', *Journal of Pediatrics*, **100**(2), pp. 209–12.

FROSTIG, M. (1963) *Developmental Test of Visual Perception*, Palo Alto, Consulting Psychologists Press.

GADDES, W. H. and CROCKETT, D. J. (1975) 'The Spreen-Benton aphasia tests, normative data as a measure of normal language development', *Brain and Language*, **2**, pp. 257–80.

GARDNER, M. F. (1979) *Expressive One-Word Picture Vocabulary Test*, Novato, Academic Therapy Publications.

GREVILLE, K. A. and KEITH, W. J. (1978) 'The effectiveness of two infant hearing screening programmes in New Zealand', *Scandinavian Audiology*, **7**, 139–45.

HASLAM, R., ALLEN, J., DORSEN, M., KANOFSKY, D., MELLITS, D. and NORRIS, D. (1977) 'The sequelae of Group B haemolytic streptococcal meningitis in early infancy', *American Journal of Diseased Child*, **131**, pp. 845–9.

JADAVJI, T., BIGGAR, W. and GOLD, R. (1986) 'Sequelae of acute bacterial meningitis children treated for 7 days', *Pediatrics*, **78**(1), pp. 21–5.

KANKKUNEN, A. (1982) 'Pre-school children with impaired hearing in Goteborg, 1964–1980', *Acta Oto-Laryngologica*, Supplement 391, pp. 1–35.

KEANE, W., POTSIC, W., ROWE, L, and KONKLE, D. (1979) 'Meningitis and hearing loss in children', *Archives of Otolaryngology*, **15** pp. 39–44

MCCARTHY, J. J. and KIRK, S. A. (1961) *Illinois Test of Psycholinguistic Abilities*, Urbana, Institute for Research on Exceptional Children.

MARTIN, J. A. M. (1982) 'Aetiological factors relating to childhood deafness in the European Community', *Audiology*, **21**, pp. 149–58.

MARTIN, J. A. M., BENTZEN, O., COLLEY, J. HENNEBERT, D., HOLM, C., IURATO, S., DE JONGE, G., MCCULLEN, O., MEYER, M., MOORE, W. and MORGAN, A. (1981) 'Childhood deafness in the European Community', *Scandinavian Audiology*, **10**, pp. 165–74.

NADOL, J. (1978) 'Hearing loss as a sequela of meningitis', *Laryngoscope*, **88**, pp. 738–55.

PAPPAS, D. (1985) *Diagnosis and Treatment of Hearing Impairment in Children: A Clinical Manual*, London, Taylor & Francis.

PARVING, A. (1985) 'Hearing disorders in childhood, some procedures for detection, identification and diagnostic evaluation', *International Journal of Pediatric Otorhinolaryngology*, **9**, pp. 31–57.

REYNOLDS, D.W., STAGNO, S., STUBBS, K., DAHLE, A.J., LIVINGSTONE, M.M., SAXON, S.S. and ALFORD, C.A. (1974) 'Inapparent congenital cytomegalovirus infection with elevated cord IgM levels', *New England Journal of Medicine*, **290**, pp. 291-6.

SCHOEMAN, J., HEWLETT, R. and DONALD, P. (1988) 'MR of childhood tuberculous meningitis', *Neuroradiology*, **30**, pp. 473-7.

SELL, S. (1987) '*Haemophilus influenzae* type B meningitis: Manifestations and long-term sequelae', *Pediatric Infectious Diseases Journal*, **8**, pp. 775-8.

SELL, S., MERRELL, R., DOYNE, E. and ZIMSKY, E. (1972a) 'Long-term sequelae of *Haemophilus influenzae* meningitis', *Pediatrics*, **49**(2), pp. 206-11.

SELL, S., WEBB, W., PATE, J. and DOYNE, E. (1972b) 'Psychological sequelae to bacterial meningitis: 2 controlled series', *Pediatrics*, **49**(2), pp. 212-16.

SMYTH, V. (1984) 'Successful auditory brainstem evoked response testing and test-age relationships in difficult-to-test children', *Australian Paediatric Journal*, **40**, pp. 115-17.

SMYTH, V., O'CONNELL, B., PITT, R., O'CALLAGHAN, M. and SCOTT, J. (1988) 'Audiological management in the recovery phase of bacterial meningitis', *International Journal of Pediatric Otorhinolaryngology*, **15**, pp. 79-86.

SPROLES, E.T., AZARRAD, J., WILLIAMSON, C. and MERRILL, R.E. (1969) 'Meningitis due to *Haemophilus influenzae*: Long-term sequelae', *Journal of Pediatrics*, **75**, pp. 782.

SWARTZ, M. (1984) 'Bacterial meningitis: More involved than just the meninges', *New England Journal of Medicine*, **310**, pp. 912-14.

TAYLOR, H.G., MICHAELS, R., MAZUR, P., BAUER, R. and LIDEN, C. (1984) 'Intellectual, neuropsychological and achievement outcomes in children 6-8 years after recovery from *Haemophilus influenzae* meningitis', *Pediatrics*, **74**(2), pp. 198-205.

TEJANI, A., TOBIAS, B. and SAMBURSKY, J. (1982) 'Long-term prognosis after *H. influenzae* meningitis: prospective evaluation', *Developmental Medicine and Child Neurology*, **24**, pp. 338-43.

THIRINGER, K., KANKKUNEN, A. LIDEN, G. and NIKLASSON, A. (1984) 'Perinatal risk factors in the aetiology of hearing loss in preschool children', *Developmental Medicine and Child Neurology*, **26**, pp. 799-807.

TOMLIN, A. (1989) 'Demographic characteristics of handicapping childhood hearing loss in Queensland: 1950 to 1988', Master of Audiology Thesis, University of Queensland.

VAN DONGEN, H.R. and VISCH-BRINK, E.G. (1988) 'Naming in aphasic children: Analysis of paraphasic errors', *Neuropsychologia*, **26**, pp. 629-32.

VAN HOUT, A., EVRARD, P. and LYON, G. (1985) 'On the positive semiology of acquired aphasia in children', *Developmental Medicine and Child Neurology*, **27**, pp. 231-41.

VAN HOUT, A. and LYON, G. (1986) 'Wernicke's aphasia in a 10-year-old boy', *Brain and Language,* **29**, pp. 268-85.

WALD, E.R., BERGMAN, I., TAYLOR, H.G., CHIPONIS, D., PORTER, C. and KUBEK, K. (1986) 'Long-term outcome of Group B streptococcal meningitis', *Pediatrics*, **77**, pp. 217-21.

WECHSLER, D. (1974) *Manual for the Wechsler Intelligence Scale for Children—Revised*, New York, Psychological Corporation.

Chapter 5

Linguistic Status Following Acute Cerebral Anoxia in Children

Bruce E. Murdoch and Anne E. Ozanne

Introduction

A continuous and adequate supply of oxygen to the brain is essential for the maintenance of normal brain function. According to Bell (1980), although the brain constitutes only about 2 per cent of the total body weight of the adult, it accounts for approximately 20 per cent of the oxygen consumption of the entire body. In the nursing infant and in children up to 4 years of age, the proportion of the total body oxygen consumption accounted for by the brain rises to over 30 per cent (McIlwain, 1955). To provide the necessary oxygen, approximately 15 per cent of the cardiac output is received by the adult brain, equivalent to around 45 ml of blood per 100 g per minute. In children, the cerebral perfusion rate is even higher, being about twice that of the adult brain (McIlwain, 1966).

Anoxia is the condition in which the oxygen levels in the body tissues fall below physiological levels (i.e. below the level required to maintain normal function) as a result of either an absence or deficiency of oxygen. The supply of oxygen to the brain is dependent upon two factors, the level of cerebral flood flow and the oxygen content of the blood. Anything causing a drop in either of these two factors may lead to cerebral anoxia. Nerve cells or neurones are particularly susceptible to anoxia since they have an obligatory, aerobic, glycolytic metabolism. Consequently, any period of prolonged cerebral anoxia can lead to permanent brain damage (anoxic encephalopathy) which may in turn be associated with the production of a range of neurological disorders, amongst which speech and language deficits may be included.

The neurological deficits that may occur following cerebral anoxia are determined to a large extent by the length of the anoxic period. These deficits may range from no deficit, to mild intellectual impairment, to a pure vegetative state, and at worst, death. The eventual degree of clinical recovery is determined by whether or not satisfactory resuscitation can be achieved before permanent brain damage ensues. Patients with acute cerebral anoxia have been reported to recover without clinical functional sequelae if tissue oxygenation is restored within 1–2 minutes (Bell, 1980). It should be noted, however, that the exact duration of anoxia that separates recovery of the neural tissue on the one hand and extensive permanent brain damage on the other, has not been critically defined in man (Plum, 1973). According to Bell (1980), under normal circumstances, anoxia lasting more than 4 minutes causes destruction of neurons in the brain, especially in the cerebral cortex, hippocampus and cerebellum. Similarly, Brierly (1972) stated that in cases of cardiac arrest, under normal conditions complete clinical recovery is unlikely if the period of arrest is more than 5–7 minutes. Neuronal death has been reported to follow cerebral anoxia lasting more than 10 minutes (Weinberger *et al.*, 1940).

Certain parts of the brain are selectively vulnerable to the effects of cerebral anoxia. Consequently, the maximum period of anoxia compatible with recovery varies in different areas of the brain. The most vulnerable areas are the so-called 'watershed' or 'border-zone' regions of the cerebral hemispheres in that they receive their vascular supply from the most distal branches of the cerebral arteries. In contrast, those regions of the brain concerned with autonomic (vegetative) functions, such as the brainstem, appear to be the most resistant areas to anoxic damage.

Anoxic encephalopathy may result from any condition that causes the oxygen supply to the brain to become inadequate. It is therefore a potential outcome in any person subjected to general anaesthesia, a severe episode of hypotension (low blood pressure), cardiac arrest, suffocation, near-drowning, status epilepticus, carbon monoxide poisoning, barbiturate intoxication and hypoglycaemic coma.

Types of Anoxia

Four different major causes of anoxia are commonly recognized in the literature including: anoxic (hypoxic) anoxia; anaemic anoxia; stagnant anoxia and metabolic or toxic anoxia. In that all of these four types of anoxia may occur in children and are known to cause brain damage (see Sites of Anoxic Brain Damage below), it is conceivable that any of them might also lead to the production of acquired speech and language disorders.

Anoxic anoxia involves an absence or reduction (hypoxic anoxia) of oxygen in the lungs as a result of either respiratory insufficiency or a lack of oxygen in the inhaled air. This type of anoxia may result from events which include, among others, accidental suffocation, strangulation, near-drowning, exposure to high altitudes, accidents in anaesthesia and exposure to places with inadequate ventilation. Respiratory insufficiency may occur, especially in children, from spasm of the respiratory muscles in status epilipticus. This condition, involving a rapid succession of epileptic fits without intervals of consciousness, may cause brain damage as a result of the cerebral anoxia that arises from the respiratory insufficiency. Although many individuals make an uneventful recovery from status epilepticus, others who survive may be left with permanent intellectual or neurological deficits resulting from the associated anoxic encephalopathy.

Anaemic anoxia is caused by a reduction in the oxygen-carrying capacity of the blood which, in turn, results in an insufficient amount of oxygen carried to the brain. The reduction on oxygen-carrying capacity may be the result of either an insufficient level of haemoglobin in the blood (e.g. in pernicious anaemia) or carbon monoxide poisoning. Haemoglobin has a much higher affinity for cabon monoxide than for oxygen. Consequently the presence of carbon monoxide in the inhaled air reduces the oxygen levels in the blood by more effectively competing with oxygen for the binding sites on the haemoglobin molecule.

Both anaemic anoxia and anoxic anoxia lead to a deficiency in the oxygenation of the blood (hypoxaemia) which in turn causes problems in the intracellular oxidation of glucose for energy by the brain cells (hypoxidosis). Schwedenberg (1959) referred to this condition as hypoxaemic hypoxidosis.

Any interruption to the blood supply to the brain causes stagnant anoxia. This type of anoxia is divided into two subtypes: ischaemic and oligaemic. Ischaemic cerebral anoxia results from either localized or generalized arrest of the blood supply to the brain, as may occur following cerebrovascular accidents involving blockage or rupture of one of the cerebral arteries (see Ch. 1) or following cardiac arrest. Oligaemic anoxia is caused by either a localized or generalized reduction in cerebral blood flow, as may occur, for instance, in association with systemic arterial hypotension (i.e. a generalized drop in blood pressure).

Factors that interfere with oxygen consumption by brain cells or which have direct toxic effects on nervous tissue lead to metabolic or toxic anoxia. These factors include, among others, hypoglycaemia (low blood glucose levels) and cyanide poisoning. Hypoglycaemia occurs idiopathically in some infants or may also occur as a result of an excess of insulin administered for the treatment of diabetes mellitus. Cyanide poisoning severely reduces the energy state of the brain in the presence of normal supplies of oxygen by interfering with the oxidative enzymes of the nerve cells. In addition, however, it also induces respiratory failure. Consequently, the brain damage resulting from exposure to cyanide not only occurs as a result of its direct effects on the brain tissues but also from secondary effects on respiration and circulation.

Sites of Anoxic Brain Damage

As indicated earlier, some parts of the brain have been reported to be more susceptible to the damaging effects of anoxia than others (Adams, 1963; Graham, 1977). Studies based on either pathological examination of the brains of victims of anoxia at post mortem or the findings of computed tomographic (CT) scans have shown that brain lesions resulting from cerebral anoxia may involve both the grey and white matter of the brain (Brierley, 1972; Brucher, 1967; Graham, 1977). Grey matter involvement may include damage to the cerebral and cerebellar cortex, the hippocampus, the basal ganglia, the thalamus and various brainstem nuclei. Damage to the white matter (anoxic leucoencephalopathy) may take the form of both diffuse changes in the white matter including demyelination, as well as circumscribed areas of total necrosis. The diffuse white matter changes occur predominantly in the centrum semiovale (Brucher, 1967).

According to studies of cases of anoxia of different origins, such as those reported by Brucher (1967) and Richardson *et al.* (1959), the clinical signs and the anatomical location of anoxic brain lesions are fundamentally the same for all types of anoxia. Although to a large extent this appears to be true, some subtle differences in the topography of lesion sites associated with the different types of cerebral anoxia have been reported. These subtle differences will become evident in the following discussion.

Anoxic lesions involving the cerebrum most commonly involve the border-zones of the cerebral cortical and subcortical arterial circulation (Adams *et al.*, 1966; Graham, 1977), with damage often being most severe in the parieto-occipital region, which represents the common border-zone between the territories of the anterior, middle and posterior cerebral arteries. Although anoxic lesions of the cerebral cortex are usually bilateral, they may be asymmetrical and, especially where the anoxia is the result of systemic arterial hypotension, even unilateral in some cases, the pattern of anoxic damage often being determined in such cases by the presence of atheroma and variations in the calibre of the vessels comprising the circle of Willis (Graham, 1977).

Involvement of the basal ganglia in lesions induced by cerebral anoxia is variable. Several CT studies of patients with anoxic lesions, including those resulting from accidental suffocation (Murdoch *et al.*, 1989), carbon monoxide poisoning (Murray *et al.*, 1987; Zeiss and Brinker, 1988), cardiorespiratory arrest (Murray *et al.*, 1987) and hydrogen sulphide inhalation (Matsuo *et al.*, 1979) have shown the presence of symmetrical lesions involving the lenticular nucleus bilaterally. In some reports, concomitant bilateral involvement of the head of the caudate nucleus has also been demonstrated. For example, in the case of anoxic brain damage following accidental suffocation reported by Murdoch *et al.* (1989), the CT scan showed a bilateral symmetrical decrease in attenuation in the head of the caudate nucleus in addition to bilateral damage to the lenticular nucleus (Figure 5.1).

Graham (1977) reported variations in the involvement of the basal ganglia depending on the type of anoxia involved. In cases of ischaemic cerebral anoxia following cardiac arrest, Graham (1977) noted that the associated basal ganglia lesions most commonly involved the outer halves of the head and body of the caudate nucleus and the outer portions of the putamen with occasional damage to the globus pallidus. In patients with oligaemic anoxic brain damage resulting from a major and abrupt

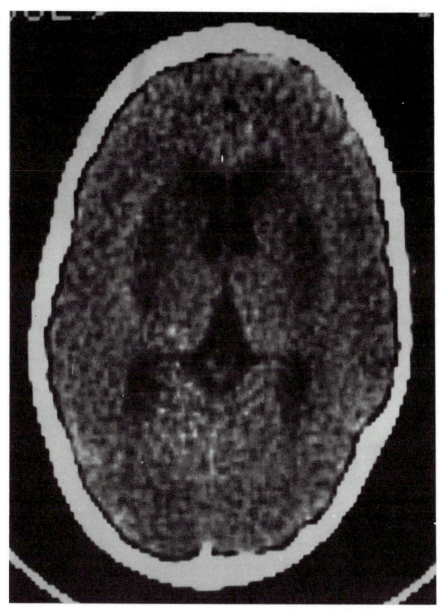

Figure 5.1   CT scan showing bilateral hypodense changes in the head of the caudate nucleus and lenticular nucleus consistent with cerebral anoxia in a 13-year-old boy 5 weeks after accidental suffocation

drop in blood pressure followed by a rapid return to normal blood pressure, however, Graham (1977) reported that the components of the basal ganglia that were damaged most frequently involved the head of the caudate nucleus and the upper parts of the putamen. Although the globus pallidus may be damaged by any type of cerebral anoxia, there is a particular predilection for infarction of this structure in carbon monoxide poisoning.

As in the case of the cerebrum, anoxic damage to the cerebellum most frequently involves the border-zones between the distributions of the major cerebellar arteries (e.g. between the superior and posterior-inferior cerebellar arteries). Damage to the cerebellum appears to be a common finding in all types of cerebral anoxia (Graham, 1977).

Adams *et al.* (1966) reported that, although anoxic damage to the brainstem nuclei may occur following an episode of ischaemic anoxia (e.g. cardiac arrest), it is usually not present subsequent to oligaemc anoxia. Further, these investigators reported that anoxic damage to the brainstem nuclei is more severe in young children and infants than adults.

Not all types of cerebral anoxia appear to cause damage to the thalamus. Thalamic lesions induced by cerebral anoxia appear to be most severe following oligaemic anoxia resulting from a drop in blood pressure, with a slow onset but of long duration (Adams *et al.*, 1966; Graham, 1977). Although present in most cases, involvement of the hippocampus in anoxic brain damage is also variable.

Clearly, the lesions identified in cases of anoxic encephalopathy are in a position to cause speech and language problems. In adults, lesions in the arterial border-zone of the dominant cerebral cortex have been linked to the occurrence of transcortical aphasia (Benson, 1979). The term 'transcortical aphasia' is used to describe a group of aphasic syndromes characterized by retention of repetition out of all proportion compared with other language functions. Further, lesions of the striatocapsular region have been reported to be associated with the occurrence of speech and language disorders in adults (Alexander and Lo Verme, 1980; Murdoch *et al.*, 1986) and children (Aram *et al.*, 1983).

Aram *et al.* (1983) documented the presence of language difficulties, but not dysarthria, in a 7-year-old girl who had an acquired vascular lesion in the putamen, anterior limb of the internal capsule and the lateral aspect of the head of the caudate nucleus. After an initial period of mutism, oral apraxia and moderate comprehension difficulties, the child gradually regained expressive language by going through the stages of using phrases, short sentences and simple sentences until 6 months after the cerebrovascular accident (CVA) she had fully regained her verbal language abilities. Severe anomia, in that she was unable to name on confrontation, was also present in the early stages, but it too resolved after passing through a stage of semantic paraphasias and word-finding difficulties. Her written language skills at 6 months after the accident showed reading to be at her appropriate grade level, although minor spelling difficulties were noted. Five years after the accident, however, she presented with major learning problems including reading difficulties.

Four other children with subcortical lesions studied by Aram *et al.* (1989) also presented with reading problems. All four children had lesions involving the head of the caudate nucleus and the anterior limb of the internal capsule and three of them also showed speech and language problems. One of the three children presented with global language problems in auditory comprehension, word retrieval and expressive syntax. The presence of a motor speech impairment was also indicated by his impaired articulation skills and slow diadochokinetic rate and a memory problem was also noted. A second subject reported by Aram *et al.* (1989) presented with similar language problems; however, his speech was described as having a mild dysarthric quality. Again verbal memory was poor. The third subject presented with only a persistent word-retrieval problem and a mild to moderate fluency disorder, which only became evident after the CVA. The findings in these three cases led Aram *et al.* (1989) to hypothesize a relationship between language and reading function and left subcortical structures in children. Such subcortical structures (e.g. the head of the caudate nucleus) have also been noted as a site of anoxic damage.

Mechanisms of Anoxic Brain Damage

The pathological mechanisms involved in the genesis of anoxic brain lesions are complex. Brucher (1967) identified four principal factors that may be involved including: hypoxidosis, oedema, circulatory disorders and histotoxic action.

Hypoxidosis refers to the basic disruption to intracellular metabolism that occurs in neurons as a result of cerebral anoxia. One theory proposed to explain the topography of focal anoxic brain lesions that has gained some acceptance in the literature suggests that the pattern of lesions observed in patients who have suffered anoxia is determined by a process of selective cellular vulnerability (pathoclisis). According to this theory, tissue hypoxidosis induces the necrosis of neurons in certain susceptible regions of the brain where the nerve cells are more vulnerable to the effects of anoxia. The basis of this vulnerability is not clear. Some authors have suggested that it is metabolically mediated (Helgason *et al.*, 1987). Others, however, such as Környey (1963), believe that the areas of the brain most sensitive to anoxia present a particular type of arterial irrigation which makes them more susceptible to ischaemia. In particular the susceptible areas tend to lie at the ends of arterial distributions or in arterial border-zones.

It has been suggested that focal anoxic brain lesions are caused by compression of the cerebral arteries against the cranium as a result of cerebral oedema (Lindenberg, 1955). Anoxia causes disruption of the walls of the brain capillaries, leading to an increase in the permeability of the blood-brain barrier. Consequently fluid and macromolecules pass from the blood into the parenchyma of the brain leading to cerebral oedema. As a result of the increased volume that it produces, it has been suggested that the resulting cerebral oedema causes an intracranial hypertension which in turn leads to compression of various cerebral blood vessels (Lindenberg, 1955, 1963). Lindenberg (1955) proposed compression of the anterior choroidal artery as a result of cerebral oedema as a possible mechanism to explain basal ganglia necrosis secondary to cerebral anoxia. According to Lindenberg, therefore, the determining factor in the topography of anoxic lesions is not a selective cellular vulnerability but rather a capillary stasis caused by arterial compression.

In recent years Lindenberg's proposal has been refuted by the findings of several studies which have shown that the distribution of brain lesions following anterior choroidal artery occlusion are not entirely consistent with the distribution of lesions observed in patients who have suffered an anoxic episode (Helgason *et al.*, 1987; Murray *et al.*, 1987). For one thing, although the posterior limb of the internal capsule is damaged in cases of anterior choroidal artery occlusion (Helgason *et al.*, 1986), it is not usually involved in anoxic encephalopathy. Further, as pointed out by Helgason *et al.* (1987), anoxic brain damage usually involves the thalamus and other structures distant to the distribution of the anterior choroidal artery. As a consequence of their findings, Helgason *et al.* (1987) and Murray *et al.* (1987) concluded that the mechanism of damage to the basal ganglia in cases of anoxic brain damage is probably not related to compression of the anterior choroidal artery, but rather may be metabolically mediated and due to selective cellular vulnerability. Finally, as further evidence against Lindenberg's proposal, a number of investigators have reported that many patients with anoxic brain damage do not show evidence of brain swelling with associated intracranial hypotension, particularly those patients whose vital signs become stabilized after the anoxic event (Adams *et al.*, 1966; Edstrom and Essex, 1956).

The oxygen needs of the cerebral white matter are five times less than those of the grey matter (Gänshirt, 1957). Consequently, factors other than hypoxidosis are probably responsible for the production of anoxic white matter lesions. Brucher (1967) suggested that cerebral oedema following breakdown of the blood-brain barrier caused by hypoxaemia is the probable cause of the diffuse lesions of the cerebral white matter observed in patients following anoxia.

In addition to causing disorders in the permeability of the vascular walls, anoxia also has a number of other effects on the circulation that might exert secondary influences on the distribution of anoxic brain lesions. These include vasoparalysis, vasostasis and obstructions in small blood vessels either by swelling of the endothelium or possibly by vasospasms. Oedema of the endothelial cells of the cerebral capillaries has been found to result from severe and prolonged ischaemia (De Reuck and Vander Eecken, 1978). Following correction of the ischaemia (e.g. by resuscitation), the presence of capillary oedema is responsible for the production of a 'no-reflow' phenomenon (Ames *et al.*, 1968) whereby restoration of circulation to the affected area of the brain is prevented, thereby leading to infarction of that area. De Reuck and Van der Eecken (1978) proposed that focal infarctions associated with cerebral anoxia result from the 'no-reflow' phenomena rather than from arterial compression secondary to brain swelling as proposed by Lindenberg (1955).

In addition to the above mechanisms, in cerebral anoxia induced by chemical agents such as carbon monoxide or anaesthetic products it is possible that the agents, in addition to causing anoxia, also have a direct toxic action on the neurons of the brain.

Although the majority of the evidence suggests that selective cellular vulnerability represents the principal pathological mechanism underlying the genesis of anoxic brain lesions, it is possible that under different circumstances all of the mechanisms described above may contribute to the pattern of brain damage observed in patients who have experienced an anoxic episode.

Speech and Language Disorders Associated with Anoxic Encephalopathy in Children

In children, speech and language disorders have been reported to occur in association with anoxic encephalopathy resulting from near-drowning (Reilly *et al.*, 1988), accidental suffocation (Murdoch *et al.*, 1989), cardiac arrest resulting from cardiac surgery (Cooper and Flowers, 1987) and respiratory arrest (Cooper and Flowers, 1987).

Neurological and Linguistic Status Subsequent to Near-Drowning in Childhood

Although speech and hearing impairments, including dysarthria and mild dysphasia, have been reported to occur in near-drowned children secondary to anoxic encephalopathy (Pearn, 1977; Pearn *et al.*, 1979b), only one study has been reported that has specifically investigated the effects of immersion and its associated intracranial pathophysiology on speech and language skills (Reilly *et al.*, 1988).

The morbidity of immersion is both pulmonary and neurological in origin (Peterson, 1977). The neurological morbidity following immersion injury is of particular interest to speech pathologists in that it is known to be associated with the occurrence of speech and language deficits. In order to comprehend the basis of the neurological morbidity following immersion, and hence the basis of any associated speech and language deficits, it is important that the process and physiology of the near-drowning incident be understood, with particular reference to anoxia.

During the initial period of immersion, the child panics and struggles. Apnoea or breath holding occurs and the victim gasps and swallows quantities of water which enter the larynx and trachea. At this point tachycardia and arterial hypoxaemia occur, due to the presence of high carbon dioxide levels and low oxygen concentrations in the blood. Blood pressure at this time increases. A phase of secondary apnoea occurs followed by involuntary gasping under water and eventually by respiratory arrest. Arrhythmias are inevitable and, in the absence of ventilation, lead within minutes to death. Consciousness is lost within 3 minutes of involuntary submersion, almost always because of cerebral anoxia (Pearn, 1985).

Neurological deficits following immersion

Specific neurological morbidity reported to occur secondary to childhood immersion includes spastic quadriplegia (Frates, 1981), truncal ataxia, strabismus and optic atrophy (Peterson, 1977), tetraplegia (Eriksson *et al.*, 1973), upper motor neuron lesions (Fleetham and Munt, 1978), peripheral neuromuscular paralysis (Pearn *et al.*, 1979a) and athetosis (Kruus *et al.*, 1979). Although some children exhibit persistent neurological deficits following immersion, in most studies reported in the literature, the majority of near-drowning cases have been described as showing a good recovery of neurological function (Table 5.1).

Unfortunately, with the exception of the studies reported by Kruus *et al.* (1979) and Pearn (1977), none of the investigations listed in Table 5.1 provided details of the specific procedures used to assess the neurological status of the victims of near-drowning. In most instances to determine the incidence of neurological sequelae following immersion, the authors either reviewed hospital records retrospectively or administered the subjects an unspecified neurological examination. In one study, the presence or absence of neurological deficit following immersion was determined by obtaining, by way of a telephone conversation, the parents' perception of whether their child had recovered or not (Eriksson *et al.*, 1973). As a result of their failure to use detailed and specific neurological assessment procedures, it is possible that many researchers who have investigated the neurological sequelae of near-drowning may have missed the presence of subtle or mild neurological deficits. Towbin (1971) suggested that mild hypoxia results in focal or diffuse neuronal damage with consequent neurological symptoms of a minimal or latent nature. If present it is possible that subtle neurological changes occurring secondary to immersion could influence the high-level language performance of victims of near-drowning.

Pearn (1977) investigated the possible existence of subtle neurological deficits following immersion. In a large ($n = 54$) population study, he examined the neurological and psychological outcome of all childhood survivors of fresh-water immersion accident who lost consciousness in the water. Pearn's subjects were neurologically examined and psychologically tested between 3 months and 60 months after immersion by means of a full specific neurological assessment and a range of psychometric tests. Neurological examination revealed that 52 of the 54 immersion

Table 5.1 Neurological deficits reported in children following immersion

Study	Number of Subjects	Follow-up period	Assessment	Neurological Outcome	Clinical Features of Impaired Group
Eriksson *et al.* (1973)	36	2–7 years	(a) Hospital records examined; (b) Parents inter-viewed by phone.	Serious disablement = 2 Normal = 34	• Occasional reaction to light or pain; • Tetraplegic syndrome with general rigidity and dystonia.
Fandel and Bancalari (1976)	34	ND	Records reviewed	Without neurological sequelae = 24 With neurological sequelae = 4 Death = 6	Defined as persistent coma or vegetative state.
Pearn (1977)	54	3–60 months	• Neurological examination • 3 years assigned developmental quotient • Psychometric tests	Normal = 52 Severe brain deficit = 1 The remaining case had complications from a head injury	Spastic quadraplegic
Peterson (1977)	72	NS	Review of records	No detectable neurological decifit = 57 Severe anoxic Encephalopathy = 13 Moderate anoxic encephalopathy = 1	Truncal ataxia strabismus, optic atrophy

Table 5.1 Continued

Study	Number of Subjects	Follow-up period	Assessment	Neurological Outcome	Clinical Features of Impaired Group
Kruus et al. (1979)	30	6–58 months	• Interview with parents • EEG recording • Clinical neurological examination • Psychometric tests	Complete recovery (to pre-accident level) = 8 Slight neurological signs (coordination failure) = 5 Mental retardation and tetraplegic = 4 Death = 13	Decreased in IQ; no movement or speech, difficulty in swallowing, slowing in EEG, muscle hypotomia, spastic tetraplegic
Pearn et al. (1979a)	104	6–58 months	Review of case history	No significant neurological damage = 98 Neurological deficit = 0 Death = 6	—
Modell et al. (1980)	64	—	Retrospective review	Normal survival = 53 Severe brain deficit = 3 Death = 8	ND
Frates (1981)	42	—	Retrospective review of case studies	Death = 10 Normal = 27 Profound cerebral Injury = 5	Spastic quadraplegia

Table 5.1 Continued

Study	Number of Subjects	Follow-up period	Assessment	Neurological Outcome		Clinical Features of Impaired Group
Oakes *et al.* (1982)	40	Mean = 11.4 months	Review hospital	Full recovery	= 23	ND
				Severe neurological Impairment	= 7	
				Death	= 10	
Conn and Barker (1984)	140	ND	ND	Abnormal	= 9	ND
				Normal	= 105	
				Death	= 26	
Frewen *et al.* (1985)	28	6 months	Neurological examination	Good recovery	= 15	ND
				Impaired, severe	= 4	
				Impaired, mild-moderate	= 1	
				Death	= 8	
Nussbaum (1985)	51	—	ND	Complete recovery	= 19	Mental deterioration, spasticity
				Brain damage	= 14	
				Death	= 18	

NS = Not stated
ND = No details provided

189

cases had no clinically detectable evidence of motor, cerebellar, extrapyramidal, sensory (tactile) or cranial nerve dysfunction (i.e. they were neurologically normal). However, comparison of the verbal intelligence quotient scores with the performance intelligence quotient scores that were achieved on the Wechsler Preschool and Primary Scale of Intelligence (Wechsler, 1967) by 16 of the immersion cases yielded a significant difference ($p < 0.05$) of 11 points or more in five subjects. Three of the 16 children showed disparities between verbal and performance scores of greater than 15 IQ points: the term 'minimal cerebral dysfunction' is sometimes applied to this (Pearn, 1977). Also, such a discrepancy between performance IQ and verbal IQ is said to be indicative of a specific language impairment and/or a language-learning disability (Wechsler, 1974).

The presence of coma following immersion has been shown to be prognostically indicative of neurological impairment in victims of near-drowning (Modell *et al.*, 1980). Modell *et al.* (1980) retrospectively reviewed 121 cases of near-drowning and compared their neurological outcome with their neurological status on admission to hospital as determined by the neurological classification scale for victims of near-drowning (Conn and Barker, 1984). According to this scale, victims of immersion can be placed into one of three different neurological classifications: A (awake) — alert and fully conscious; B (blunted) — obtunded, stuporous but rousable with purposeful response to pain and abnormal respiration; and C (comatose) — comatose, not rousable with abnormal response to pain and abnormal respiration. Modell *et al.* (1980) reported that neurological deficit was apparent only in Group C cases. Allman *et al.* (1986) stated that no near-drowned child presenting as flaccid and comatosed on admission to hospital recovers normal neurological functioning.

Linguistic deficits following immersion

The findings of several studies have either indicated or suggested the presence of speech and language disorders in children who have experienced near-drowning. Pearn *et al.* (1979b) identified dysarthria and aphasia as potential sequelae of near-drowning incidents. In addition, as discussed earlier, the findings of Pearn (1977) were suggestive of the presence of a language impairment in children following immersion. Reilly *et al.* (1988), however, are the only authors to date to have specifically investigated and documented the linguistic abilities of near-drowned children. These researchers investigated the linguistic abilities of two groups of children who had been involved in near-drowning incidents, one group 12 months after immersion ($n = 25$) and the second group 5 years after immersion ($n = 9$). Reilly *et al.* (1988) compared the performances of the two groups on standardized language tests with the performances of appropriate controls matched for age, sex and socio-economic status. In addition Reilly and co-workers assigned each of their immersion subjects to one of the categories A, B or C of the neurological classification for victims of near-drowning (Conn and Barker, 1984) and correlated their neurological status with their language abilities.

The findings of Reilly *et al.* (1988) showed that the 12-month after immersion group was language delayed, as determined by their performance on the Sequenced Inventory of Communicative Development (Hedrick *et al.*, 1975) compared with their control group. In particular, Reilly *et al.* (1988) found that the near-drowned children had significantly lower scores than their controls for expressive language age and receptive language age when these scores were calculated as percentages of the child's chronological age.

Reilly *et al.* (1988) also reported that all their subjects in the 12-months after immersion group who were categorized as either Group A or B according to the Conn and Barker (1984) neurological scale at the time of their admission to hospital, exhibited language abilities within normal limits. In contrast, however, four of the five near-drowned cases from the 12-month after immersion group categorized as Group C did exhibit some degree of language impairment (Table 5.2).

The low level of performance of subject 5 would be anticipated from the findings of Allman *et al.* (1986), as he was the only child in the study who presented on admission to hospital in a flaccid comatose condition. Reilly *et al.* (1988) also noted that all of the Group C children, with the exception of subjects 3 and 5, had been described as 'neurologically normal' except for drooling from the mouth and the presence of a mild speech problem.

No significant differences were found by Reilly *et al.* (1988) between the language scores achieved by the immersion subjects assessed 5 years after the near-drowning incident and their controls, although it was noted by the authors that the majority of the immersion subjects in this group were categorized as Group A on the Conn and Barker (1984) scale.

Two subjects in the 5-year after immersion group were comatose at the time of their admission to hospital and were therefore categorized as Group C. One of the Group C subjects exhibited a linguistic impairment when assessed 5 years later, his

Table 5.2 *Speech and language outcome in Group C subjects in the 12-month following immersion study by Reilly* et al. *(1988)*

Subject No.	Age (months)	Receptive language age (months)	Expressive language age (months)
1	40	32	36
2	37	40	40
3	22	16	16
4	47	36	40
5	45	12	8

performance being below the 20th percentile for the receptive vocabulary, sentence-imitation and articulation subtests of the Test of Language Development — Primary (Newcomer and Hammill, 1982). The other Group C child, however, did not exhibit a linguistic problem when assessed 5 years later. This child was assessed initially by a speech pathologist 4 weeks after the immersion incident. At that time he presented with auditory processing difficulties and word-finding problems. Three months after the near-drowning incident, the child was reported as functioning within normal limits on all speech and language tests. Despite this, he presented at the hospital outpatient clinic 5 years later for investigation of suspected learning difficulties. His parents, at this time, reported that they had noted that the child was slow to learn, had a poor concentration span and exhibited auditory inattention. Subsequent assessments of the child showed normal performance on neurological examination, psychometric IQ testing and speech and language assessment. However, in the light of the presenting symptoms, Reilly *et al.* (1988) were unable to rule out the presence of an auditory processing deficit, as at that time a comprehensive audiological assessment had not been carried out. Both of these subjects had been described as 'neurologically normal' within 3 months of the near-drowning incident.

Reilly *et al.* (1988) concluded that children who are victims of near-drowning incidents, and who initially present at hospital as comatose, form a population that is at risk for impaired development of linguistic abilities.

Motor Speech Disorders in a Case of Accidental Childhood Suffocation

Murdoch *et al.* (1989) described the case of a 13-year-old boy who had suffered anoxic encephalopathy as a result of being accidentally buried under sand for approximately 20 minutes. A CT scan taken 5 weeks after the injury demonstrated the presence of bilateral striatocapsular lesions involving the lenticular nucleus and head of the caudate nucleus in each hemisphere (Figure 5.1). The topography of the lesions was consistent with the pattern observed in cases of cerebral anoxia (De Reuck and Vander Eecken, 1978). Administration of a series of speech and language tests, including the Frenchay Dysarthria Assessment (Enderby, 1983), the Apraxia Battery for Adults (Dabul, 1979) and the Western Aphasia Battery (Kertesz, 1982) over a 3-month period starting at 6 weeks post-onset revealed that the subject displayed a range of symptoms typical of aphemia (Schiff *et al.*, 1983) including a progression from initial mutism to syntactically intact verbalizations with retained ability to write and comprehend spoken language. Murdoch *et al.* (1989) concluded that the aphemia was best explained by either a disruption of the subcortical connections of the peri-Rolandic region of each hemisphere or alternatively by an impairment in speech motor planning due to direct involvement of the basal ganglia.

At the time of the initial assessment some 6 weeks after the injury, Murdoch *et al.*

(1989) described their patient as being mute but able to communicate by means of a letter board. No receptive language disturbance was evident at this time. Although his intelligibility was poor, the subject was able to vocalize in single words 7 weeks after the injury and could use short sentences by 8 weeks after his accidental burial. Murdoch *et al.* (1989) noted that when examined 12 weeks post-onset, the patient's speech contained some elements typical of hypokinetic dysarthria. In particular, an increase in speech rate reminiscent of that seen in Parkinson's disease was reported to be present during speech production. Furthermore, the patient also showed difficulty in initiating speech movements.

A Western Aphasia Battery administered 14 weeks post-onset showed the presence of intact receptive language abilities, with only a minor expressive problem being evident, probably resulting from the above mentioned concomitant dysarthria. Written language was described as being syntactically appropriate and orthographically correct, although the motor aspects of writing were abnormal. Certainly no overt aphasia was evident. The authors noted, however, that they were unable to rule out with certainty the possible presence of subtle language problems, in that the Western Aphasia Battery does not assess high-level language function. Murdoch *et al.* (1989) also noted that the subject may have shown a transient language disorder in the acute stage following suffocation which could have resolved during the 6 weeks before their initial assessment of the patient.

The findings in the above case of anoxic encephalopathy led Murdoch *et al.* (1989) to suggest that if striatocapsular structures do have a role in language, as suggested by evidence from the adult literature and in children by Aram *et al.* (1983), this role may be assumed by other brain structures in children following damage to the striatocapsular region.

Linguistic Deficits following Cardiac Arrest and Respiratory Arrest

Two cases of acquired childhood aphasia resulting from anoxic encephalopathy were described by Cooper and Flowers (1987). One case (subject 1) was a boy who suffered a cardiac arrest following cardiac surgery while the second case (subject 11) was a girl who developed anoxic encephalopathy subsequent to respiratory arrest at 8 years 4 months of age. Both children were described as being mute in the initial period post-onset. In the case of subject 11, verbal communication did not return until 6 months post-onset, while in subject 1, at the time of his discharge from hospital 2 months post-onset, no comment on the presence of communication difficulties was noted.

When assessed with a range of speech/language assessments just over 6 years post-onset, subject 1 was reported to show deficits in receptive and expressive single-word vocabulary. Cooper and Flowers (1987) also noted that, during the course of the language assessment, subject 1 appeared reticent to talk, spoke rarely and did not initiate conversation. Subject 1 scored only 29 of a possible 85 correct responses on the Boston Naming Test with the errors being described by Cooper and Flowers (1987) as being primarily semantically related, phonological or misperceptions of the picture stimulus. Word fluency was also disturbed and subject 1 was reported to have problems with arithmetic computation. His intellectual function, however, was reported to be normal although it was noted that he did attend full-time special education.

Unlike subject 1, hospital and school reports indicated that subject 11 had persistent language difficulties from the time of onset until assessed by Cooper and Flowers (1987), almost 7 years later. Based on her performance on the various language tests administered, Cooper and Flowers (1987) reported that subject 11 had deficits in receptive single-word vocabulary and production and completion of syntactical constructions. Impaired performance of the Token Test was also noted, subject 11 scoring more than two standard deviations below the mean for her peer age category. As in subject 1, problems with arithmetic computation were also present. Indeed, all areas of academic performance were said to be impaired, with the exception of reading comprehension. In terms of intellectual functioning, subject 11 was reported to fall in the low-average to borderline range and she attended special education.

The two anoxia cases described by Cooper and Flowers (1987) clearly demonstrate that anoxic encephalopathy may be associated with the occurrence of long-term linguistic deficits, even in those cases where apparent recovery of speech and language abilities occurs in the acute stage post-onset.

Summary

Although there are few reports in the literature that have related anoxic encephalopathy to the occurrence of speech and language deficits in childhood, the evidence available suggests that anoxic brain damage can cause linguistic deficits in both the acute and chronic stages post-onset. To date, speech and language disorders in childhood have only been described subsequent to anoxia resulting from events such as near-drowning, accidental suffocation and cardiac arrest. In that all types of anoxia cause fundamentally the same distribution of lesions in the brain, it could be expected, however, that anoxia resulting from any cause has the potential to induce linguistic deficits in children.

It is important, therefore, that speech pathologists recognize that any child who has experienced some type of anoxic episode, and especially those cases that initially present at hospital as comatose, are at risk of developing speech and language disorders. Although in some cases the long-term linguistic deficits that result from the anoxic encephalopathy may be sufficiently overt to be detected by parents, teachers etc., in many cases these deficits are of a subtle, subclinical or latent nature and are only evidenced by an extensive and detailed speech and language examination. Despite their subtle nature, however, these subclinical linguistic problems may manifest as impaired academic performance in later life, with affected subjects in some cases presenting many years after the anoxic injury for investigation of suspected learning difficulties. The need for speech pathologists to monitor the development of the speech and language of children who have had an anoxic episode is therefore imperative.

References

ADAMS, R. (1963) 'General discussion', in SCHADÉ, J. P. and MCMENEMEY, W. H. (Eds) *Selective Vulnerability of the Brain in Hypoxaemia*, Oxford, Blackwell Scientific Publications.

ADAMS, J. H., BRIERLEY, J. B., CONNOR, R. C. R. and TREIP, C. S. (1966) 'The effects of systemic hypotension upon the human brain: Clinical and neuropathological observations in 11 cases', *Brain*, **89**, pp. 235–68.

ALEXANDER, M. P. and LO VERME, S. R. (1980) 'Aphasia after left hemispheric intracerebral hemorrhage', *Neurology*, **30**, pp. 1193–202.

ALLMAN, F. D., NELSON, W. B., PACENTINE, G. A. and MCCOMB, G. (1986) 'Outcome following cardiopulmonary resuscitation in severe pediatric near-drowning', *American Journal of Disorders in Children*, **140**, pp. 571–5.

AMES, A., WRIGHT, R. L., KOWADA, M., THURSTON, J. M. and MAJNO, G. (1968) 'Cerebral ischaemia: The no-reflow phenomenon', *American Journal of Pathology*, **52**, pp. 437–53.

ARAM, D. M., EKELMAN, B. L. and GILLESPIE, L. L. (1989) 'Reading and lateralized brain lesions in children', in VON EULER, K. (Ed.) *Developmental Dyslexia and Dysphasia*, Hampshire, England, Macmillan Press.

ARAM, D. M., ROSE, D. F., REKATE, H. L. and WHITAKER, H. A. (1983) 'Acquired capsular/striatal aphasia in childhood', *Archives of Neurology*, **40**, pp. 614–17.

BELL, R. D. (1980) 'Metabolic encephalopathies', in ROSENBERG, R. N. (Ed.) *Neurology*, Vol.5, New York, Grune & Stratton.

BENSON, D. F. (1979) *Aphasia, Alexia and Agraphia*, New York, Churchill Livingstone.

BRIERLY, J. B. (1972) 'The neuropathology of brain hypoxia', in CRITCHLEY, M., O'LEARY, J. L. and JENNETT, B. (Eds) *Scientific Foundations of Neurology*, London, Heinemann.

BRUCHER, J. M. (1967) 'Neuropathological problems posed by carbon monoxide poisoning and anoxia', *Progress in Brain Research*, **24**, pp. 75–100.

CONN, A. W. and BARKER, G. A. (1984) 'Fresh water drowning and near-drowning – an update', *Canadian Anaesthesia Society Journal*, **31**, pp. 538–44.

COOPER, J. A. and FLOWERS, C. R. (1987) 'Children with a history of acquired aphasia: Residual language and academic impairments', *Journal of Speech and Hearing Disorders*, **52**, pp. 251–62.

DABUL, B. (1979) *Apraxia Battery for Adults*, Tigard, C.C. Publications.

DE REUCK, J.L. and VANDER EECKEN, H.M. (1978) 'Periventricular leukomalacia in adults', *Archives of Neurology*, **35**, pp. 517–21.

EDSTROM, R.F.S. and ESSEX, H.E. (1956) 'Swelling of the brain induced by anoxia', *Neurology*, **6**, pp. 118–24.

ENDERBY, P. (1983) *Frenchay Dysarthria Assessment*, San Diego, College-Hill Press.

ERIKSSON, R., FREDIN, H., GERDMAN, P. and THORSAN, J. (1973) 'Sequelae of accidental near-drowning in childhood', *Scandinavian Journal of Social Medicine*, **1**, pp. 3–6.

FANDEL, I. and BANCALARI, E. (1976) 'Near drowning in children: Clinical aspects', *Pediatrics*, **58**, pp. 573–9.

FLEETHAM, J.A. and MUNT, P.W. (1978) 'Near-drowning in Canadian waters', *Canadian Medical Association Journal*, **118**, pp. 914–17.

FRATES, R.C. (1981) 'Analysis of predictive factors in the assessment of warm water near-drowning in children', *American Journal of Diseases in Childhood*, **135**, pp. 1006–8.

FREWEN, T.C., SUMABAT, W.O., HAN, V.K., AMACHER, A.L., DEL MASTRO, R.F. and SIBBALD, W.J. (1985) 'Cerebral resuscitation therapy in pediatric near-drowning', *Journal of Pediatrics*, **104**, pp. 615–17.

GÄNSHIRT, H. (1957) *Die Sauerstoffversorgung des Gehirns und ihre Störung bei der Liquor drucksteigerung und beim Hirnödem*, Berlin, Springer.

GRAHAM, D.I. (1977) 'Pathology of hypoxic brain damage in man', *Journal of Clinical Pathology*, **30**, Suppl. 11, pp. 170–80.

HEDRICK, D.L., PRATHER, E.M. and TOBIN, A.R. (1975) *Sequenced Inventory of Communication Development*, Seattle, University of Washington Press.

HELGASON, C., CAPLAN, L.R., GOODWIN, J.A. and HEDGES, T. (1986) 'Anterior choroidal artery – territory infarction', *Archives of Neurology*, **43**, pp. 681–6.

HELGASON, C., CAPLAN, L.R., GOODWIN, J.A. and HEDGES, T. (1987) 'Bilateral basal ganglia necrosis following diffuse hypoxic-ischemic injury — a reply', *Archives of Neurology*, **44**, p. 897.

KERTESZ, A. (1982) *The Western Aphasia Battery*, New York, Grune & Stratton.

KÖRNYEY, S. (1963) 'Patterns of CNS vulnerability in CO, cyanide and other poisoning', in SCHADÉ, J.P. and MCMENEMEY, W.H. (Eds) *Selective Vulnerability of the Brain in Hypoxaemia*, Oxford, Blackwell Scientific Publications.

KRUUS, S., BERGSTROM, L., SUUTARINEN, T. and HYVONEN, R. (1979) 'The prognosis of near-drowned children', *Acta Paediatrica Scandinavica*, **68**, pp. 315–22.

LINDENBERG, R. (1955) 'Compression of brain arteries as pathogenetic factor for tissue necrosis and their areas of predilection', *Journal of Neuropathology and Experimental Neurology*, **14**, pp. 223–43.

LINDENBERG, R. (1963) 'Patterns of CNS vulnerability in acute hypoxaemia, including anaesthesia accidents', in SCHADÉ, J.P. and MCMENEMEY, W.H. (Eds) *Selective Vulnerability of the Brain in Hypoxaemia*, Oxford, Blackwell Scientific Publications.

MCILWAIN, H. (1955) *Biochemistry and the Central Nervous System*, London, Churchill Livingstone.

MCILWAIN, H. (1966) *Biochemistry and the Central Nervous System*, 3rd ed, London, Churchill Livingstone.

MATSUO, F., CUMMINS, J. W. and ANDERSON, R. E. (1979) 'Neurological sequelae of massive hydrogen sulfide inhalation', *Archives of Neurology*, **36**, pp. 451–2.

MODELL, J. H., GRAVES, S. A. and KUCK, E. J. (1980) 'Near-drowning: Correlation of level of consciousness and survival', *Canadian Anaesthetics Society Journal*, **27**, pp. 211–15.

MURDOCH, B. E., CHENERY, H. J. and KENNEDY, M. (1989) 'Aphemia associated with bilateral striato-capsular lesions subsequent to cerebral anoxia', *Brain Injury*, **3**, pp. 41–9.

MURDOCH, B. E., THOMPSON, D., FRASER, S. and HARRISON, L. (1986) 'Aphasia following nonhaemorrhagic lesions in the left striato-capsular region', *Australian Journal of Human Communication Disorders*, **14**, pp. 5–21.

MURRAY, R. S., STENSAAS, S. S., ANDERSON, R. E. and MATSUO, F. (1987) 'Bilateral basal ganglia necrosis following diffuse hypoxic-ischaemic injury', *Archives of Neurology*, **44**, p. 897.

NEWCOMER, P. L. and HAMMILL, D. D. (1982) *Test of Language Development: Primary*, Texas, Pro-ed.

NUSSBAUM, E. (1985) 'Prognostic variables in nearly-drowned comatose children', *American Journal of Diseases in Childhood*, **139**, pp. 1058–9.

OAKES, D. D., SHERCK, J. P., MALONEY, J. R. and CRANE–CHARTERS, A. (1982) 'Prognosis and management of victims of near drowning', *Journal of Trauma*, **22**, pp. 544–8.

PEARN, J. H. (1977) 'Neurologic and psychometric studies in children surviving freshwater immersion accidents', *Lancet*, **i**, pp. 7–9

PEARN, J. H. (1985) 'Pathophysiology of drowning', *Medical Journal of Australia*, **142**, pp. 586–8.

PEARN, J. H., BART, R. D. and YAMAOKA, R. (1979a) 'Neurologic sequelae after childhood near drowning: a total population study from Hawaii', *Pediatrics*, **64**, pp. 187–91.

PEARN, J. H., DE BUSE, P., MOHAY, H. and GOLDEN, M. (1979b) 'Sequential intellectual recovery after near-drowning', *Medical Journal of Australia*, **1**, pp. 463–4.

PETERSON, B. (1977) 'Morbidity of childhood drowning', *Pediatrics*, **59**, pp. 364–5.

PLUM, F. (1973) 'The clinical problem: How much anoxia-ischemia damages the brain?', *Archives of Neurology*, **29**, pp. 359–60.

REILLY, K., OZANNE, A. E., MURDOCH, B. E. and PITT, W. R. (1988) 'Linguistic status subsequent to childhood immersion injury', *Medical Journal of Australia*, **148**, pp. 225–8.

RICHARDSON, J. C., CHAMBERS, R. A. and HEYWOOD, P. M. (1959) 'Encephalopathies of anoxia and hypoglycemia', *Archives of Neurology*, **1**, pp. 178–90.

SCHIFF, H. B., ALEXANDER, M. P., NAESER, M. A. and GALABURDA, A. M. (1983) 'Aphemia: Clinical anatomic correlations', *Archives of Neurology*, **40**, pp. 720–7.

SCHWEDENBERG, T. H. (1959) 'Leukoencephalopathy following carbon monoxide asphyxia', *Journal of Neuropathology and Experimental Neurology*, **18**, pp. 597–608.

TOWBIN, A. (1971) 'Organic causes of minimal brain dysfunction', *Journal of the American Medical Association*, **217**, pp. 1207–14.

WECHSLER, D. (1967) *Wechsler Pre-School and Primary Scale of Intelligence*, New York, The Psychological Corporation.

WECHSLER, D. (1974) *Wechsler Intelligence Scale for Children*, New York, The Psychological Corporation.

WEINBERGER, L. M., GIBBON, M. H. and GIBBON, J. H. (1940) 'Temporary arrest of the circulation to the central nervous system: 1. Physiological effects', *Archives of Neurology and Psychiatry*, **43**, p. 615.

ZEISS, J. and BRINKER, R. (1988) 'Role of contrast enhancement in cerebral CT of carbon monoxide poisoning', *Journal of Computer Assisted Tomography*, **12**, pp. 341–3.

Chapter 6

Linguistic Problems Associated with Childhood Metabolic Disorders

Anne E. Ozanne, Bruce E. Murdoch and Helen L. Krimmer

Introduction

Abnormal body metabolism can cause disturbances in brain development and function. Systemic metabolic disorders for instance, such as inborn errors of metabolism, can lead to the accumulation of metabolites in the bloodstream and body tissues which may cause structural changes in the brain leading to a decline in intellectual function and, in some cases, speech and language disorders. Inborn errors of metabolism that have been reported to cause speech/language disorders include phenylketonuria (Ozanne *et al.* in press), galactosaemia (Waisbren *et al.*, 1983) and Wilson's disease (Berry *et al.*, 1974). In addition to inborn errors of metabolism, speech/language disorders have also been reported to occur in association with impaired intellectual function resulting from disruption of normal brain development in cases of congenital hypothyroidism (Dussault *et al.*, 1980).

Inborn Errors of Metabolism Causing Speech/Language Disorders

Phenylketonuria

Clinical characteristics

Phenylketonuria is an inborn error of metabolism resulting from an absence of the hepatic (liver) enzyme phenylalanine hydroxylase that converts phenylalanine (an essential amino acid) into tyrosine. As a result of the deficiency in this enzyme system, phenylalanine (as well as other metabolites of phenylalanine such as phenylketones), normally present in only small amounts, accumulates in the blood as well as in the cerebrospinal fluid and tissues, and is excreted in the urine as phenylpyruvic acid in greater than normal amounts.

Phenylketonuria is inherited as an autosomal recessive disorder and occurs in approximately 1 in every 10 000–20 000 births. In past years, phenylketonuria has accounted for approximately 1 per cent of institutionalized mentally deficient persons (Rosenberg and Pettegrew, 1980). The condition is most common in Caucasians and is rare in some racial groups, including the African, Jewish and Japanese populations.

At birth, infants with phenylketonuria may appear normal although an increased frequency of vomiting and a poor appetite have been noted. In that melanin is formed from tyrosine, most children with phenylketonuria have reduced pigmentation in their skin, hair and eyes. Consequently, the majority have fair skin, blonde hair and blue eyes. Phenylketonuria in the offspring of people with darker heritage may be red-haired or brunette. The occurrence of phenylketonuria is suspected on the basis of the presence of phenylpyruvic acid in the urine. A transient green colour is produced when ferric chloride is added to urine containing excessive levels of phenylpyruvic acid. In that this test is not reliable until the infant is approximately 4–6 weeks of age, however, the early confirmation of phenylketonuria is dependent on the detection of elevated serum phenylalanine levels. The most commonly used screening test for phenylketonuria is the Guthrie technique. In this, a drop of the infant's blood is placed on a specific type of filter paper and the levels of various amino acids (including phenylalanine) determined by a microbiological method.

Most, if not all, of the manifestations of phenylketonuria are accounted for by the disruption of normal body processes caused by the accumulation of phenylalanine and its metabolites. Although largely symptom-free at birth, children with phenylketonuria, if left untreated, eventually manifest a number of abnormal signs and symptoms. The most important clinical characteristic of untreated phenylketonuria is severe mental retardation. Signs of mental retardation usually become evident clinically after the first 6 months of life, although the process may begin at an earlier stage and go undetected until this time. According to Rosenberg and Pettegrew (1980), when not treated infants with phenylketonuria lose approximately five IQ points each 10 weeks and ultimately 96–98 per cent of them have an IQ of less that 50. Although the specific mechanism that produces the decline in mental abilities is unknown, it would appear that interference with the structural development of the brain, rather than a direct effect on performance, is responsible. It has been suggested that the mental decline is caused by a neurotoxic agent that has an inhibiting effect on development before myelinization of the brain is complete. Histologically, the white matter of the brain of children with phenylketonuria shows the greatest alteration, with the white matter of the cerebral hemispheres, optic tracts and cerebellum being more affected than the brainstem white matter. The lesions in the white matter range from spongy degeneration to profound demyelinization with accompanying gliosis. Brain lipids are reduced, especially the galactolipids associated with myelin. Occasional loss of neurons in the cerebral cortex and grey matter of the cerebellum may also occur with heterotopia (displacement of parts) and laminar disruption.

In addition to mental retardation, other signs and symptoms often exhibited by children with untreated phenylketonuria include: eczematoid dermatitis (rash in the body folds), an aromatic, musty odour associated with the presence of phenylacetic acid in the sweat and urine, seizures, abnormal electroencephalographic activity, hyperactivity, erratic and unpredictable behaviour, including temper tantrums, slowness in attaining motor milestones, motor performance habits (e.g. chewing on an arm), and insufficient head growth. Neurological examination usually shows no specific abnormalities, although in some cases a little spasticity may be evident without corticospinal signs.

Treatment of phenylketonuria involves elimination from the diet of those foods that contain high concentrations of phenylalanine. Dietary management appears to be most effective when initiated shortly after birth. It has been suggested that in those cases where a phenylalanine-restricted diet is commenced early in infancy (before 3 months of age) and maintained during the period of most rapid myelinization, damage to the central nervous system is averted. Clinically, it has been observed that very young children with phenylketonuria who are placed on low phenylalanine diets while normal (i.e. before the onset of seizures, mental decline etc.) and who have blood phenylalanine levels maintained at near normal levels, appear to develop mentally at a normal rate. Despite their IQ measurements being within normal limits, however, there is evidence to suggest that the IQs of these children are significantly lower than those of their parents, siblings or non-sibling controls (Berry *et al.*, 1979; Netley *et al.*, 1984). It is uncertain, however, how long it is necessary to maintain the treatment to ensure development of maximal intellectual capacity. There is a feeling that children with phenylketonuria should remain on a low phenylalanine diet during the period when the brain is still undergoing myelinization and is, therefore, most susceptible to damage. Consequently, treatment may be required for the first 3–6 years of life or more. It is important, however, that intellectual and behavioural monitoring continue after the diet is discontinued. In that a decline in cognitive functioning and even language skills has been documented in some children who have been routinely taken off their low phenylalanine diet (Koch *et al.*, 1984; Seashore *et al.*, 1985; Waisbren *et al.*, 1980), dietary control in some countries is continued for the first 8 years of life.

In older children with phenylketonuria, initiation of a low phenylalanine diet has been found to reduce the occurrence of seizures and skin rashes and to improve the level of pigmentation. Only modest improvements in behaviour, however, have been observed in these children. Furthermore, initiation of diets after brain damage has occurred does not reverse the process but may, if begun early enough, limit its progress. It is important therefore that phenylketonuria be detected early. The lack of symptoms in the neonatal period, however, makes this early detection difficult. Routine screening is therefore needed to detect affected infants.

Overall, with early neonatal diagnosis and appropriate dietary therapy, and with monitoring of behaviour and intellectual abilities, the prognosis of children with phenylketonuria is good. Without early dietary treatment, however, the prognosis is very poor.

Linguistic deficits associated with phenylketonuria

Little information regarding the linguistic skills of children with phenylketonuria is available. Early reports described the presence of speech and language disorders in children in association with intellectual handicap (Boehme and Theile, 1972). Since the introduction of low phenylalanine diets, however, the speech and language skills of children with phenylketonuria have been assumed to be within normal limits, in line with their intellectual functioning.

Gross measures of language such as verbal IQ scores have, in fact, been found to be superior to performance IQ scores in some studies (Koff *et al.*, 1977; Pennington and Smith, 1983), while in other studies no notable difference between the verbal and performance IQ scores of children with early treated phenylketonuria was evident (Koch *et al.*, 1982, 1984; Seashore *et al.*, 1985). Recently neuropsychological assessments, aimed at detecting subtle cognitive defects in children with phenylketonuria and normal intelligence, have found deficits in visuospatial and conceptual tasks but minimal impairment on language tasks (Pennington *et al.*, 1985). These conclusions, however, have been based on language asssessment using neuropsychological tasks, such as word fluency tasks, rather than linguistic tests. Both these types of findings would lead one to suspect that children with early-treated phenylketonuria do not present with language impairments.

Some authors have suggested, however, that speech and language disorders do occur in children with phenylketonuria. Vogel (1985: 342) stated that 'diet-treated phenylketonuria homozygotes often show a slight weakness in verbal abilities', but provided no further details. To date, only two studies have reported on the speech and language skills in children with early-treated phenylketonuria using linguistic assessments. Melnick *et al.* (1981) assessed 12 children with phenylketonuria between 4 months and 6 years of age. All children had normal intelligence. The children were assessed using the Bzoch-League Receptive-Expressive Emergent Language Scale (Bzoch and League, 1971), the Peabody Picture Vocabulary Test (Dunn, 1965), the Developmental Sentence Score (Lee, 1974a), mean length of utterance (Brown, 1973), the Northwestern Syntax Screening test (Lee, 1974b), the Goldman–Fristoe Test of Articulation (Goldman and Fristoe, 1969) and the digit span subtest of the Stanford–Binet. Using the test percentile ratings for each child, Melnick *et al.* (1981) identified children who scored below the tenth percentile as having a speech and/or language disorder. By using this criterion, Melnick *et al.* (1981) found that 50 per cent of their subjects showed a speech or language impairment; however, there was no particular pattern of linguistic deficit that could be said to be associated with phenylketonuria. Two of their subjects presented with articulation disorders four with receptive and six with expressive language problems. One child presented with all three areas of linguistic deficit; three subjects had both receptive and expressive language impairments while one subject had expressive syntax and articulation deficits while one other had only expressive syntactical delays. After speech and language therapy, the one case with the expressive only problem was remediated, while two other cases had acquired age-appropriate receptive but not expressive skills. All other cases continued to exhibit persistent speech and/or language impairment. Despite the lack of commonality of presenting speech and language deficits, Melnick *et al.* (1981) did find that all the children who presented with linguistic deficits also had poor auditory memory skills.

A study by Ozanne *et al.* (in press) assessed a similar group to Melnick *et al.* (1981); the subjects were between 7 months and 3 years 11 months of age, with normal intelligence. The subjects with phenylketonuria were assessed using the Sequenced Inventory of Communication Development (SICD) (Hedrick *et al.*, 1978) with similar results to those reported by Melnick *et al.* (1981). Thirty-six per cent (i.e. four of 11) of the subjects with phenylketonuria examined by Ozanne and co-workers were considered language-impaired. Since the SICD does not use percentile scores or gives guidelines for the identification of language impairment, the authors used the criterion of a language age which was 75 per cent or below of the subject's chronological age, to identify children whom they considered to have language impairment.

When the language skills of the subjects with phenylketonuria of Ozanne and co-workers were compared as a group, however, with a group of children matched for age and sex, no significant difference in language abilities was found between the two groups. The authors suggested that the wide variation in language skills observed in both groups of subjects accounted for this lack of a significant difference. The wide variation in language abilities was, in turn, attributed to the fact that all the children were in the period of maximum language growth when large individual differences may occur. Using their criterion for identifying language impairment in the group of children with phenylketonuria, Ozanne *et al.* (in press) noted that two of the subjects in the control group could also be classified as having a language problem. In that both Melnick *et al.* (1981) and Ozanne *et al.* (in press) assessed children with normal intelligence, it could be said that the young children with phenylketonuria who presented as having a language impairment exhibited a specific language disorder rather than a language impairment as part of a general cognitive impairment, or that the language impairment was one of the first symptoms of a developing cognitive deficit. Longitudinal studies are required to investigate this further.

When a second group of 18 subjects with phenylketonuria, between 5 and 16 years of age, were studied by Ozanne *et al.* (in press), again no significant difference was noted between the subjects with phenylketonuria and their matched controls in the language scores, as measured on the Test of Language Development (TOLD)

(Hammill *et al.*, 1987; Hammill and Newcomer, 1982; Newcomer and Hammill, 1987) series of language tests. This group of subjects was also assessed using the Fisher–Logemann Test of Articulation Competence (Fisher and Logemann, 1971) which also failed to distinguish the subjects with phenylketonuria from their control group. This time the criterion used by Melnick *et al.* (1981) (i.e. score below the tenth precentile) was used to identify any child who had a language impairment. No child in the study had an articulation/phonological disorder. Three children with phenylketonuria, but no control subjects, were identified as being language impaired. Like Melnick *et al.*'s subjects there was no consistent pattern of linguistic deficit. When the language quotients of the subjects with phenylketonuria were ranked as shown in Table 6.1 a trend showing a relationship between language and intelligence quotient could be observed.

A stronger trend, however, can be seen in the relationship between language quotient and dietary compliance. All the subjects in both groups with phenylketonuria

Table 6.1 Ranked individual language quotients, dietary compliance ratings and IQ scores of subjects with phenylketonuria studied by Ozanne et al. (in press)

Subject No.	LQ	DC	FIQ	VIQ	PIQ
1	123	good	126φ		
14	122	good	107	113	100
9	120	good	101	106	98
3	119	good	110φ		
6	116	fair	107	108	105
12	111	fair	109	114	102
11	105	good	91	108	80
18	103	good	91	95	91
7	98	fair	118	118	114
2	94	fair	95φ		
15	93	fair	105	105	106
5	92	fair	107φ		
8	92	fair	92φ		
10	92	poor	92	91	94
13	89	poor	85	90	78
16	74 +	poor	88	90	88
17	68 +	poor	75	81	72
4	56 +	poor	65	65	67

LQ = Language quotient measured on TOLD tests
+ = Language quotient measured below tenth percentile
DC = Dietary compliance
FIQ = Full IQ measure
VIQ = Verbal IQ score
PIQ = Performance IQ score
φ = IQ assessed using Stanford–Binet

studied by Ozanne *et al.* (in press) were still currently on a low phenylalanine diet. Dietary compliance had been rated 'good', 'fair' or 'poor' by the dietitian, at the clinic these subjects attended, based on serum phenylalanine levels in the blood measured on each visit to the clinic. All three subjects with language impairment had amongst the lowest IQ scores in this group of subjects and all had a poor dietary rating. While the number of children with phenylketonuria with language impairment is too small to make definitive statements, individual data does suggest that in older children, particularly those with poor dietary control, speech and language deficits may be part of a decline in cognitive functioning.

The clinical implications from the limited research data available does suggest that as a group children with early-treated phenylketonuria do not have speech and language deficits, but rather that there are individual children with phenylketonuria (perhaps between 30 and 50 per cent) who do present with specific language disorders before 5 years of age. As there is no common pattern of linguistic deficit each child must be assessed and treated on an individual basis. Therefore regular monitoring of the speech and language skills of all young children with phenylketonuria and parent education programmes by speech and language pathologists should become a routine part of the functioning of the clinic. For older children with phenylketonuria it appears that those most at risk may be those who have difficulties maintaining their diet. Further studies of subjects with phenylketonuria presenting with language impairment are required to confirm this finding and to clarify the relationship between language abilities and cognitive functioning including auditory memory abilities.

Galactosaemia

Galactosaemia is an inborn error of carbohydrate metabolism in which, due to the absence or deficiency of the enzyme galactose-1-phosphate uridyl transferase, the body is unable to utilize the sugars galactose and lactose. Under normal circumstances, lactose (milk sugar) is broken down in the epithelium of the intestine to galactose and glucose. The galactose is then transported to the liver where it is converted into galactose-1-phosphate which in turn reacts with uridine diphosphate glucose (UDP-glucose) to form UDP-galactose. This substance is then transformed into glucose-1-phosphate. In galactosaemia, the conversion of galactose-1-phosphate to UDP-galactose is blocked due to the enzyme deficiency. Consequently, galactose-1-phosphate accumulates in the body tissues. Diagnosis is made on the basis of galactosuria, increased levels of galactose in the blood or by demonstration of the absence or deficiency of galactose-1-phosphate uridyl transferase in the erythrocytes.

The disease is inherited as an autosomal recessive disorder and occurs in approximately 1 in every 25 000–35 000 births. As in phenylketonuria, infants with galactosaemia may appear to be normal at birth. Symptoms tend to manifest, however, shortly after birth when the infant is exposed to large amounts of galactose derived from the lactose in the mother's milk. The toxic manifestations of galactosaemia are thought to result from the accumulation of galactose-1-phosphate. The major symptoms of the condition when the infant is exposed to galactose include cataract formation, hepatosplenomegaly (enlargement of the liver and spleen), nutritional failure and, most importantly, mental retardation. Jaundice may also occur in some cases and the hepatosplenomegaly may progress to cirrhosis of the liver if galactose ingestion continues for a prolonged period. Speech and language difficulties have also been reported to occur in children with galactosaemia (Jan and Wilson, 1973; Komrower and Lee, 1970; Lee, 1972).

Treatment of galactosaemia involves the elimination of galactose from the diet (i.e. removal of all milk and galactose-containing foods). With the exception of mental retardation which is permanent once established, maintenance of a galactose-free diet may cause reversal of many of the other clinical symptoms of galactosaemia or, in some cases, at least halt their progression. Even total exclusion of galactose from the diet, however, does not ensure the absence of all pathology (Gitzelmann and Steinmann, 1984).

Newborn screening programmes for galactosaemia have been implemented in many parts of the world on the premise that early detection and treatment may reduce the occurrence of the negative outcomes of this condition. As in the case of phenylketonuria, the screening process for galactosaemia involves collection of a blood sample, via a heel-prick onto filter paper, from every newborn child during the first week of life.

Varying degrees of success for galactosaemia screening programmes have been reported in the literature. Gitzelmann and Steinmann (1984) reported that although early- and well-treated children with galactosaemia show satisfactory general health and growth and make reasonable but suboptimal intellectual progress, they are, none the less, prone to developing speech deficits, ovarian failure and visual perceptual difficulties and in some cases exhibit social maladjustment. Similarly, the results of a study by Waisbren *et al.* (1983) showed that early-treated children with galactosaemia are at risk for developing speech and language difficulties. They found that all eight of their early-treated galactosaemic children exhibited delays or early speech difficulties and that all except one developed subsequent language problems. Waisbren *et al.* (1983) did not specify the tests used to assess the children's language. In addition, their criterion for a deficit has been questioned by some authors (Hayes *et al.*, 1986). 'A deficit is defined as one standard deviation below the mean on tests with standardized norms or 1 year below chronological age on tests with age norms' (Waisbren *et al.*, 1983: 76). Hayes *et al.* (1986: 238) concluded that 'in the absence of information on the tests and the children's scores, there is insufficient information to support the authors' conclusions'.

In contrast to the findings of Waisbren *et al.* (1983), Hayes *et al.* (1988) provided preliminary data indicating that neonatal screening and careful management results in improved outcomes for children with galactosaemia. In particular these authors found that while children with galactosaemia diagnosed before the introduction of neonatal screening had intellectual development in the low average to moderately handicapped range, children with galactosaemia diagnosed subsequent to the introduction of neonatal screening appeared to be developing normally. In addition, although most (5 of 7) of the children in their pre-screening group presented with speech and language difficulties, only one child (1 of 6) in their screened group presented with a speech and language deficit, this latter child showing mild expressive language and moderate articulation delays. The expressive language was reported to be characterized by immature syntax. In addition, Hayes *et al.* (1988) indicated that the speech of this child was affected by a phonological processing disorder which involved stopping and idiosyncratic palatization of fricatives.

In summary, although reports in the literature before the introduction of neonatal screening programmes have included speech and language disorders amongst the various outcomes of galactosaemia (Jan and Wilson, 1973; Komrower and Lee, 1970; Lee, 1972), at present the chances of early-treated children with galactosaemia developing speech and language problems is uncertain, with conflicting evidence having been reported to date. Further research is therefore needed to establish the long-term outcomes of early-treated galactosaemia. Until such time as these outcomes are clarified, however, all children with galactosaemia should be considered as having the potential to develop speech and language problems and therefore the development of their speech and language skills should be monitored.

Wilson's Disease (Hepato-Lenticular Degeneration)

Wilson's disease is a rare, inborn error of metabolism inherited as an autosomal recessive disorder. The condition is characterized by progressive degenerative changes in the brain and liver resulting from a deficiency in the body's ability to process dietary copper. As a consequence of this deficiency copper accumulates in the tissues of the body, especially in the brain, liver and cornea of the eye. The basal ganglia are the most severely affected parts of the brain, although smaller amounts of copper may also be deposited in the cerebellum, brainstem and parts of the cerebrum. Of the basal ganglia, the corpus striatum is most involved, with a greater degree of damage occurring in the putamen than in the caudate nucleus. Cirrhosis of the liver also occurs and the deposition of copper in the eye gives a greenish-brown colour to the cornea (Kayser–Fleisher rings).

Two separate neurological pictures characterize Wilson's disease, an acute form and a more chronic form. The acute form usually has an onset around puberty and is characterized by dystonia. It is this form of the disorder that involves paediatric clinicians and will, therefore, be described more fully here. The more chronic form, on the other hand, usually manifests around 19–35 years of age. It has a slowly progressive course and is characterized by a tremor and rigidity.

The initial symptoms of the acute form of Wilson's disease vary from mild slowing of voluntary movements to dysarthria and mental changes. The latter includes problems with memory and concentration as well as mild personality changes such as increased irritability and emotional lability. In terms of the disturbances in speech, Berry *et al.* (1974) described a mixed ataxic-hypokinetic-spastic dysarthria as a feature of Wilson's disease. Dystonia appears as a later symptom and serves to differentiate the acute form from the more chronic form. Ultimately, deterioration of intellectual function becomes evident. The face may become mask-like and drooling is common.

The course of the acute form is progressive unless treatment is provided. The rate of progress varies greatly and partial remissions and exacerbations may occur in some cases. Untreated Wilson's disease is invariably fatal. Treatment involves restricting the intake of dietary copper and use of D-penicillamine to reduce the blood copper levels. Rosselli *et al.* (1987) showed the improvement of one case with Wilson's disease on neuropsychological assessment after treatment with D-penicillamine. Similar improvements have also been documented by Hach and Hartung (1979). In a recent study, Lang and co-workers (see Lang, 1989) investigated the long-term neuropsychological outcome of 15 subjects with Wilson's disease after long-term treatment with D-penicillamine. They found, when compared with a control group, that the patients with Wilson's disease had mild deficits on divergent naming tasks and visuospatial/logical processing but not on auditory memory tasks (Lang, 1989). It is possible, therefore that speech and language pathologists may be involved with patients with Wilson's disease in both the acute form for dysarthria and after treatment of the chronic form for naming difficulties.

Other Metabolic Disorders Causing Speech/Language Disorders

Hypothyroidism

Clinical characteristics

Thyroid hormones are important regulators of the metabolic activity of the body. An adequate supply of thyroid hormone is also necessary for the normal development of the nervous system, especially during the first few months after birth. Consequently, an absence or deficiency of thyroid hormone during this period has a profound effect on brain development. In particular, thyroid deficiency in the first year of life leads to inadequate brain cell and dendritic development (de Escobar *et al.*, 1983) leading to a reduction in the intellectual potential of the affected child (Frost, 1986; Frost *et al.*,

1979). Speech/language disorders have been reported in association with the depressed intellectual abilities of hypothyroid children (Dussault *et al.*, 1980).

Congenital hypothyroidism can result from congenital absence of the thyroid gland, thyroid hypoplasia (underdevelopment of the thyroid gland) or, less commonly, from an enzymatic defect in the production of thyroid hormones. If left untreated, congenital hypothyroidism leads to cretinism, a classical clinical syndrome in which the affected individual exhibits marked mental retardation and deficiency in intellect as well as retarded skeletal growth and maturation. The child, termed a cretin, has a large head, short limbs, puffy eyes, a thick and protruding tongue, excessively dry skin, a lack of motor coordination (ataxia) and a low IQ (often below 75).

In recent years, early detection through neonatal screening and prompt treatment with replacement thyroid hormone in the first weeks of life has greatly improved the mental and physical prognosis of children with congenital hypothyroidism. As a consequence of such action, the incidence of classical cretinism has declined. Despite this several studies have shown that especially in those cases where either the diagnosis and treatment was delayed for several weeks after birth or where the patients were negligent in adhering to the treatment programme (i.e. neglected to take medication), the average IQ of children treated for hypothyroidism is one to two standard deviations below that of matched controls (Birrell *et al.*, 1983; Hulse, 1984). In addition, these children may also exhibit a range of neurological problems, including difficulties with coordination and balance, abnormal limb tone and reflexes, abnormal fine motor movement, speech problems, squints and marked behavioural disturbances (Frost, 1986; Hulse, 1984).

It would appear, therefore, that amongst children with congenital hypothyroidism, speech and language disorders may be related to a child's intellectual ability and/or neurological functioning.

Linguisitic deficits associated with hypothyroidism

As mentioned above, children who receive treatment for congenital hypothyroidism within the first three months of life develop intellectual functioning within the normal range (Frost, 1986; Glorieux *et al.*, 1985; Moschini *et al.*, 1986; Murphy *et al.*, 1986; New England Congenital Hypothyroidism Collaborative, 1985). Yet there are still some children who do not reach their full potential and present with less than average cognitive and/or neurological functioning. This then has implications for the speech/language pathologist dealing with such children. In this section we will discuss what factors in a child relate to poor prognosis, whether there is any evidence for specific linguistic deficits outside of depressed intellectual ability, and what are the implications of poor neurological outcome.

Some studies (Glorieux *et al.*, 1985; Rovet *et al.*, 1987) have shown that despite

IQ scores being within normal limits, children with hypothyroidism as a group have significantly lower IQ scores than their siblings or a group of matched controls. Such a difference, however, has not been found in the group of hypothyroid children studied by the New England Congenital Hypothyroidism Collaborative (1985). The distribution of the IQ scores obtained from children with congenital hypothyroidism reflects the distribution seen in the normal population (Frost, 1986). Some authors report an increase in IQ scores over time (Frost, 1986). One of the factors which relates to a poor prognosis for cognitive functioning in a child with congenital hypothyroidism is, as mentioned above, non-compliance with treatment. Other factors include perinatal and/or socio-emotional problems (Moschini *et al.*, 1986) such as: socio-economic status (Dussault *et al.*, 1980); delay in treatment (Sack et al., 1986) although this effect has disappeared with the advent of neonatal screening procedures, and the absence of thyroid tissue in the child (Murphy et al., 1986; Sack *et al.*, 1986). Children born without any thyroid tissue (athyrotic) have been found to have a poorer performance on intelligence tests than children who have reduced thyroid function (ectopic), even though there is often a delay in diagnosis in the ectopic group. Again this effect seems to have disappeared since the introduction of neonatal screening (Glorieux *et al.*, 1985; Sack *et al.*, 1986).

Glorieux *et al.* (1988) examined pretreatment factors that could predict the consistently lower performance of certain children in the group of 150 children with congenital hypothyroidism included in their longitudinal study. Thirteen subjects who had IQ scores below or equal to 90 were found to differ from the other subjects only on their initial thyroxine (T_4) values and their bone maturation score. Glorieux *et al.* (1988) then tested these parameters as predictive factors for cognitive development. They concluded that initial thyroxine values of less than 2 g per day, and bone maturation scores (calculated by measuring the surface areas of the ossification centres of the knee) of less than $0.05cm^2$, could be used for early identification of children with congenital hypothyroidism whose prognosis was poor.

The factors discussed above therefore affect the cognitive abilities of children with congenital hypothyroidism. These same factors can be said to affect some speech and language skills as part of an overall cognitive delay in this same group of children. Information relating specifically to the speech and language skills seen in children with congenital hypothyroidism, however, is not readily available to clinicians as, to date, no study designed to describe the linguistic abilities of children with congenital hypothyroidism has been reported. While we can predict poor linguistic outcome associated with poor cognitive prognosis, an examination of cognitive profiles which include information on verbal abilities must be used to predict specific linguistic deficits until the results of appropriate research becomes available. The few studies, however, that do report separate verbal scores on the WISC-R, the Gesell Developmental Test or the Griffiths Mental Developmental Scales would indicate that most subjects with congenital hypothyroidism obtained verbal scores within a ten point range of either their global IQ or performance IQ scores (Frost and Parkin, 1986; Glorieux *et al.*, 1988).

Moschini *et al.* (1986) noted that language scores of children with congenital hypothyroidism did not show any change over the ages of 6 months to 3 years as measured on the Brunet-Lezine Test (no reference available). However, examination of individual scores show that although the group mean did not change, the range of scores did. At 18, 24 and 36 months of age the individual language scores showed the greatest range of scores of all developmental scales. Again in two cases of children with congenital hypothyroidism the verbal scores appeared to be lower than the global developmental quotient. Moschini *et al.* (1986) felt that perinatal risks and socio-emotional conditions accounted for all children with congenital hypothyroidism who had low developmental quotients. Therefore, as in children with phenylketonuria there may be individual children who exhibit specific linguistic deficits. In some cases, however, this may relate to factors other than those directly resulting from congenital hypothyroidism.

Also like children with phenylketonuria it would appear that the majority of language impairments seen in children with congenital hypothyroidism are associated with a decreased intellectual ability and as such are affected by those risk factors that have been documented as indicating a poor cognitive prognosis. Some studies are available to support this hypothesis. Glorieux *et al.* (1988) found a significantly lower verbal IQ score on the WISC-R and the Griffiths Mental Developmental Scales in a group of children with low T_4 values and retarded bone maturation before treatment. A study by Rovet *et al.* (1987) also reported similar results in a group of children with congenital hypothyroidism, who had delayed skeletal maturity. In this study the children were assesssed on a yearly basis and compared with another group of children with congenital hypothyroidism, but with normal skeletal maturity. At 12 months of age there was no difference between the two groups; however, by 2 years of age the children with delayed skeletal maturity scored significantly lower on all scales of the Griffiths Developmental Scales, including Hearing and Speech, even though all individual scores were within normal limits. There was no difference between groups at 2 years of age on the Receptive or Expressive Scales of the Reynell Developmental Language Scales (RDLS) (Reynell, 1977). At 4 years of age, the RDLS scores for both the receptive and expressive language scales were significantly lower for the children with congenital hypothyroidism with delayed skeletal development, as were the scores on the McCarthy Scales of Children's Abilities. By 5 years of age only the language comprehension scores on the RDLS and the motor subscore on the McCarthy Scales were significantly lower. The 5-year-old children with delayed skeletal development also scored significantly lower on the WISC-R quotients of full IQ and performance IQ (but not verbal IQ) and the WISC-R subtests, vocabulary geometric design and block design. Lower scores were also obtained on the Beery Buktenica Development Test of Motor Integration. This led Rovet *et al.* (1987) to conclude that children with congenital hypothyroidism who have delayed skeletal maturity have specific deficits in neuromotor, perceptual and language aspects of intellectual functioning. Since it was the RDLS comprehension score and the vocabulary subtest of the WISC-R which were significantly lower it may be that these language scores only represent a generalized cognitive deficit rather than a specific linguistic deficit. Therefore more research into the linguistic abilities of children with congenital hypothyroidism is required before definitive statements can be made about specific language deficits, even in the group of children with congenital hypothyroidism and delayed bone maturation.

The other aspect of congenital hypothyroidism which may result in communication disorders is neurological impairments which are often noted in the literature. Several studies report motor impairments in children with congenital hypothyroidism when compared with matched controls (Murphy *et al.*, 1986; New England Congenital Hypothyroidism Collaborative, 1985; Rovet *et al.*, 1987). As yet no studies have assessed articulation or oromotor skills in children with congenital hypothyroidism.

Hypotonia was evident in 73 per cent of the hypothyroid cases studied by Moschini *et al.* (1986) when examined at 33 ± 12 days of age. Nineteen per cent of the cases studied by Moschini *et al.* (1986) also presented with feeding problems. Feeding problems were also reported by Thompson *et al.* (1986); 10 per cent were in the ectopic gland group and 44 per cent were in the athyrotic group.

Frost and Parkin (1986) listed the major neurological problems in subjects with congenital hypothyroidism including: poor fine motor coordination, squints, and nystagmus and speech impairment in both children and adults. They reported that 22 per cent of children and 18 per cent of adults had received speech therapy, and 38 per cent of children and 28 per cent of adults presented with dysarthria. Furthermore 37 per cent of the children and 26 per cent of adults with congenital hypothyroidism had three or more signs of cerebellar dysfunction (i.e. 'intention tremor, dysdiadochokinesis, poor coordination, ataxia, abnormalities of balance and Romberg's sign, dysarthria, nystagmus') (Frost and Parkin, 1986: 483). Frost (1986) suggested that the cerebellum may be affected *in utero* by thyroxine deficiency causing motor coordination to be more affected than cognitive functioning even if early treatment is available.

Therefore the role of the speech/language pathologist in cases of congenital hypothyroidism may be in monitoring language development and conducting parent education programmes, especially for those children with risk factors for a poor prognosis. A greater involvement, however, may be required with the hypothyroid cases that present with impaired neurological functioning at the early stages in the area of feeding and later in the treatment of their dysarthria.

References

BERRY, W. R., DARLY, F. L. ARONSON, A. E. and GOLDSTEIN, N. P. (1974) 'Dysarthria in Wilson's disease', *Journal of Speech and Hearing Research*, **17**, pp. 167–83.

BERRY, H. K., O'GRADY, D. J., PERLMUTTER, L. J. and BOFINGER, M. K. (1979) 'Intellectual development and academic achievement of children early treated for phenylketonuria', *Developmental Medicine and Child Neurology*, **21**, pp. 311–20.

BIRRELL, J., FROST, G. J. and PARKIN, J. M. (1983) 'The development of children with congenital hypothyroidism', *Development Medicine and Child Neurology*, **25**, pp. 502–11.

BOEHME, G, and THEILE, H. (1972) 'Speech disorders in phenylketonuria', *Deutsch Gesundheitsw*, **27**, pp. 561–3.

BROWN, R. (1973) *A First Language*, Cambridge Ma. Northwestern University Press.

BZOCH, K. R. and LEAGUE, R. (1971) *Assessing Language Skills in Infancy*, Tallahassee, Anhinga Press.

DE ESCOBAR, G. M., RUIZ-MARCOS, A. and REY, DEL F. E. (1983)'Thyroid hormone and the development brain', in Dussault, J. H. and Walker, P. (Eds.) *Congenital Hypothyroidism*, New York, Marcel Dekker.

DUNN, L. M. (1965) *Peabody Picture Vocabulary Test*, Minnesota, American Guidance Service.

DUSSAULT, J. H., LETARTE, J., GLORIEUX, J. MORRISSETTE, J. and GUYDA, H. (1980) 'Psychological development of hypothyroid infants at age 12 and 18 months experience after neonatal screening', in Burrows, G. N. (Ed.) *Neonatal Thyroid Screening*, New York, Raven Press.

FISHER, H. B. and LOGEMANN, J. A. (1971) *The Fisher–Logemann Test of Articulation Competence*, Chicago, The Riverside Publishing Company.

FROST, G. J. (1986) 'Aspects of congenital hypothyroidism', *Child Care, Health and Development*, **12**, pp. 369–75.

FROST, G. J., PARKIN, J. M. and ROWLEY, D. (1979) 'Congenital hypothyroidism', *Lancet* **ii**, p. 1026.

FROST, G. J., and PARKIN, J. M. (1986) 'A comparison between the neurological and intellectual abnormalities in children and adults with congenital hypothyroidism', *European Journal of Pediatrics*, **145**, pp. 480–4.

GITZELMANN, R. and STEINMANN, B. (1984) 'Galactosemia; How does long–term treatment change outcome', *Enzyme*, **32**, pp. 37–46.

GLORIEUX, J., DESJARDINS, M., LETARTE, J., MORISSETTE, J. and DUSSAULT, J. H. (1988) 'Useful parameters to predict the eventual mental outcome of hypothyroid children', *Pediatric Research*, **24**, pp. 6–8.

GLORIEUX, J., DUSSAULT, J. H., MORISSETTE, J., DESJARDINS, M., LETARTE, J. and GUYDA, H. (1985) 'Follow-up at ages 5 and 7 years on mental development in children with hypothyroidism detected by Quebec Screening Program', *Journal of Pediatrics*, **107**, pp. 913–15.

GOLDMAN, R. and FRISTOE, M. (1969) *Goldman Fristoe Test of Articulation*, Circle Pines, American Guidance Service.

HACH, B. and HARTUNG, M. L. (1979) 'The effect of penicillamine on the mental disorders associated with Wilsons's Disease', *Nervenarzi*, **50**, pp. 115–20.

HAMMILL, D.D., BROWN, V.L., LARSEN, S.C. and WIEDERHOLT, J.L. (1987) *Test of Adolescent Language-2: A Multidimensional Approach to Assessment*, Texas, Pro-ed.

HAMMILL, D.D. and NEWCOMER, P.L. (1982) *Test of Language Development — Intermediate*, Texas, Pro-ed.

HAYES, A., ELKINS, J., FRASER, D., BOWLING, F., CLAGUE, A., KRIMMER, H. and MARRINAN, A. (1986) 'Galactosaemia: A preventable form of mental retardation?' *Australia and New Zealand Journal of Developmental Disabilities*, **12**, pp. 235–41.

HAYES, A., BOWLING, F.G., FRASER, D., KRIMMER, H.L., MARRINAN, A. and CLAGUE, A.E. (1988) 'Neonatal screening and an intensive management programme for galactosaemia: Early evidence of benefits', *Medical Journal of Australia*, **149**, pp. 21–5.

HEDRICK, D.L., PRATHER, E.M. and TOBIN, A.R. (1978) *Sequenced Inventory of Communication Development*, Seattle, University of Washington.

HULSE, J.A. (1984), 'Outcome for congenital hypothyroidism', *Archives of Disease in Childhood*, **59**, pp. 23–30.

JAN, J.E. and WILSON, R.A. (1973) 'Unusual late neurological sequelae in galactosaemia', *Developmental Medicine and Child Neurology*, **15**, p. 72.

KOCH, R., AZEN, C., FRIEDMAN, E.G. and WILLIAMSON, M. (1982) 'Preliminary report on the effects of diet discontinuation in PKU', *Journal of Pediatrics*, **100**, pp. 870–5.

KOCH, R., AZEN, C., FRIEDMAN, E.G. and WILLIAMSON, M.L. (1984) 'Paired comparisons between early treated PKU children and their matched sibling controls on intelligence and school achievement test results at eight years of age', *Journal of Inherited Metabolic Disorders*, **7**, pp. 86–90.

KOFF, E., BOYLE, P. and PEUSCHEL, S.M. (1977) 'Perceptual-motor functioning in children with phenylketonuria', *American Journal of Diseases in Children*, **131**, pp. 1084–7.

KOMROWER, G.M. and LEE, D.H. (1970) 'Long-term follow-up galactosemia', *Archives of Disordered Child*, **45**, p. 367.

LANG, C. (1989) 'Is Wilson's disease a dementing condition?' *Journal of Clinical and Experimental Neuropsychology*, **14**, pp. 569–70.

LEE, D.H. (1972) 'Psychological aspects of galactosemia', *Journal of Mental Deficiency Research*, **16**, pp. 173.

LEE, L. (1974a) *Developmental Sentence Analysis*, Evanston, Northwestern University Press.

LEE, L. (1974b) *The Northwestern Syntax Screening Test*, Evanston, Harvard University Press.

MELNICK, C.R., MICHALS, K.K. and MATALON, R. (1981) 'Linguistic development of children with phenylketonuria and normal intelligence', *Journal of Pediatrics*, **98**, pp. 269–72.

MOSCHINI, L., COSTA, P., MARINELLI, E., MAGGIONI, G., SORCINI CARTA, M., FAZZINI, G., DIODATO, A., SABINI, G., GRANDOLFO, M.E., CARTA, S., PORRO, G., PAOLELLA, A., CORDIALE, S. and BRINCIOTTI, M. (1986) 'Longitudinal assessment of children with congenital hypothyroidism detected by neonatal screening,' *Helvetia Paediatricia Acta*, **41**, pp. 415–24.

MURPHY, G., HULSE, J.A., JACKSON, D., TYRER, P., GLOSSOP, J., SMITH, I. and GRANT, D. (1986) 'Early treated hypothyroidism: development at 3 years', *Archives of Disease in Childhood*, **61**, pp. 761–5.

NETLEY, C., HANLEY, E. B. and RUDNER, H. L. (1984) 'Phenylketonuria and its variants: Observations on intellectual functioning,' *Canadian Medical Association Journal*, **131**, pp. 751–5.

NEW ENGLAND CONGENITAL HYPOTHYROIDISM COLLABORATIVE (1985) 'Neonatal hypothyroidism screening: status of patients at 6 years of age,' *Journal of Pediatrics*, **107**, pp. 915–18.

NEWCOMER, P. L. and HAMMILL, D. D. (1987) *Test of Language Development — Primary.* Austin, Pro Ed.

OZANNE, A. E., KRIMMER, H. and MURDOCH, B. E. 'Speech and language skills in children with early treated phenylketonuria,' *American Journal on Mental Retardation* (In press).

PENNINGTON, B. F. and SMITH, S. D. (1983) 'Genetic influence on learning disabilities and speech and language disorders,' *Child Development*, **54**, pp. 369–87.

PENNINGTON, B. F., VAN DOORNICK, W. J., MCCABE, L. L. and MCCABE, E. R. B. (1985) 'Neurological deficits in early treated phenylketonuric children', *American Journal of Mental Deficiency*, **89**, pp. 467–75.

REYNELL, J. (1977) *Reynell Developmental Language Scales — Revised*, Oxford, NFER Publishing Company Ltd.

ROSENBERG, R. N. and PETTEGREW, J. W. (1980) 'Genetic diseases of the nervous system,' in Rosenberg R.N. (Ed.) *Neurology*, Vol.5, New York, Grune and Stratton.

ROSSELLI, M., LORENZANA, P., ROSSELLI, A. and VERGARA, I. (1987) 'Wilson's disease, a reversible dementia: Case Report,' *Journal of Clinical and Experimental Neuropsychology*, **9**, pp. 399–406.

ROVET, J., EHRLICH, R. and SORBARA, D. (1987) 'Intellectual outcome in children with fetal hypothyroidism,' *Journal of Pediatrics*, **110**, pp. 700–4.

SACK, J., ELICER, A., SOFRIN, R., THEODOR, R. and COHEN, B. (1986) 'Influence on psychological development of early treatment of congenital hypothyroidism detected by neonatal screening: a controlled study', *Israel Journal of Medical Sciences*, **22**, pp. 24–8.

SEASHORE, M. R., FRIEDMAN, E., NOVELLY, R. A. and BAPAT, V. (1985) 'Loss of intellectual function in children with phenylketonuria after relaxation of dietary phenylalanine restriction,' *Pediatrics*, **75**, pp. 226–32.

THOMPSON, G. N., MCCROSSIN, R. B., PENFOLD, J. L., WOODROFFE, P., ROSE, W. A. and ROBERTSON, E. F. (1986) 'Management and outcome of children with congenital hypothyroidism detected on neonatal screening in South Australia,' *Medical Journal of Australia*, **145**, pp. 18–22.

VOGEL, F. (1985) 'Phenotypic deviations in heterozygotes of phenylketonuria (PKU),' *Progress in Clinical and Biological Research*, **177**, pp. 337–49.

WAISBREN, S. E., NORMAN, T. R., SCHNELL, R. R. and LEVY, H. L. (1983) 'Speech and language deficits in early-treated children with galactosaemia,' *Journal of Pediatrics*, **102**, pp. 75–7.

WAISBREN, S. E., SCHNELL, R. R. and LEVY, H. L. (1980) 'Diet termination in children with phenylketonuria: A review of psychological assessments used to determine outcome,' *Journal of Inherited Metabolic Diseases*, **3**, pp. 149–53.

Chapter 7

Communicative Impairments in Neural Tube Disorders

Bruce E. Murdoch, Anne E. Ozanne and Veronica Smyth

Introduction

During the early weeks of pregnancy, the central nervous system (CNS), including both the brain and spinal cord, develops from a hollow cylinder of cells called the neural tube. Congenital malformations of the nervous system which arise from defective formation of the neural tube in the embryo are referred to as neural tube disorders. In that failure of the neural tube to form properly also causes disruption of supportive tissues such as bone, muscle and connective tissue, as well as producing abnormalities in the central nervous system, neural tube disorders also cause defects in overlying structures such as the vertebrae and cranium. The aetiological factor or factors which cause neural tube disorders in humans have not been clearly defined, although both genetic and environmental factors have been implicated (Simpson, 1976). Overall the incidence of neural tube disorders is approximately 2.6 per 1000 total single births.

Neural tube disorders can involve anatomical deformities in either the brain or spinal cord. The major types of neural tube disorders include anencephaly, encephalocele and spina bifida. The more severe types of neural tube disorders, such as anencephaly, are incompatible with extra-uterine life. Consequently children with this disorder do not form part of the clinical caseloads of speech pathologists and will, therefore, be mentioned only briefly here. Less severe neural tube disorders, however, such as several forms of spina bifida are compatible with extra-uterine life. Although extra-uterine life is possible, some of these less severe neural tube disorders may cause functional disabilities manifest as a variety of neurological problems which may include, amongst others, impaired intellectual abilities and communication deficits.

Spinal Cord Abnormalities

Spina Bifida

Spina bifida, which literally translated means 'bifid spine', is a term used to refer to a number of different neural tube disorders involving defective fusion of structures dorsal to the spinal cord. Females are affected more commonly than males in a ratio of approximately 1.3 : 1 (Anderson and Spain, 1977). Overall the incidence of spina bifida varies from 1 to 2 per 1000 live births (Anderson and Spain, 1977; Knowlton *et al.*, 1985). Although spina bifida may occur anywhere along the length of the vertebral column, it is most common in the lower thoracic, lumbar and sacral regions.

Depending on the involvement of the underlying meninges and spinal cord, several different types of spina bifida are recognized. These include: spina bifida occulta and spina bifida cystica (including spina bifida with meningocele and spina bifida with myelomeningocele, and spina bifida with myeloschisis). Of the different types of spina bifida, occulta is the most common followed by spina bifida with myeloschisis. Many of the infants with the latter condition, however, are born dead or die within a few days of birth from infection of the spinal cord.

In its simplest form (spina bifida occulta), spina bifida involves a failure of the bilateral dorsal laminae of the vertebrae to fuse in the midline to form a single spinous process. As a result of this failure, two unfused halves of the vertebral arch remain as short spines on either side of the midline. The defect may not, however, be limited to abnormal growth of the neural arches, but may also involve the meninges, especially in those cases where the defect in the vertebral column is large. In such cases the meninges may herniate through the defect in the vertebral column to form a large fluid-filled cyst on the child's back. Such a condition is called spina bifida cystica.

Spina Bifida Occulta

Spina bifida occulta, the most common but least serious form of spina bifida, involves an absence of the spinous process of one or more vertebrae. The vertebral defect, usually located in the lumbosacral region, is covered by postvertebral muscles and skin and in most cases is not evident from the surface. Occasionally, however, a small tuft of hair or fatty tumour may be present over the defect (Figure 7.1).

In that the spinal cord and nerve roots lie in their normal position in the vertebral canal and are therefore not damaged, spina bifida occulta is usually symptomless, with no neurological or musculoskeletal abnormalities being present. Consequently, spina bifida occulta is also not usually associated with the occurrence of speech/language or hearing deficits. Often the condition is only detected by chance when radiographs are taken of the vertebral column.

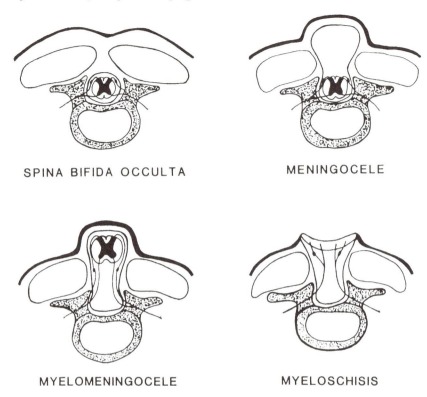

SPINA BIFIDA OCCULTA   MENINGOCELE

MYELOMENINGOCELE   MYELOSCHISIS

Figure 7.1 Diagrammatic sketches showing the major types of spina bifida and the commonly associated malformations of the nervous system

Spina Bifida with Meningocele

In this type of spina bifida the meninges protrude through the defect in the vertebral column to form a cystic swelling covered by skin, usually in the lumbosacral region of the child's back. The spinal cord and cauda equina, however, remain in their normal position in the vertebral canal (Figure 7.1) and therefore function normally. As a result there may be no abnormal neurological signs present in children with spina bifida with meningocele and, as in the case of spina bifida occulta, communication disorders are an unlikely occurrence. The meningocele can be repaired surgically.

Spina Bifida with Myelomeningocele

Spina bifida with myelomeningocele is another form of spina bifida cystica and is the type of spina bifida most likely to cause communication disorders. It differs from spina bifida with meningocele in that in addition to the meninges the spinal cord or cauda equina also protrude through the defect in the vertebral column and adhere to the inner surface of the meningeal cyst (Figure 7.1). The cystic swelling in this case is covered by a thin membrane which is easily ruptured and is present in most cases in the lumbar and lumbosacral regions.

Menelaus (1980) reported that myelomeningocele occurs in 94 per cent of cases of spina bifida cystica. In Australia, myelomeningoceles occur with a frequency of 0.95 per 1000 births (Simpson, 1976). Unlike the two types of spina bifida described above, spina bifida with myelomeningocele does cause a variety of neurological impairments including: paralysis or paresis of the lower limbs, sensory loss (anaesthesia), autonomic disturbances including bladder and bowel incontinence and urine retention, mental and emotional disturbances, and an unusual system of usage and delivery of speech ('cocktail party speech').

The segmental level of the lesion determines the area of anaesthesia and which muscles are affected. In general, a child with a myelomeningocele will be unable to move the muscles receiving their nerve supply from the spinal cord below the level of the lesion. The most severely physically handicapped children with myelomeningocele are those with lesions at or above the third lumbar vertebra who are totally paraplegic (Anderson and Spain, 1977; Smith, 1965). Cases with lesions at or below the fourth lumbar vertebra suffer from paralysis of some, but not all, of the muscles of the hips, knees and feet. Children with lesions at the first and second sacral vertebrae may have adequate function of the hips but have paralysis of the feet. Least handicapped are children with lesions at or below the third sacral vertebra. Although these latter children may have normal function of the lower limbs, they may be incontinent (Smith, 1965). Overall, between 30 to 50 per cent of all children with a myelomeningocele show a total paraplegia while most others have significant locomotor problems (Anderson and Spain, 1977). Children with severe functional impairment may require a wheelchair for mobility.

In addition to motor problems, damage to the spinal cord in cases of myelomeningocele results in anaesthesia in parts of the body receiving their nerve supply from the spinal cord below the level of the lesion (Anderson and Spain, 1977). Anaesthesia of the lower limbs may lead to the development of pressure sores and increases the child's susceptibility to burns and frostbite because the child feels no discomfort for extremes of temperature.

Menelaus (1980) reported that only 7 per cent of persons with myelomeningocele have normal urinary and bowel control. Urinary control is generally achieved through intermittent self-catheterization or urinary diversion. Management of bowel incontinence is achieved through developing regular habits of elimination with the use of suppositories. Urinary incontinence increases the risk of urinary tract infection and kidney damage.

Some of the neurological deficits shown by children suffering from spina bifida with myelomeningocele are the direct consequence of the spinal cord defect, while others arise from hindbrain anomalies or deformities. One complication often associated with myelomeningocele that has important clinical consequences is hydrocephalus. Approximately 72 per cent of children with spina bifida develop hydrocephalus (Menelaus, 1980). In infants the bones of the skull are not fused. Consequently, as a result of the accumulation of cerebrospinal fluid (CSF), the heads of infants with untreated hydrocephalus expand without necessarily causing much damage to the brain itself. In older children, however, where the skull bones have fused increased intracranial pressure resulting from the increase in volume of CSF causes compression and damage to the brain, and if not relieved leads to impaired control of the movements of the upper and lower limbs, ocular defects and progressive loss of sight and eventually to cognitive and communication impairments. Apart from death in the first few weeks of life, of which hydrocephalus is a major cause, the major significance of the presence of hydrocephalus is that the long-term problems of myelomeningocele, including impaired communicative and intellectual abilities, are, for the greater part, due to the effects of hydrocephalus on the brain. For instance, research suggests that hydrocephalus and its complications are the primary associated features of children with spina bifida who show evidence of decreased cognitive skills (Knowlton *et al.*, 1985).

The occurrence of hydrocephalus in children with myelomeningocele is largely accounted for by two structural anomalies: the Arnold–Chiari hindbrain malformation and stenosis of the aqueduct of Sylvius. In some spina bifida children both of these abnormalities may occur. Arnold–Chiari malformation often coexists with myelomeningocele. The malformation consists of a caudal displacement of the hindbrain involving projection of components of the medulla oblongata, cerebellum, choroid plexus and fourth ventricle through the foramen magnum into the spinal canal. As a consequence of this caudal displacement, the circulation of CSF is blocked at the foramina of the fourth ventricle leading to the accumulation of fluid in the ventricular system of the brain.

As in the case of spina bifida with meningocele, children with myelomeningocele can be treated surgically. The cyst is opened and the spinal cord or nerves are freed and carefully replaced in the vertebral canal. Full recovery of function, however, rarely if ever occurs. Associated hydrocephalus, if present, may be controlled by insertion of either a ventriculoperitoneal shunt or a ventriculoatrial shunt which reduce the abnormally high cerebrospinal fluid pressure and maintain normal intracranial pressure by draining fluid away from the ventricles of the brain. Complications of shunting procedures include occasional obstruction of the catheter due to growth of the child, infection, blockage of the shunt and disconnection of the shunt (Anderson and Spain, 1977). Not every child with hydrocephalus, however, requires surgical treatment. In some cases the hydrocephalus becomes 'arrested' in that the amount of CSF produced becomes balanced with the amount of CSF absorbed. In such children, the head stops growing at an abnormal rate.

Spina Bifida with Myeloschisis (Myelocele)

This type of spina bifida results from a failure of the neural tube to close, usually in the lumbosacral region (Figure 7.1). Consequently the spinal cord appears on the surface of the child's back as a raw area in the configuration of the wide-open neural plate. CSF discharges from the central canal of the spinal cord onto the surface of this raw patch. In that microorganisms have easy access to the exposed CNS, the chance of survival of infants with this condition is slight.

Brain Abnormalities

Anencephaly

Anencephaly is a severe condition that occurs in approximately 1 in every 1000 births and results from a failure of the neural tube to close at the cranial end. As a result the cerebral hemispheres are absent and the cranial vault fails to form. Laurence and Weeks (1971) reported that anencephaly occurs four times more often in females than males. Anencephaly is not compatible with sustained extra-uterine life and is, therefore, not related to the occurrence of communication deficits.

Encephalocele

Encephalocele occurs in approximately 1 in every 2000 births and involves the protrusion of a portion of the brain and meninges through a defect in the skull (cranium bifidum) (Figure 7.2). The defect is always in the midline and occurs most commonly in the occipital region. The condition is often accompanied by hydrocephalus.

If the protruding meningeal sac contains only CSF, the brain remaining within the cranium, the condition is called cranial meningocele. In some cases the cranial defect may be repaired.

Audiological Manifestations in Spina Bifida

While the myelodysplasias described above occur amongst the most common developmental defects of the CNS, there have been relatively few significant clinical studies detailing the audiological status of children with such lesions, with or without associated hydrocephalus. However, improvements in valve-regulated shunt insertion methods would in any event relegate studies other than contemporary reports to a position of redundancy and their interpretation largely irrelevant. Similarly as Bigler (1988) reported, brain imaging (computed tomography (CT) and magnetic resonance imaging (MRI) technology) now enables far more accurate CNS examination than in the past, which will facilitate more meaningful clinical investigation in the future as these techniques provide an *in vivo* method of assessing ventricular size and the presence of cortical destruction.

Peripheral Auditory Pathway Function

Peripheral hearing loss does not occur generally in spina bifida and although published studies occasionally indicate the presence of hearing loss in sample populations, details are sparse. For example Billard *et al.* (1986) in their study of 77 spina bifida children with hydrocephalus, reported one case of deafness, without detailing the subject's characteristics. Dorman *et al.* (1984) reported normal speech perception in a $16\frac{1}{2}$-year-

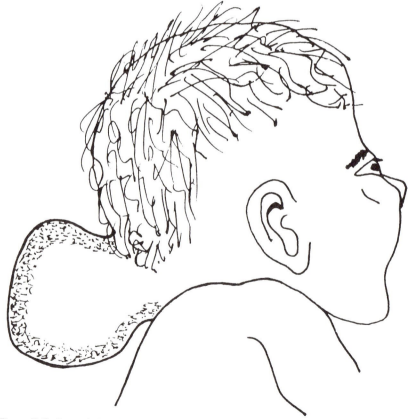

Figure 7.2 Encephalocele

old male with a lumbar (L-1) level lesion with unshunted spontaneous arrest of hydrocephalus before 12 months of age. However, the assessment used by Dorman *et al.* (1984) was part of a neuropsychological test battery which did not include formal or standard calibration audiological test procedures in determining speech perception ability. Hearing loss has, however, been reported to occur in association with hydrocephalus in children (de L. Costello *et al.*, 1988; Fernell *et al.*, 1988). Fernell *et al.* (1988) followed a population-based series of 68 full-term infants with infantile hydrocephalus in which their audiological results indicated two children with moderate (41–55 dBHLA) hearing impairment, one further child with total hearing loss and two other children who were untestable because of severe mental retardation. The child with total hearing loss was multiply handicapped. De L. Costello *et al.* (1988) found a very small incidence of sensorineural hearing loss in very pre-term infants, but nevertheless regarded their results as indicating a tendency for significant hearing loss among children with either ventricular dilation or hydrocephalus/cerebral atrophy.

Routine clinical assessment of a paediatric spina bifida cohort ($n = 16$) by one of the present authors (V.S.), using standardized pure-tone audiological procedures, indicated the presence of peripheral hearing sensitivity within normal range in 15 subjects. In addition one subject, $3\frac{1}{2}$ years of age, unable to be tested via play audiometry techniques, provided behavioural responses using conditioned orienting response audiometry, which were consistent with functionally normal peripheral hearing sensitivity. Such results support the notion of non-involvement of the peripheral auditory system in neural tube disorders.

On the other hand an interesting and novel application of acoustic remittance measurements and acoustic stapedial reflex-induced tympanic membrane displacement was reported by Marchbanks *et al.* (1987). These researchers monitored the effects of changes in intracranial fluid pressure on cochlear fluid pressure following ventriculolumbar peritoneal shunt operations by means of a sensitive time-base capable of resolving tympanic membrane displacements as small as 10^{-9} litres. In the absence of middle ear pathology, pre- and post-operative differences in reflex tympanic membrane displacement could be used to infer changes in the perilymphatic pressure of the inner ear as a result of pressure fluctuations of the CSF. The study was performed on only three subjects, therefore the conclusions are in the nature of a pilot study. Since the transfer of fluid pressure from CSF to perilymph depends largely on cochlear aqueduct patency which is variable, and more usually, subject to early closure, the Marchbanks *et al.* (1987) technique and its interpretation appears confounded, as it seems to require an assumption of aqueduct patency which is therefore unlikely to be met. However, despite this drawback, refinement of the technique in the future may prove to be useful clinically. At the present time an absence of studies implicating the cochlea in hydrocephalus tends to suggest that the peripheral end organ is remote from and unaffected by raised intracranial pressure in neural tube disorders.

The presence of retrocochlear lesions has been suggested audiologically in patients and with Arnold–Chiari malformations, where abnormal auditory adaptation has been noted clinically. However, no research results are available and no studies currently appear to have investigated the peripheral differential audiological test battery profiles associated with neural tube dysfunction.

Central Auditory Pathway Function

Electrophysiological Studies and Neuroaudiology

The neuropathology of posterior neural tube closure defects reported by Gilbert *et al.* (1986) included: (1) spinal cord malformations in addition to the meningomyelocele, and (2) brainstem maldevelopment — distortion, incomplete development (hypoplasia, aplasia or defective myelinization) of cranial nerve nuclei, olivary and basal pontine nuclei and tegmentum, and various developmental anomalies as indicated in Table 7.1 which affect the ventricles, cerebellar, cerebral and other discrete structures. The authors suggested that in those severely impaired children who succumbed in infancy, first, the primary aetiology was not identified, second, their conditions were consistent with a wide spectrum of anomalies of which the presenting physical malformations were features only, and third they did not conform to any theoretical aetiological pattern currently espoused. Other authors have also reported a similar range of neuropathologies in association with neural tube deficits (Warkany and O'Toole, 1981).

It would seem therefore that owing to the possibility of diffuse sites of pathological foci even the most accurate measurable estimates of central auditory pathway function are unlikely to produce evidence of absolute site of lesion involvement. In this context, evoked potential studies have provided consistent

Table 7.1 CNS Gross and microscopic neuropathological post-mortem examination of 25 paediatric patients who had meningomyelocele, hydrocephalus and the Arnold–Chiari malformation. (Collated from Gilbert et al., 1986)

Developmental anomalies	Incidence %
Obstruction of CSF flow within the ventricular system	92
Disorder of migration of cortical neurons	92
Cerebellar dysplasia	72
Brainstem malformation — disorder of myelinization	44
Hypoplasia or aplasia of cranial nerve nuclei	20
Fusion of the thalami	16
Agenesis of the corpus callosum	12
Complete or partial agenesis of the olfactory tract and bulb	8

evidence of auditory brainstem dysfunction across a range of neural tube disorders and types of lesion and pathological outcome. Table 7.2 lists studies representative of auditory brainstem response (ABR) investigations since 1984, which have been concerned with such lesions and outcomes.

The Docherty *et al.* (1987) study reported normal auditory brainstem-evoked potentials in subjects with shunted hydrocephalus due to aqueduct stenosis ($n = 2$) and secondary to intracranial haemorrhage ($n = 2$) but abnormal auditory brainstem evoked potentials in spina bifida aperta (myelocele) subjects with hydrocephalus ($n = 18$). Peripheral hearing sensitivity was normal in all subjects. The auditory brainstem abnormalities seen most often were Jewett Wave V-III and Wave V-I interpeak latency prolonged beyond three standard deviations, suggesting the likelihood of higher pons and lower midbrain dysfunction. Docherty and co-workers suggested that the ABR should be used cautiously as a monitoring device in ventriculoperitoneal shunt procedures because they concluded that the underlying brainstem structure was likely to be malformed producing abnormal responses independently of raised levels of intracranial pressure.

On the other hand, Holliday *et al.* (1985) reported ABR changes (reduced interpeak latencies) in a full-term infant with myelomeningocele, Arnold–Chiari II malformation and shunted hydrocephalus following posterior surgical decompression, with ABR Wave V-I interpeak latencies returning to within normal range 6 days after surgery.

Kraus *et al.* (1984) examined the incidence and nature of ABR abnormalities in hydrocephalus patients from congenital and acquired bases and compared these

Table 7.2 *Auditory brainstem-evoked response studied in children with neural tube-related hydrocephalus*

Authors	Subject n	Classification	ABR Abnormality
Kraus *et al.* (1984)	40	Hydrocephalus due to congenital abnormalities, meningitis or intercranial haemorrhage	yes
Holliday *et al.* (1985)	Case study	Arnold–Chiari	yes
Lütschg *et al.* (1985)	27	Myelomeningocele	yes
Ducati *et al.* (1986)	26	Adequeductal stenosis} Hydrocephalus}	yes (19 subjects)
Docherty *et al.* (1987)	18 4	Myelomeningocele Hydrocephalus only	yes no
Venkataramana (1988)	20} 8}	Congenital hydrocephalus only} with meningomyelocele}	19 subjects

abnormalities with those of other non-hydrocephalus subjects with CNS disorders which commonly manifest ABR abnormalities. Their results supported the contention that hydrocephalus was responsible for auditory brainstem pathway abnormality but the authors did not exclude the possibility that congenital brainstem abnormalities may have been responsible for the observed ABR dysfunction in some cases. The authors also speculated that alterations to the tissue medium, through which the evoked potentials are normally volume conducted, may have contributed to the results observed. Their major observations were Wave I-V prolongation in 33 per cent of hydrocephalus subjects compared with 18 per cent of the remainder and ABR threshold abnormalities including 'no response' in 70 per cent of hydrocephalus subjects with this 'no response' incidence being three times greater than in other groups of patients who frequently show ABR abnormalities (e.g. multiple handicap and following bacterial meningitis).

The ABR threshold estimates were derived from ascending incremental click stimulus presentation using a presentation rate of 20 clicks per second. It is possible that such an ascending protocol coupled with such a click rate, may have contributed to threshold estimations slightly less accurate than can be obtained using a descending click presentation with a 10 or 11 clicks per second presentation rate, which tends to enhance threshold identification in auditory brainstem-evoked recordings. Furthermore, 29 subjects in the Kraus *et al.* (1984) study were less than 3 years of age and 9 subjects were between 3 and 11 years of age and it is not reported in the study whether an incidence of conductive pathology may have been found in this subject group, since they would be considered potentially to be at risk for middle ear disease, on the basis of age alone. The presence of middle ear disease is known to affect ABR thresholds, latencies and morphology, even to the extreme results of 'no response' (Smyth *et al.*, in press).

Lütschg *et al.* (1985) studied 27 myelomeningocele paediatric patients, 17 of whom required shunts; the remaining 10 had never shown evidence of increased intracranial pressure. Subjects were subgrouped into two additional categories, those with and those without clinically detectable cranial nerve defects. Results were compared with normal control subjects. Again the major finding was Wave V-I interpeak prolongation and prolonged absolute Wave V latency in the neural tube-disordered subject group. Subjects with shunted hydrocephalus and cranial nerve defects were most prolonged, subjects without hydrocephalus produced the shortest latencies in the experimental group, but these latencies were still longer than the normal control group values. However, their absolute values in msecs ($WV = \overline{X}5.96$, S.D. 0.15: $WV\text{-}I = \overline{X}4.18$, S.D. 0.28) would be considered clinically normal in most settings. Children with clinical signs of inspiratory stridor gave the most abnormal ABR responses. The authors concluded that the traction theory could explain the presence of stridor, in that Wave V was prolonged in the presence of a normal Wave I in all instances. Consequently, elongation of the brainstem from the cochlear nucleus to the inferior colliculus was considered a possible reason for the prolonged Wave V ABR. Traction theories have been proposed by a number of authors, for example Lütschg *et al.* (1985) noted the hypothesis and Charney *et al.* (1987) discuss its effects. The traction theory regards spinal cord tethering as a cause of the displaced brainstem being pulled virtually into the cervical spinal canal thereby causing traction on the lower cranial nerves.

Ducati *et al.* (1986) suggested that deteriorating changes in the ABR with time may reflect an increase in supratentorial pressure in hydrocephalic children, with good correlations existing between clinical neurological status and the ABR. It is of interest that in four subjects in their study, abnormalities in the ABR were elicited only in sensitized conditions (that is, using an increased click presentation rate of 70 clicks per second, compared with a standard rate of 11 clicks per second). This should be noted since it is considered that clinicians generally do not incorporate sensitized condition studies into their audiological test battery as a routine, and as a result may overlook occult abnormality in the ABR. (Note: this is in contrast to the need for low level click rate presentation in determining ABR thresholds, discussed previously.)

The Venkataramana *et al.* (1988) study is important as it focused on clinically diagnosed subjects with congenital hydrocephalus alone (Group A, *n* = 12) and congenital hydrocephalus with meningomyelocele (Group B, *n* = 8) all of whom were given both CT scan and ABR testing before and after shunt surgery. The preoperative prospective study confirmed the presence of abnormally prolonged absolute Wave V latencies in 75 per cent of children, prolonged Wave V-I interpeak latency in 45 per cent of children and Wave III-I and Wave V-III prolongation each in 35 per cent of children. Three children had absent Wave IV and Wave V. No ABR difference appeared to exist between Group A and Group B. Postoperative monitoring indicated a return to normal within 4–5 months of the ABR response in 50 per cent of subjects. Improvement in interpeak latency, although still beyond normal range was noted in 20 per cent of subjects. In four subjects interpeak latency increased after the operation. CT scanning of the four subjects revealed shunt block and slipped shunt tube in two subjects and bilateral subdural haematoma in the other two subjects. Serial monitoring of all subjects after surgery indicated improvement of Wave III-I latencies, which correlate with caudal brainstem function which recovered the earliest (within 1 month) and rostral brainstem conduction evidenced by Wave V-III latency recovering at a later date. The ABR changes observed correlated with a reduction in ventricular size.

Subjects with abnormal morphology before surgery had postoperative results as follows:

Subject 4   — Recovery of all Wave peaks.

Subject 9   — Recovery of all Wave peaks except Wave IV left (although it could be suggested that Wave IV is subject to electrode montage artefact and may not be clinically significant).

Subject 11 — No ABR right, before surgery, but normal ABR right and left after surgery.

Subject 12 — Wave V only before surgery on the left, but Wave I-II-III present and Wave V absent after surgery on the left.

Subject 13 — Right absent Waves beyond Wave III before surgery, left normal ABR after surgery. Right normal before surgery. Left absent beyond Wave III after surgery.

Venkataramana *et al.* (1988) postulated that proximity of the upper brainstem to the ventricular system may account for Wave V involvement, which appeared more sensitive to change than any other ABR feature in these intriguing and somewhat challenging results. The degree of ventricular dilation on CT scan did not correlate with degree of ABR abnormality but appeared to correlate with ABR improvement in latency and morphology after surgery. The sensitivity of the ABR in this study appeared to relate specifically to intracranial pressure and shunt status.

Gilbert *et al.* (1986) completed autopsy studies on 25 children under 2 years of age who had died with meningomyelocele, the Arnold–Chiari malformation and hydrocephalus. They reported a wide range of CNS malformations including hypoplasia or aplasia of cranial nerve nuclei, obstruction to CSF flow, cerebellar dysplasia, disorder of migration of cortical neurons, fusion of the thalami, corpus callosum agenesis and olfactory tract and bulb agenesis. These anomalies were considered to be developmental defects. Brainstem malformation at the level of the olivary complex indicated hypoplasia/aplasia and there was a marked reduction in the neuronal populations of the hypoglossal and dorsal vagal nuclei. The most common brainstem abnormality was defective myelinization, which was identified in 44 per cent of autopsied subjects.

The functional ABR abnormalities reported in the literature are consistent with such defects. Gilbert and co-workers also reported dysplasia in cerebellar and cerebral cortex structures and associated ventricular system malformation, especially of the aqueduct. Thus their range of malformations encompassed virtually the whole of the CNS. Unfortunately the study gave no indication of case history status which could have provided useful rehabilitative information. For example, the developmental quotient status, behavioural maturational level and cognitive developmental abilities achieved by this subject group, up to their time of death (which was reported as being a mean of 22.4 months of age), was not documented. The fact that the group had succumbed to their condition suggests that the neuropathology observed may have been in excess of the 'average' degree of dysfunction, and thus have been likely to have been representative of the extreme higher end of the range of dysfunction in neuropsychological terms.

Middle- and long-latency cognitive and auditory evoked potentials and electroencephalographic findings in adult hydrocephalus have been studied, with the results generally indicating abnormalities. In a paediatric study, Saukkonen (1988) reported 98 per cent of children with hydrocephalus (mean 2 years of age) to have an abnormal EEG before shunting. However, there has been no significant recent work published in the area of evoked response audiometry using middle- or long-latency protocols in paediatric hydrocephalus or related populations. This fact undoubtedly reflects the uncertainty felt by many clinicians concerning the reliability of middle- and long-latency auditory evoked potentials in paediatric applications. Normative studies are currently lacking and commercial equipment has not been available on a widespread basis to facilitate such studies.

Neuropsychological and neuroaudiological studies

The results of neuropsychological studies investigating the communicative abilities of children with neural tube disorders have typically demonstrated both cognitive and perceptual motor deficits. Attentional deficits (Horn *et al.*, 1985) and memory deficits (Cull and Wyke, 1984) are also documented.

Bigler (1988) in a set of case studies indicated the most common finding of neuropsychological function in hydrocephalus to be a lack of significant correlations between neuropsychological test batteries and neuroanatomy as identified by MRI studies, and although verbal deficits were often less evident than perceptual-based skill deficits, neuropsychological impairment was not predictable but rather characterized by variability.

Renier *et al.* (1988) in a prospective study of 108 prenatal hydrocephalic children, reported a lack of correlation between medical studies and treatment and functional intellectual outcome; however, they did observe a relationship between final postoperative ventricular size and final IQ, with children with normal ventricles performing better than others. The overall mean IQ achieved was 55, with normal IQ achieved in 28 per cent of subjects. Twenty-nine per cent of children in this study attended normal schools. Behavioural reports indicated mild or indeed non-existent behavioural problems in 46 per cent of subjects. Shunt infection proved to carry the poorest prognostic outcome of final IQ.

In a frequently-cited study, Op Heij *et al.* (1985) found no correlations between IQ outcome and degree of primary non-obstructive, non-progressive hydrocephalus in infancy, but performance IQ deficit was more affected by the degree of hydrocephalus than full IQ. The group reported verbal-performance differences in their subjects, with a verbal IQ better than performance IQ (mean difference of 6.9 ± 0.8). Despite this relative strength in verbal IQ, speech development correlated best with the lower overall full IQ level.

Dorman *et al.* (1985) used the Halstead–Reitan and Luria–Nebraska neuropsychological test batteries with adolescent spina bifida subjects and found the Halstead–Reitan speech sounds perceptual testing to be achievable in 29 of 33 subjects in contrast to cerebral palsy and muscular dystrophy subjects where 25 of 47 subjects were unable to perform the task. Non-verbal auditory perception, using the Luria–Nebraska tests appeared deficit prone and memory was another possible deficit area identified in one of the case studies. It was of interest, however, that the subject's musical sense was intact.

Shaffer *et al.* (1985) tested 159 children born with myelomeningocele, using a range of psychological tests and found no significant differences in verbal IQ when compared with normative profiles, whereas performance IQ was significantly reduced. However, a significant subtest score difference was found for digit span, suggesting the presence of memory problems (which could be auditorily based [V.S.]). The WISC factors (i.e. verbal comprehension ability (VCA) and freedom from distractibility (FFD)) produced contrasting outcomes, with the VCA being within normal range, whereas the FFD was significantly lower ($P < .001$) than normative expectancy.

WISC verbal scores were significantly superior to performance scores in children with infantile hydrocephalus (Fernell *et al.*, 1988). Similar results were also found by Billard *et al.* (1986), although they reported that four of the hydrocephalic children had a higher performance IQ than verbal IQ because of expressive language disorders. In one of these four children there was a left sylvian porencephaly, in another there was deafness and the remaining two had marked congenital ventricular dilation. Billard *et al.* (1986) also reported an incidence of deficit function in syntactical comprehension and attention, with disorders noted in 40 per cent of the hydrocephalic subjects in their study.

Aspects of language development in young children with hydrocephalus were studied by Dennis *et al.* (1987). Their tests included aspects of auditory processing via rhyming and immediate memory for sentences. Results were not uniform but there was a trend suggesting that intraventricular hydrocephalus disrupted rhyming functions and word-finding lexical access activities. Sentence recall results produced a significant regression effect with both intraventricular and extraventricular hydrocephalus. The authors concluded that the individual with intraventricular hydrocephalus would be at risk for deficits in central aspects of language involving linguistic content and form and suggested that the verbal memory system was vulnerable to disturbances of intracranial pressure. It is possible that the deficits described were in part attributable to functional central auditory pathway deficits or dysfunction, affecting auditory storage, retrieval and recall. Such factors have not been examined in neural tube disorders.

Further evidence of possible central auditory pathway involvement can be found in the frequent references to attentional problems in various hydrocephalus and spina bifida groups (Knowlton *et al.*, 1985). Such problems may be seen in specific auditory selective attention dysfunction where figure-ground discrimination tasks and ability to attend to relevant stimuli are poor. No recent studies, specifically of perceptual function, involving such tasks have been published although Horn *et al.* (1985) addressed the problem in the visual perceptual domain using a classification task. Their results indicated that spina bifida/hydrocephalus subjects were susceptible to the presence of irrelevant visual stimuli.

An alternative methodology to that of neuropsychology involves the use of speech audiometry as a neuroaudiological diagnostic procedure in assessing central auditory pathway function. Jerger (1987) used her Pediatric Speech Intelligibility test (PSI) in a validation study of children with central nervous system lesions including subject A with surgically resolved hydrocephalus, and subject B with an extra-axial porencephalic cyst and associated hydrocephalus and ventriculoperitoneal shunting with multiple revisions. Subject A with a resolved CNS lesion produced PSI results consistent with normal central auditory processes, whereas subject B produced PSI results consistent with brainstem auditory pathway dysfunction and in addition showed abnormal crossed and uncrossed reflexes with sound stimulus to the ipsilateral ear (with reference to the site of pathology) and normal crossed and uncrossed reflexes with sound to the contralateral ear (with reference to the site of pathology). The same subject B showed an abnormal performance-intensity function (PI) for the words and sentences in the PSI battery when material was presented to the ipsilateral ear. Thus as Jerger (1987: 309) pointed out the 'principle of ipsilateral ear effects in extra-axial brainstem lesions' appeared to apply to subject B. The findings of further work carried out in this area by one of the present authors provided support for this principle, where the use of the PSI test battery with the spina bifida cohort referred to earlier (V.S.) indicated the presence of brainstem auditory dysfunction but normal temporal lobe auditory area function in paediatric subjects ($n = 16$).

The existence of brainstem auditory dysfunction consistently appears to be predictable from tasks involving difficult ipsilateral competing message tasks where adverse or negative signal to noise (or message to competition) ratio tasks are finely adjusted by the audiologist. The subject invariably appears unable to 'squelch' the background noise presented to the ipsilateral ear (ICM condition) but has little difficulty if the competition is presented to the opposite ear (CCM condition). Thus this observation is analogous to the behavioural phenomena observed whereby spina bifida subjects are reported to experience selective attention problems and high levels of distractibility. One may hypothesize that such behavioural indices may be a feature of brainstem auditory pathway dysfunction. In Jerger's (1987) study, subjects with non-auditory CNS lesions, with non-involvement of the auditory temporal lobe and auditory brainstem areas, produced normal ICM and CCM results. Subjects with temporal lobe (auditory) lesions or thalamic lesions produced normal ICM and abnormal CCM results.

Hanson and Graves (1987) reported that children with myelomeningoceles appear to have learning disabilities associated with auditory attention deficit disorders which are more pronounced in patients with shunts. Other investigators have reported decreased attention span. Billard *et al.* (1986) found 42 per cent of 77 subjects (of whom 19 were spina bifida) to have behaviours consistent with inattention, distraction, impulsivity and restlessness, although their results do not apportion the contribution of the spina bifida subjects to this percentage figure.

In summary, there is a paucity of information available at present to document central auditory pathway functional performance in neural tube disorders. Whilst ABR data are relatively the most comprehensive and widely reported, methodology often differs between studies, leading to difficulties in extrapolation and comparisons, and reports remain in isolated pockets of the literature as discrete units of information. Middle-latency and long-latency auditory evoked-potential studies are rarely reported in a manner relevant to audiological issues. Central auditory speech tests have not been applied with any rigour to the population under discussion here; however, in view of the nature of the most common behavioural abnormalities reported in the literature on children with neural tube disorders, central auditory processing dysfunction should be considered as a high priority area in educational audiological research, as the identification of specific central auditory pathway deficit disorders has implications for their educational management.

Cognitive Deficits in Spina Bifida Children

A large number of studies show that the normal distribution of IQ is not seen in the spina bifida population. Instead, the distribution curve is skewed toward the lower end of the IQ range with a peak of scores below average (Anderson and Spain, 1977; Badell-Ribera *et al.*, 1966; Mapstone *et al.*, 1984; Ruchert *et al.*, 1986; Shurtleff *et al.*, 1975; Spain, 1974; Tew and Laurence, 1975). Several factors have been related to this decreased cognitive functioning. These include: the complications of shunting (Mapstone *et al.*, 1984); the presence of seizures (Dennis *et al.*, 1981); the level of the lesion (Hunt and Holmes, 1975), social class (Scherzer and Gardner, 1970; Soare and Raimondi, 1977), and ventriculitis and meningitis (Billard *et al.*, 1986; Hunt and Holmes, 1975; Lorber and Segall, 1961; McLone *et al.*, 1982). The most significant factor, however, is the presence of hydrocephalus (Badell-Ribera *et al.*, 1966; Billard *et al.*, 1986; Hagberg and Sjorgen, 1966; McLone *et al.*, 1982; Soare and Raimondi, 1977; Spain, 1974).

As indicated earlier, studies of cognitive deficits in spina bifida children with hydrocephalus have reported a 10 to 20 point difference between verbal and performance IQ scores (Anderson and Spain, 1977; Billard *et al.*, 1986; Dennis *et al.*,

1981). The performance IQ score is the lower because of poor visuospatial skills (Billard *et al.*, 1986; Ruchert *et al.*, 1986).

Linguistic Abilities of Spina Bifida Children

Poor cognitive functioning is only one of the factors affecting the communication skills of children with spina bifida. Other factors which may pre-dispose these children to impairments in speech and/or language skills include: poor attending behaviours; hypersensitivy to auditory, tactile and visual stimuli; difficulties in visual-motor coordination, spatial orientation and figure-ground perception; limitations in gross and fine motor skills; and long illnesses or hospitalizations (Williamson, 1987). Therefore any assessment or treatment procedure for communication skills used with children with spina bifida must take into account the individual child's level of functioning in each of these areas.

Descriptions of the linguistic abilities of children with spina bifida are less conclusive than those on cognitive functioning. One reason for this is that some studies in this area have concentrated on children with hydrocephalus, of whom only some were children with spina bifida, in a manner similar to that evident in the above discussion of audiological manifestations in spina bifida.

Phonology

In general, most authors report a low incidence of phonological disorders in children with spina bifida (Spain, 1974). In a number of studies Tew found less than 10 per cent of children with spina bifida and hydrocephalus had difficulties with speech production (Tew, 1979; Tew and Laurence, 1972, 1975, 1979). In contrast to this low incidence, Khan and Soare (1975) reported phonological impairment in 65 per cent of their hydrocephalic subjects. Henderson *et al.* (1989) studied the linguistic abilities of children with spina bifida and hydrocephalus, most of whom had intellectual handicaps and all of whom lived in residential care, and reported that five of the nine subjects had phonological impairment. In two of these cases the level of phonological development was consistent with their language and cognitive skills; while in two more cases phonological development was only comparable with their language level and was below their cognitive level. In one case phonological skills were in advance of other language skills. All phonological processes used by these nine children with spina bifida were reported by Henderson *et al.* (1989) to be developmental rather than disordered in nature.

Receptive Language

A number of researchers have reported receptive language deficits in children with spina bifida (Anderson and Spain, 1977; Billard *et al.*, 1986; Menelaus, 1980). In several studies receptive language scores were in advance of expressive language scores but both were below chronological age (Tew, 1979; Tew and Laurence, 1979; Spain, 1974). This pattern was also found in five of the eight children with spina bifida with language impairment studied by Henderson *et al.* (1989). Two other cases studied by these latter authors, however, had the reverse pattern (i.e. expressive skills in advance of receptive skills) and one case presented with both skills at the same level.

Very little information is presented relating receptive language skills to intellectual functioning, in children with spina bifida. Khan and Soare (1975), however, reported scores of receptive vocabulary as measured on the Peabody Picture Vocabulary Test (Dunn, 1965) were commensurate with IQ scores. This was not the case with the children studied by Henderson *et al.* (1989) as all of their spina bifida subjects with language impairment scored in the range +1 to −1 percentile ranks on the Peabody Picture Vocabulary Test — Revised (Dunn and Dunn, 1981) irrespective of their intellectual functioning. Other factors such as occular deficits, attentional deficits, visuospatial impairments and the effect of hospitalization and institutionalization must be considered in these subjects. Horn *et al.* (1985), however, reported that their subjects performed as well as controls on vocabulary comprehension tasks until irrelevant background stimuli were introduced. While some children with spina bifida may perform well on picture vocabulary tasks, according to Swisher and Pinsker (1971) they perform more poorly on comprehension and reasoning tasks.

Dennis *et al.* (1987) suggested that poor comprehension and reasoning may not be directly related to the condition of spina bifida but rather to the hydrocephalus and factors related to that. In their study of 75 hydrocephalic children between 5 and 22 years of age, Dennis and co-workers assessed five domains of language and compared the performance of the hydrocephalic children with that of a control group. Thirty were children with spina bifida. Fourteen had intraventricular hydrocephalus associated with myelomeningocele, two had extraventricular hydrocephalus also associated with myelomeningocele, while the remaining 14 had an unspecified type of hydrocephalus associated with myelomeningocele. Thirty-four medical variables and verbal (VIQ) and performance intelligence quotients (PIQ) were then related to the performance of the hydrocephalic subjects on the language tests. From this Dennis *et al.* (1987: 614) concluded that the hydrocephalic brain provided 'an adequate but not ideal substrate for the acquisition of language', and that all language domains were not equally affected.

For both comprehension tasks (comprehension of grammar and metalinguistic awareness) assessed by Dennis *et al.* (1987), hydrocephalic subjects improved less well with increasing age than the normal control group. On the comprehension of grammar task this delayed improvement with age was true for both the number of items correct and the response time taken. The presence of intraventricular hydrocephalus particularly disrupted the development of the language skill measured by the number of items correct on this task. Metalinguistic awareness was measured on a number of features but only the detection of surface structure anomalies developed less well in the hydrocephalic subjects as age increased. This test score was found to relate to both the verbal and performance IQ scores. This was particularly so for the Lexical Anomaly Identification and the Optional Anomaly Identification scores which were accounted for by moderate amounts of variability in the VIQ scores. On this test the best predictor of a poor performance was being female. As stated before, there is a larger number of females who have spina bifida. Therefore the receptive language deficits reported in children with spina bifida may be multi-factorial in aetiology stressing the need for assessment of the individual child with spina bifida on a number of different aspects of comprehension, and with regard to the medical, cognitive, social and perceptual factors operating within that child.

Expressive Language

Contrary to the majority of children with developmental language disorders, Parsons (1968) found no difference in morphemic development in a group of children with spina bifida when compared with a group of controls. This apparent morphological ability would be in line with statements that children with spina bifida have well-developed syntax compared with other language skills (Anderson and Spain, 1977; Swisher and Pinsker, 1971; Tew, 1979) in that their syntactic skills are within normal limits for chronological age (Schwartz, 1974; Spain, 1974; Tew and Laurence, 1979). Anderson and Spain (1977) suggested that it was this ability to use complex syntax that was one of the reasons that children with spina bifida appear to have normal verbal ability. An imitation task, for different grammatical constructions, given to hydrocephalic children by Dennis *et al.* (1987) demonstrated that intraventricular and extraventricular hydrocephalus both predicted a poor sentence imitation score. This score also appeared to be related to VIQ but not PIQ. Although a poor performance score was predicted by hydrocephalus, this poor performance did not occur if shunt treatment had been implemented.

Some researchers also state that expressive vocabulary is generally well developed in children with spina bifida (Billard *et al.*, 1986; Spain, 1974). Tew (1979) reported that the vocabulary score on the WPPSI was the highest of all the subtest scores while Ingram and Naughton (1962) found their hydrocephalic subjects to have vocabulary scores superior to their 'general psychometric status'. Normal vocabulary acquisition and normal performance on a vocabulary learning task have also been reported (Parsons, 1968; Schwartz, 1974). The presence of shunts was shown by Anderson and

Spain (1977) to adversely affect vocabulary scores, with only one third of the group with shunts having vocabulary scores within normal limits.

Despite these reports of normal vocabulary development, descriptions of the language of children with spina bifida and hydrocephalus has been described as meaningless and lacking content (Hadenius *et al.*, 1962; Ingram and Naughton, 1962; Swisher and Pinsker, 1971; Tew and Laurence, 1975, 1979). Below average scores for the content subtests of the Reynell Developmental Language Scales (Reynell, 1977) have also been reported (Spain, 1974; Tew, 1979). Dennis *et al.* (1987) also found that semantic lexical access measured on the Word Finding Test (Wiegel-Crump and Dennis, 1986) improved less with age in the children with hydrocephalus than in the control group. This lexical access ability appeared to relate moderately to VIQ. Poor scores on both the semantic and visual lexical accessing conditions of the Word Finding Test were reported in children with intraventricular hydrocephalus.

Shunt treatment in children with hydrocephalus, moreover, predicted a poor performance on the automaticity of language as assessed on the Automatized Naming Test (Denckla and Rudel, 1974). Errors made by the children with hydrocephalus studied by Dennis *et al.* (1987) on this test were Serial Order errors such as perseveration, anticipation and incorrect sequencing of items. The only language skill which was specifically affected by the presence of spina bifida, in the hydrocephalic subjects studied by Dennis *et al.* (1987), was verbal fluency as measured on Automatized Naming Test (i.e. the time it took the subject to name the 300 items).

Therefore some expressive language deficits have been identified in children with spina bifida; however, in some cases this relates to the presence of hydrocephalus, the type of hydrocephalus or the treatment of the hydrocephalus. In that different language skills were related to VIQ and PIQ in varying amounts and that the level of relationship was only moderate, Dennis *et al.* (1987: 615) considered that any cognitive deficits produced by hydrocephalus could not fully account for all language deficits, as it appeared 'that the language tests tapped functions other than those involved in intelligence'. Therefore hydrocephalus was shown to produce some specific linguistic deficits but the only one specifically related to the condition of spina bifida was poor verbal fluency. As stated by a number of authors, however, despite what appears to be good development of expressive language in children with spina bifida, they lack the ability to use language appropriately (Anderson and Spain, 1977; Billard *et al.*, 1986; Horn *et al.*, 1985; Schwartz, 1974; Spain, 1974; Swisher and Pinsker, 1971; Tew and Laurence, 1979).

'Cocktail Party Syndrome'

The term 'cocktail party syndrome' refers to the use of language that has been noted in some children with hydrocephalus, both with and without the presence of spina bifida.

It is described as a chatty, superficial quality of the children's discourse. Various labels have been used to try and capture the essence of this inappropriate language usage. Some terms used in the literature are: chatterboxes and blethuers (Ingram and Naughton, 1962), shallow intellect (Laurence and Coates, 1962), dysverbal (Badell-Ribera *et al.*, 1966) and hyperverbal (Spain, 1974). The term most frequently used in the literature, however, is 'cocktail party syndrome', a term coined by Hadenius *et al.* (1962). Some definitions of 'cocktail party syndrome' commonly cited are 'a good ability to learn words and talking without knowing what they are talking about' (Hadenius *et al.*, 1962: 118); 'their spontaneous verbal behaviour is superficial and lacking in appropriateness to the situation at hand' (Fleming, 1968: 74); 'they show a characteristic pattern for language with good syntax but poor comprehension and inability to use language creatively' (Spain, 1974: 779). This characteristic pattern of language abilities was refined into two sets of criteria to aid in the diagnosis of 'cocktail party syndrome'. One set of criteria was developed by Tew (1979) and the other by Schwartz (1974) (Table 7.3).

The prevalence of 'cocktail party syndrome' reported in the literature has ranged from 0 per cent (Khan and Soare, 1975) to 40 per cent (Tew and Laurence, 1979). The most commonly reported figure, however, is around 28 per cent. This figure stands whether the children have spina bifida (Diller *et al.*, 1966; Spain, 1974) or myelomeningocele with and without hydrocephalus (Tew and Laurence, 1972). Several factors appear to influence the presence of 'cocktail party syndrome'. These factors include: low intellectual functioning (Tew and Laurence, 1972, 1979; Spain, 1974); multiple physical handicaps (Tew and Laurence, 1979), younger age group (Tew and Laurence, 1979), shunted hydrocephalus (Spain, 1974), and female sex (Tew and Laurence, 1972, 1979).

Table 7.3 Criteria for identification of cocktail party syndrome

---

Tew (1979)
- perseveration of response
- an excessive use of social phrases in conversation
- an overfamiliarity in manner
- irrelevant introduction of personal experience into conversation
- fluent and normally well articulated speech

[four of these criteria must be met]

Schwartz (1974)
- excessive verbalization
- performance IQ lower than verbal IQ
- inflection and stress patterns resembling adult speech
- spontaneous utterances out of context
- use of automatic phrases and cliches
- utterances often in the form of verbal commands and inappropriate questions
- good articulation

Likewise, many explanations of the underlying cause of 'cocktail party syndrome' have been postulated. These include: subtle brain damage (Laurence and Coates, 1962), self-stimulation (Diller *et al.*, 1966), reinforcement of hyperverbal behaviour by parents (Diller *et al.*, 1966; Swisher and Pinsker, 1971; Tew, 1979; Tew and Laurence, 1979), attention-seeking behaviour to gain adult attention in hospital (Tew, 1979; Tew and Laurence, 1979), or poor ability at monitoring verbal output (Dennis *et al.*, 1987).

Despite the development of behavioural descriptions and criteria as described earlier to diagnose 'cocktail party syndrome', few empirical studies have been able to qualitatively or quantitatively demonstrate its true nature. Those studies which have addressed the issue of hyperverbality have measured the number of words per turn/response (Diller *et al.*, 1966; Fleming, 1968), the total number of words (Fleming, 1968; Swisher and Pinsker, 1971), and type:token ratio (Henderson *et al.*, 1989; Swisher and Pinsker, 1971). The study by Swisher and Pinsker (1971) was the only study to find an increase in the number of words used by children with spina bifida when compared with a group of controls or normative data. All of the above authors, however, commented on the inappropriateness of the language usage observed in their group of subjects. Billard *et al.* (1966) found their subjects not to be too excessive but merely irrelevant, while Fleming (1968: 81) felt that the 'personal and socially aggressive nature of their spontaneous conversation' made her hydrocephalic subjects appear more verbose.

It would be expected that the inappropriateness of the language observed in children with spina bifida could be demonstrated using a pragmatic language assessment, most of which have been developed since the publication of the studies cited. In addition, such a pragmatic analysis should identify behaviours described in the literature as being associated with 'cocktail party syndrome' such as: irrelevant responses, difficulty staying on topic, over familiarity of manner, prosodic features and superficiality of output (Diller *et al.*, 1966; Fleming, 1968; Schwartz, 1974; Tew, 1979). Based on this assumption Henderson *et al.* (1989) assessed a group of children with spina bifida who were most likely to exhibit 'cocktail party syndrome' (i.e. they had intellectual handicaps, lived in residential care, had moderate to severe physical disabilities and had hydrocephalus) using the Pragmatic Protocol (Prutting and Kirchner, 1987). The children were all between 6 and 13 years of age. Pragmatic deficits were found in seven of the nine subjects studied (Figure 7.3). Subject 1, who had pragmatic skills within normal limits, did not present with a language disorder and had normal intellectual functioning.

As can be seen from Figure 7.3 the notion that some of the children with spina bifida exhibit inappropriate language behaviour is supported by this study, as between four and fourteen inappropriate pragmatic behaviours were identified in each of the subjects presenting with pragmatic deficits. Some of these behaviours would have been predicted from the literature, for example, speech pair act analysis, topic selection, topic introduction, topic maintenance, turn-taking response and prosody. The

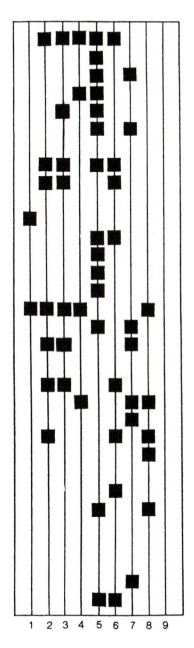

VERBAL ASPECTS
Speech pair act analysis

Variety of speech acts

Topic selection

Topic introduction

Topic maintenance

Topic change

Turntaking initiation

Turntaking response

Turntaking repair revision

Turntaking pause time

Turntaking interruption/overlap

Turntaking feedback to speaker

Turntaking adjacency

Turntaking contingency

Turntaking quantity/conciseness

Specificity/accuracy

Cohesion

Varying communicative style

PARALINGUISTIC ASPECTS
Intelligibility

Vocal intensity

Vocal quality

Prosody

Fluency

NONVERBAL ASPECTS
Physical proximity

Physical contacts

Body posture

Front/leg and hand/arm movements

Gestures

Facial expression

Eye gaze

1 2 3 4 5 6 7 8 9

Figure 7.3 Inappropriate pragmatic parameters on the pragmatic protocol for individual subjects with spina bifida (from Henderson et al., 1989)

difficulties noted on specificity and accuracy would support Dennis *et al.*'s (1987) findings re poor verbal fluency in children with spina bifida or poor word finding skills in children with intraventricular hydrocephalus. It may also relate to the low receptive vocabulary scores also found in the Henderson *et al.* (1989) subjects. Despite confirmation of the descriptive symptoms of 'cocktail party syndrome' seen in this group of subjects, no individual subject met the criteria of either Tew (1979) or Schwartz (1974) for the identification of 'cocktail party syndrome'. Further research is obviously required to refine these descriptive terms and to ascertain the pragmatic profiles of children with comparable linguistic and/or cognitive skills, and to utilize that information for the purpose of evaluating the underlying mechanisms operating in hydrocephalic children.

References

ANDERSON, E. M. and SPAIN, B. (1977) *The Child with Spina Bifida*, London, Methuen.

BADELL-RIBERA, A., SHULMAN, K. and PADDOCK, N. (1966) 'The relationship of nonprogressive hydrocephalus to intellectual functioning in children with spina bifida cystica,' *Pediatrics*, **37**, pp. 787–93.

BIGLER, E. D. (1988) 'The neuropsychology of hydrocephalus,' *Archives of Clinical Neuropsychology*, **3**, pp. 81–100.

BILLARD, C., SANTINI, J. J., GILLET, P., NARGEOT, M. C and ADRIEN, J. L. (1986) 'Long term intellectual prognosis of hydrocephalus with reference to 77 children,' *Paediatric Neuroscience*, **12**, pp. 219–25.

CHARNEY, E. B., RORKE, L. B., SUTTON, L. N. and SCHUT, L. (1987) 'Management of Chiari II complications in infants with myelomeningocele,' *Journal of Pediatrics*, **3**, pp. 364–71.

CULL, C. and WYKE, M. A. (1984) 'Memory functions of children with spina bifida and shunted hydrocephalus,' *Developmental Medicine and Child Neurology*, **26**, pp. 177–83.

DE L.COSTELLO, A. M., HAMILTON, P. A., BAUDIN, J., TOWNSEND, J., BRADFORD, B. C., STEWART, A. L. and REYNOLDS, E. O. R. (1988) 'Prediction of neurodevelopmental impairment at four years from brain ultrasound appearance of very preterm infants,' *Developmental Medicine and Child Neurology*, **30**, pp. 711–22.

DENCKLA, M. B. and RUDEL, R. (1974) 'Rapid 'automatized' naming of pictures, objects, colors, letters and numbers by normal children,' *Cortex*, **10**, pp. 186–202.

DENNIS, M. E., FITZ, L. R., NETLEY, C. T., SUGAR, J., HARWOOD-NASH, D. C. F., HENDRICK, E. B., HOFFMAN, H. J. and HUMPHREYS, R. P. (1981) 'The intelligence of hydrocephalic children,' *Archives of Neurology*, **38**, pp. 607–15.

DENNIS, M. E., HENDRICK, B., HOFFMAN, H. J. and HUMPHREYS, R. P. (1987) 'Language of hydrocephalic children and adolescents,' *Journal of Clinical and Experimental Neuropsychology*, **9**, pp. 593–621.

DILLER, L., PADDOCK, N., BADELL-RIBERA, A. and SWINYARD, C. A. (1966) 'Verbal behaviour in spina bifida children,' in Swinyard, C. A. (Ed.) *Comprehensive Care of Children with Spina Bifida Manifesta*, Rehabilitation Monograph No.31, New York, Institute of Rehabilitation.

DOCHERTY, T. B., HERBAUT, A. G. and SEDGWICK, E. M. (1987) 'Brainstem auditory evoked potential abnormalities in myelomeningocoele in the older child,' *Journal of Neurology, Neurosurgery and Psychiatry*, **50**, pp. 1318–22.

DORMAN, C., LAATSCH, L. K. and HURLEY, A. D. (1985) 'The applicability of neuropsychological test batteries for the assessment of the congenitally brain disordered,' *The International Journal of Clinical Neuropsychology*, **7**, pp. 111–17.

DUCATI, A., CENZATO, M., LANDI, A., SINA, C. and VILLANI, R. (1986) 'Evaluation of brainstem function using acoustic evoked potentials in 26 patients harbouring a CSF shunt for non-tumoral aqueductal stenosis hydrocephalus,' *Journal of Neurosurgical Sciences*, **30**, pp. 61–6.

DUNN, L. M. (1965) *Peabody Picture Vocabulary Test*, Circle Pines, MN, American Guidance Service.

DUNN, L. M. and DUNN, L. M (1981) *Peabody Picture Vocabulary Test — Revised*, Minnesota, American Guidance Service.

FERNELL, E., HAGBERG, B., HABGERG, G., HULT, G. and VON WENDT, L. (1988) 'Epidemiology of infantile hydrocephalus in Sweden: A clinical follow-up study in children born at term,' *Neuropediatrics*, **19**, pp. 135–42.

FLEMING, C. P. (1968) 'The verbal behaviour of hydrocephalic children,' *Developmental Medicine and Child Neurology*, Suppl.15, pp. 74–82.

GILBERT, J. N., JONES, K. L., RORKE, L. B., CHERNOFF, G. F. and JAMES, H. E. (1986) 'Central nervous system anomalies associated with meningomyelocele, hydrocephalus and the Arnold–Chiari malformation: Reappraisal of theories regarding the pathogenesis of posterior neural tube closure defects,' *Neurosurgery*, **18**(5), pp. 559–64.

HADENIUS, A., HAGBERG, B., HYTTNAS-BENSCH, K., and SJOGREN, I. (1962) 'The natural prognosis of infantile hydrocephalus,' *Acta Pediatrica Scandinavica*, **51**, pp. 117–18.

HAGBERG, B. and SJORGEN, I. (1966) 'The chronic brain syndrome of infantile hydrocephalus: A follow-up study of 63 spontaneously arrested cases,' *American Journal of Diseases of Children*, **112**, pp. 189–96.

HANSON, R. R. and GRAVES, M. R.(1987) 'Current concepts: Care and habilitation of the child with myelomeningocele. A multi-disciplinary approach,' *Journal of Mississippi State Medical Association*, **28**, pp. 145–50.

HENDERSON, S., MURDOCH, B. and OZANNE, A. (1989) 'Speech and language disorders in children with spina bifida', paper presented at the Annual Conference of the Australian Association of Speech and Hearing, Perth, Australia.

HOLLIDAY III, P. O., PILLSBURY, D., KELLY, D. L. and DILLARD, R (1985) 'Brainstem auditory evoked potentials in Arnold–Chiari malformation: Possible prognostic value and changes with surgical decompression,' *Neurosurgery*, **16**, pp. 48–53.

HORN, D. G., LORCH, E. P., LORCH, R. F. and CULATTA, B. (1985) 'Distractibility and vocabulary deficits in children with spina bifida and hydrocephalus,' *Developmental Medicine and Child Neurology*, **27**, pp. 713–20.

HUNT, G. M. and HOLMES, A. E. (1975) 'Some factors relating to intelligence in treated children with spina bifida cystica,' *Developmental Medicine and Child Neurology*, **17**, (Suppl. 35), pp. 65–70.

INGRAM, T. T. S. and NAUGHTON, J. A. (1962) 'Paediatric and psychological aspects of cerebral palsy associated with hydrocephalus,' *Developmental Medicine and Child Neurology*, **4**, pp. 287–91.

JERGER, S. (1987) 'Validation of the pediatric speech intelligibility test in children with central nervous system lesions,' *Audiology*, **26**, pp. 298–311.

KHAN, A. V. and SOARE, P. (1975) 'Intelligence, speech and language development of hydrocephalic children,' *Developmental Medicine and Child Neurology*, **17**, pp. 116–17.

KNOWLTON, D. D., PETERSON, K. and PUTBRESE, A. (1985) 'Team management of cognitive dysfunction in children with spina bifida,' *Rehabilitation Literature*, **46**, pp. 259–63.

KRAUS, N., OZDAMAR, O., HEYDEMANN, P. T., STEIN, L. and REID, N. L. (1984) 'Auditory brainstem responses in hydrocephalus patients,' *Electroencephalography and Clinical Neurophysiology*, **59**, pp. 310–17.

LAURENCE, K. M. and COATES, S. (1962) 'The natural history of hydrocephalus: Detailed analysis of 182 inoperated cases,' *Archives of Disease in Childhood*, **37**, pp. 345–62.

LAURENCE, K. M. and WEEKS, R. (1971) 'Abnormalities in the central nervous system,' in Norman, A. P. (Ed.) *Congenital Abnormalities in Infancy*, 2nd ed., Oxford, Blackwell Scientific Publications.

LORBER, J. and SEGALL, M. (1961) 'Bacterial meningitis in spina bifida cystica,' *Archives of Disease in Childhood*, **37**, pp. 300–8.

LÜTSCHG, J., MEYER, E. and JEANNERET-ISELI, C. (1985) 'Brainstem auditory evoked potentials in meningomyelocele,' *Neuropediatrics*, **16**, pp. 202–4.

MARCHBANKS, R. J., REID, A., MARTIN. A. M., BRIGHTWELL, A. P. and BATEMAN, D. (1987) 'The effect of raised intercranial pressure on intracochlear fluid pressure: Three case studies,' *British Journal of Audiology*, **21**, pp. 127–30.

MAPSTONE, T. B., REKATE, H. L., NULSEN, F. E., DIXON, M. S., GLASER, N. and JAFFE, M. (1984) 'Relationship of CSF shunting and IQ in children with myelomeningocele: A retrospective analysis,' *Child's Brain*, **11**, pp. 112–18.

MCLONE, D. G., CZYZEWSKI, D., RAIMONDI, A. J. and SOMERS, R. C. (1982) 'Central nervous system infections as a limiting factor in the intelligence of children with myelomeningocele,' *Pediatrics*, **70**, pp. 338–42.

MENELAUS, M. B. (1980) *The Orthopaedic Management of Spina Bifida Cystica*, 2nd ed., New York, Churchill Livingstone.

OP HEIJ, C. P. M. O., RENIER, W. O. and GABREËLS, F. J. M. (1985) 'Intellectual sequelae of primary non-obstructive hydrocephalus in infancy: Analysis of 50 cases,' *Clinical Neurology and Neurosurgery*, **87**, pp. 247–53.

PARSONS, J. G. (1968) 'An investigation into the verbal facility of hydrocephalic children with special reference to vocabulary, morphology and fluency,' *Developmental Medicine and Child Neurology*, **10**, (Suppl. 16), pp. 109–10.

PRUTTING, C. A. and KIRCHNER, D. M. (1987) 'A clinical appraisal of the pragmatic aspects of language,' *Journal of Speech and Hearing Disorders*, **52**, pp. 105–19.

RENIER, D., SAINTE-ROSE, C., PIERRE-KAHN, A. and HIRSCH, J. F. (1988) 'Pre-natal hydrocephalus: Outcome and prognosis,' *Child's Nervous System*, **4**, pp. 213–22.

REYNELL, J. (1977) *Reynell Developmental Language Scales — Revised,* Oxford, NFER Publishing Company Ltd.

RUCHERT, N., HANSEL-FRIEDRICH, G. and WOLFF, G. (1986) 'Assessment of intelligence of school-aged children with spina bifida under hospital supervision,' in Voth D. and Glees, D. (Eds) *Spina Bifida — Neural Tube Defects*, New York, De Gruyter, pp. 283–91.

SAUKKONEN, A. L. (1988) 'Electroencephalographic findings in hydrocephalic children prior to initial shunting,' *Child's Nervous System*, **4**, pp. 339–43.

SCHERZER, A. L. and GARDNER, G. G. (1970) 'Studies of the school age child with meningomyelocele: 1. Physical andintellectual development,' *Pediatrics*, **47**, pp. 424–30.

SCHWARTZ, E. R. (1974) 'Characteristics of speech and language development in the child with myelomeningocele and hydrocephalus,' *Journal of Speech and Hearing Disorders*, **39**(4), pp. 465–8.

SHAFFER, J., FREIDRICH, W. N., SHURTLEFF, D. B. and WOLF, L. (1985) 'Cognitive and achievement status of children with myelomeningocele,' *Journal of Pediatric Psychology*, **10**(3), pp. 325–36.

SHURTLEFF, D. B., KRONMAL, R. and FOLTZ, E. L. (1975) 'Follow-up comparison of hydrocephalus with and without myelomeningocele,' *Journal of Neurosurgery*, **42**, pp. 61–8.

SIMPSON, D. (1976) 'Congenital malformations of the nervous system,' *Medical Journal of Australia*, **1**, pp. 700–2.

SMITH, E. D. (1965) 'Spina bifida and the total care of spinal myelomeningocele,' Illinois, Charles C. Thomas.

SMYTH, V., SCOTT, J. and TUDEHOPE, D. 'The utility of the auditory brainstem response as a screening procedure,' *International Journal of Pediatric Otorhinolaryngology* (in press).

SOARE, P. L. and RAIMONDI, A. J.(1977) 'Intellectual and perceptual motor characteristics of treated myelomeningocele children,' *American Journal of Diseases of Children*, **131**, pp. 199–204.

SPAIN, B. (1974) 'Verbal and performance ability in preschool children with spina bifida,' *Developmental Medicine and Child Neurology*, **16**, pp. 773–80.

SWISHER, L. P. and PINSKER, E. J. (1971) 'The language characteristics of hyperverbal, hydrocephalic children,' *Developmental Medicine and Child Neurology*, **13**, pp. 746–55.

TEW, B. (1979) 'The "cocktail party syndrome" in children with hydrocephalus and spina bifida,' *British Journal of Disorders of Communication*, **14**, pp. 89–101.

TEW, B. and LAURENCE, K. (1972) 'The ability and attainments of spina bifida patients born in South Wales between 1956–1962,' *Developmental Medicine and Child Neurology*, **14**, (Suppl. 27), pp. 124–31.

TEW, B. and LAURENCE, K. M. (1975) 'The effects of hydrocephalus on intelligence, visual perception and school attainment,' *Developmental Medicine and Child Neurology*, **17**, (Suppl. 35), pp. 129–34.

TEW, B. and LAURENCE, K. M. (1979) 'The clinical and psychological characteristics of children with the 'cocktail party' syndrome,' *Zeitschrift für Kinderchirurgie und Grenzbegiete*, **28**, pp. 360–7.

VENKATARAMANA, N. K., SATISHCHANDRA, P., HEGDE, A. S., REDDY, G. N. N. and DAS, B. S. (1988) 'Evaluation of brainstem auditory evoked responses in congenital hydrocephalus,' *Child's Nervous System*, **4**, pp. 334–8.

WARKANEY, J. and O'TOOLE, B. A. (1981) 'Experimental spina bifida and associated malformations,' *Child's Brain*, **8**, pp. 18–30.

WIEGEL-CRUMP, C. A. and DENNIS, M. (1986) 'Development of word finding,' *Brain and Language*, **27**, pp. 1–23.

WILLIAMSON, G. C. (1987) *Children with Spina Bifida*, Baltimore, Paul H. Brookes

Chapter 8

Speech and Language Disorders in Childhood Brain Tumours

Lisa J. Hudson

Introduction

Brain and spinal tumours are the second most common childhood cancer after leukaemia in Australia, Europe, North America and Japan (Parkin *et al.*, 1988). In particular, tumours located in the posterior fossa (i.e. infratentorial tumours involving the cerebellum, fourth ventricle and/or brainstem) occur more commonly in childhood than supratentorial neoplasms, accounting for up to 70 per cent of all paediatric intracranial neoplasms (Farwell *et al.*, 1977; Gjerris, 1978; Hooper, 1975; Kadota *et al.*, 1989; Russell and Rubinstein, 1989; Segall *et al.*, 1985). However, it has been reported that supratentorial tumours have a higher incidence in children less than 3 years of age (Jooma and Kendall, 1982; Tadmor *et al.*, 1980).

Due to the prevalence of posterior fossa tumours in childhood, a large proportion of the literature on paediatric intracranial neoplasms has centred on tumours involving the cerebellum, fourth ventricle and/or brainstem. Consequently, this chapter aims to review the types and prognoses of posterior fossa tumours, the management of such tumours and the implications of the tumours for speech and language abilities.

Types of Posterior Fossa Tumours

The most common posterior fossa tumours are astrocytomas, medulloblastomas and ependymomas. In a sample of 115 childhood posterior fossa tumour cases studied by Matson (1956), 30 per cent had astrocytomas, 31 per cent had medulloblastomas and 12 per cent had ependymomas. Farwell *et al.* (1977) reviewed 467 cases of paediatric intracranial tumour which included astrocytomas (28 per cent), medulloblastomas (25 per cent) and ependymomas (9 per cent). Similarly, the 72 cases of paediatric brain tumours reviewed by Koh *et al.* (1985) consisted of 23 grade 1 and 2 astrocytomas (32 per cent), 11 (16 per cent) glioblastomas (grade 3 and 4 astrocytomas), 18 medulloblastomas (25 per cent), and three ependymomas (4 per cent). In this latter study, eight astrocytomas and eight glioblastomas were located supratentorially, while all other tumours were situated in the posterior fossa.

Parkin *et al.* (1988) reported a world-wide study which involved the collaboration of cancer registries from over 50 countries. Overall, astrocytomas represented 30–50 per cent of all childhood central nervous system (CNS) tumours, medulloblastomas approximately 20 per cent and 5–15 per cent were ependymomas.

Astrocytoma

An astrocytoma is a neoplasm derived from and composed of astrocytes. It can occur above or below the tentorium cerebelli; however, infratentorial astrocytomas are more common in children. Astrocytomas of the posterior fossa arise from the cerebellum and are referred to as cerebellar astrocytomas. In patients less than 20 years of age, there is a tendency for astrocytomas to originate in the lateral lobe of the cerebellum as opposed to the vermis (i.e. midline) of the cerebellum (Geissinger and Bucy, 1971; Gol and McKissock, 1959; Mabon *et al.*, 1950; Russell and Rubinstein, 1989).

Cerebellar astrocytomas are often circumscribed and tend to be predominantly cystic, containing one or more sacs of clear yellow or brown fluid. These tumours are amenable to complete surgical excision as brainstem invasion is rare (Delong and Adams, 1975). Malignant transformation (anaplasia) of cystic cerebellar astrocytomas is uncommon.

Eighty-two per cent of the 75 cases of cerebellar astrocytoma reviewed by Gol (1963) were of the cystic type, while the remaining 18 per cent were solid astrocytomas. Gol described three forms of cystic astrocytoma: (1) a neoplastic cyst where the neoplasm lined all the walls of the cyst, (2) a cyst where the walls consisted of non-malignant glial tissue and the tumour was concentrated in a nodule of vascular tumour tissue protruding from the wall of the cyst, and (3) a tumour which is polycystic in nature.

Klein and McCullough (1985) also detailed three forms of astrocytoma: (1) a tumour with a large cyst and a mural tumour nodule (most favourable for total surgical removal), (2) a solid tumour containing visible small cysts, and (3) a uniformly solid tumour. Solid tumours are more frequently positioned in the midline and are therefore associated with an increased risk of brainstem involvement. Solid tumours may display diffusely infiltrative edges, and they are particularly prone to anaplastic changes and recurrence in adult patients. Fortunately, 68–86 per cent of childhood cerebellar astrocytomas are cystic in nature (Gol, 1963; Gol and McKissock, 1959; Lee *et al.*, 1989).

As well as being described as cystic or solid, astrocytomas are also referred to as juvenile or diffuse. Juvenile astrocytomas, as their name suggests, tend to appear during the first decade of life while diffuse astrocytomas usually arise in adolescence. Juvenile astrocytomas are compact, clearly demarcated tumours, while diffuse astrocytomas infiltrate the surrounding brain tissue and are more prone to anaplastic change than the juvenile type. Juvenile and diffuse forms of astrocytoma are not directly correlated to the cystic and solid types discussed earlier (Gjerris and Klinken, 1978). Approximately 75 per cent of childhood cerebellar astrocytomas are of the juvenile type, the remaining 25 per cent being diagnosed as diffuse (Davis and Joglekar, 1981; Gjerris and Klinken, 1978).

Astrocytomas are usually assigned a grade from 1 to 4 according to their level of malignancy, with grade 1 being benign and grade 4 highly malignant. Most cerebellar astrocytomas are low grade (Gol and McKissock, 1959; Kadota *et al.*, 1989; Naidich and Zimmerman, 1984); however, grade 3 and 4 astrocytomas do occur and are referred to as glioblastomas. Glioblastomas are rare in the cerebellum and spinal cord (Koh *et al.*, 1985).

Age at onset

While it is recognized that cerebellar astrocytomas are primarily a disease of childhood, a specific age at onset has not been identified. Gol (1963) reviewed 75 astrocytoma cases and observed a peak incidence of astrocytoma in boys during the first 5 years of life after which a slow decline in the number of diagnoses being made was noted. Girls up to 10 years of age presented with astrocytomas after which an abrupt decline in the incidence was recorded. Geissinger and Bucy (1971) reported the average age at diagnosis of astrocytoma cases to be 8 years 9 months, while Delong and Adams (1975) determined an age range of 5–9 years after reviewing the literature, but found the majority of their own ten cases to be between 9 and 16 years of age. Davis and Joglekar (1981) studied 43 patients with cerebellar astrocytomas and found an average age at surgery of 12 years 6 months with a range of 4 years 4 months to 30 years 11 months.

The varying age ranges listed above may be attributed to a failure by the various authors to consider specific astrocytoma types in their analyses. Gjerris and Klinken (1978) found that juvenile astrocytomas occurred between birth and 9 years of age while diffuse astrocytomas arose later, between 10 and 14 years of age. Lee *et al.* (1989) reviewed 37 cases of supratentorial and infratentorial juvenile astrocytomas determining a mean age at onset of 7.1 years. Although this finding is in accordance with that of Gjerris and Klinken (1978), eight (22 per cent) of the patients reviewed by Lee *et al.* (1989) were diagnosed when older than 10 years of age.

It has been suggested that the age ranges documented in the literature may be influenced by advances in technology. Tadmor *et al.* (1982) compared the ages of children diagnosed with intracranial neoplasms before the introduction of computed tomography (CT) with the ages of those diagnosed with the aid of CT. There was a highly significant increase in the detection of brain tumours in children less than 6 years of age and in children older than 12 years when CT was used. However, the authors warned that differences in the population structure, fluctuations in the birth rate and alterations in the prevalence of aetiological factors may also have contributed to the changes in age at diagnosis.

Thus children with posterior fossa astrocytoma presenting at clinics for the treatment of associated speech and language deficits could be expected to vary in age from infancy through to adolescence.

Male : Female ratio

A consistent difference between male and female incidences of astrocytoma occurrence has not emerged in the literature. Although Gol and McKissock (1959), Gol (1963), and Koh *et al.* (1985) reported a slightly higher incidence in males, other authors have not found a significant difference between the incidence in the two sexes (Davis and Joglekar, 1981; Delong and Adams, 1975; Lee *et al.*, 1989; Mabon *et al.*, 1950; Naidich and Zimmerman, 1984; Parkin *et al.*, 1988; Wallner *et al.*, 1988).

Clinical symptoms

The presenting signs and symptoms of any posterior fossa tumour type are largely due to increased intracranial pressure which results from the mass effect of the tumour itself, associated oedema and obstruction to the flow of cerebrospinal fluid (CSF). Destruction or compression of brain tissue may also underly many of the signs and symptoms observed (Tew *et al.*, 1984). Symptoms associated with the presence of a brain tumour may be non-specific or localizing. Non-specific symptoms (e.g. headache, nausea) could be caused by many other childhood illnesses and do not necessarily suggest neurological damage, while localizing symptoms (e.g. ataxia, nystagmus) imply nervous system involvement.

Symptoms associated with posterior fossa tumours include bifrontal headache, nausea and vomiting, gait disturbance, depressed cerebral function (manifested as apathy and irritability), neck stiffness or neck pain, dizziness, papilloedema (oedema of the optic discs due to impairment of the venous drainage from the optic nerve and retina subsequent to increased intracranial pressure), squint and nystagmus, alteration of muscle tone, tendon reflex changes, dorsiflexor plantar response, tilting the head away from the side of the tumour, visual impairment and paresis of the limbs (Delong and Adams, 1975; Gol, 1963; Kadota *et al.*, 1989; Matson, 1956; Tew *et al.*, 1984). Facial weakness and deafness are rare but have been reported (Delong and Adams, 1975). While seizures may be the presenting symptom in childhood supratentorial neoplasms (Hirsch *et al.*, 1989), seizures have not been reported in association with tumours of the posterior fossa.

Davis and Joglekar (1981) noted an average symptom duration of 2 years 4 months before intervention in 43 cases of cerebellar astrocytoma. Delay in the diagnosis of paediatric intracranial tumours has been discussed by Matson (1956) and Delong and Adams (1975). They suggested that childhood brain tumours occur when the brain is inadequately developed so that the initial symptoms are non-specific and appear similar to those caused by non-nervous diseases. In addition, children are unable to describe the symptoms or recall their onset. The relatively slow rate at which astrocytomas proliferate may also prolong the progression of symptoms.

Medical prognosis

Cerebellar astrocytomas are usually low grade and associated with a favourable post-operative prognosis. Tumour recurrence is rare, although recurrences have been reported to occur from 7 to 48 years after surgery (Bernell *et al.*, 1972; Kleinman *et al.*, 1978; Ushio *et al.*, 1987). Metastatic spread through the cerebrospinal pathway is also rare but has been documented (Auer *et al.*, 1981). Despite a widespread belief in the benign nature of astrocytomas, Hoshino *et al.* (1988) suggested that the proliferative potential of low grade astrocytomas may actually be dangerously high. Their 47 subjects were from 2 to 68 years of age at surgery, with 17 patients less than 15 years of age. Approximately 40 per cent of the low grade astrocytomas had a higher proliferative potential and carried a far worse prognosis than histologically similar tumours with low proliferative potential. In other words, some low grade astrocytomas followed a benign course, while others behaved like malignant astrocytomas. The need to evaluate the growth characteristics of an astrocytoma before making treatment and prognostic decisions was therefore stressed by Hoshino *et al.* (1988).

Matson (1956) reported that 32 of the 34 children with astrocytoma in his sample had survived from a few months to 7 years after surgery. Twenty-four (75 per cent) were asymptomatic or had only a minimal degree of ataxia in one or more extremities. Eight (25 per cent) had residual neurological disturbances including ataxia, cranial nerve palsies and impairment of vision. Although speech deficits might be expected in association with these signs, the presence of such deficits were not mentioned by Matson (1956).

Of the 75 children studied by Gol (1963), all who had had complete excision of the astrocytoma were alive and well at the time of writing (66 per cent). However, of the 17 patients who underwent partial removal, five died from regrowth. Overall, 70 per cent were able to return to normal activities with no or only 'minor neurological disabilities'. The minor neurological deficits were not described.

Geissinger and Bucy (1971) considered 26 patients with an average age at astrocytoma removal of 8 years 9 months. Four patients died after surgery. The 22 remaining patients were reassessed 6 months to 31 years after the operation. Sixteen (73 per cent) of these cases showed no neurological signs on examination, four (18 per cent) had significant visual impairments, one was ataxic and one experienced neurological dysfunction severe enough to prevent a normal independent existence. The latter patient demonstrated nasal speech, ataxia in her arms, unsteady gait and impaired visual acuity.

All ten patients with grade 1 or 2 cerebellar astrocytomas described by Delong and Adams (1975) made a full recovery. Wallner *et al.* (1988) calculated the survival and freedom from progression rates of 28 children and 8 adults with juvenile astrocytoma. Twenty-two of the astrocytomas were located in the posterior fossa. Overall, the 10- and 20-year survival rates were 83 per cent and 70 per cent respectively, while the 10- and 20-year freedom from progression rates were 77 per cent and 56 per cent respectively. Complete tumour resection was possible in 12 patients, all of whom were well and free from recurrence at the time of writing. Of the 19 who underwent incomplete excision of the tumour and 4000 rads of radiation, 10- and 20-year survival rates were 81 per cent and 54 per cent, while the 10- and 20-year freedom from progression rates were 74 per cent and 41 per cent respectively. The data provided by Wallner *et al.* (1988) suggests that the extent of surgical removal is an important prognostic factor. Several authors have supported this view (Davis and Joglekar, 1981; Ilgren and Stiller, 1986; Kleinman *et al.*, 1978; Laws *et al.*, 1987).

Complete surgical excision of astrocytomas is limited by brainstem involvement and malignancy (Klein and McCullough, 1985). According to Klein and McCullough (1985), the degree of brainstem involvement and the level of malignancy place greater restrictions on surgical removal of cerebellar tumours than the size of the tumour, in that relatively extensive resection of cerebellar tumours can be performed with minimal functional loss.

Children with juvenile cerebellar astrocytomas who survived longer than 1 month after surgery have been reported to have a 94 per cent chance of long-term survival (Gjerris and Klinken, 1978), while Naidich and Zimmerman (1984) claimed children with diffuse astrocytomas had a 38 per cent chance of survival. The findings of Davis and Joglekar (1981) suggested that children whose ataxia and dysequilibrium failed to improve after initial surgery were prone to tumour recurrence.

Thus recovery from astrocytoma appears favourable, particularly when the brainstem is not involved, proliferative potential is low, the grade of malignancy is low and complete surgical resection is possible.

Medulloblastoma

Medulloblastoma is a highly malignant brain tumour whose origin is restricted to the cerebellum; however, subsequent invasion into the subarachnoid spaces, fourth ventricle and cerebrospinal pathways does occur (Aron, 1971; Deutsch and Reigel, 1980; Russell and Rubinstein, 1989). While astrocytomas tend to arise from a hemisphere of the cerebellum, medulloblastomas are usually situated in the midline (i.e. vermis) of the cerebellum (Delong and Adams, 1975; Park *et al.*, 1983; Perun *et al.*, 1987; Russell and Rubinstein, 1989; Segall *et al.*, 1985).

On CT scanning, a medulloblastoma characteristically appears as a well-defined, non-calcified, non-cystic, slightly dense inferior vermian mass that invades the back of the fourth ventricle but does not extend to the cerebellopontine angle.

Age at onset

Children have been diagnosed with medulloblastomas between 4 months and 16 years of age. Aron (1971) studied 22 children with medulloblastoma who were between 4 months and 15 years of age at the time of diagnosis; the majority of the group were diagnosed between 5 and 10 years of age. Delong and Adams (1975) noted that the majority of their subjects' medulloblastomas arose between 3 and 7 years of age. Raimondi and Tomita (1979) described the peak incidence of medulloblastoma to be between 4 months and 12 years of age with the median age at diagnosis being 4.5 years. Similarly, Park *et al.* (1983) and Russell and Rubinstein (1989) reported that the majority (81 per cent and 60 per cent respectively) of their medulloblastoma cases were diagnosed in the first decade of life. A wider age range for the onset of medulloblastoma was determined by Rivera-Luna *et al.* (1987) who studied 65 children between 1.4 and 16 years of age at diagnosis (mean 6.8 years). Consequently, as described for childhood astrocytomas, medulloblastoma patients can be expected to be diagnosed between birth and 16 years of age.

Male : female ratio

There is agreement in the literature on the higher incidence of medulloblastoma in male children. Male : female ratios which have been reported range from 1.3 : 1 to 3 : 1 (Delong and Adams, 1975; Naidich and Zimmerman, 1984; Park *et al.*, 1983; Parkin *et al.*, 1988; Raimondi and Tomita, 1979; Rivera-Luna *et al.*, 1987; Russell and Rubinstein, 1989).

Clinical symptoms

Because of the cerebellar site, the clinical symptoms of medulloblastoma are the same as those described for astrocytomas. However, the duration between the onset of symptoms and initiation of treatment tends to be much shorter (Delong and Adams, 1975; Kirsch *et al.*, 1980). This is attributed to the rapid growth and the midline position of medulloblastomas. Both these features result in early obstruction of the fourth ventricle and interruption of cerebrospinal fluid flow.

Tokars *et al.* (1979) reviewed nine medulloblastoma patients (six children and three adults) documenting the time that elapsed between the onset of symptoms and initiation of treatment. This period ranged from 1 to 10 months with a mean of 5.2 months which is considerably less than the average 2 year 4 months delay in diagnosis that Davis and Joglekar (1981) recorded for patients with astrocytomas. Similarly, Raimondi and Tomita (1979) determined symptom durations ranging from 1 month (in 50 per cent of the patients) to 1 year in the 51 patients studied, while Park *et al.* (1983) recorded clinical histories of less than 6 weeks in 51 per cent of the 144 children reviewed and less than 12 weeks in 76 per cent of the group.

Medical prognosis

The outlook for children with medulloblastoma is improving due to advances in technology such as the advent of CT and operating microscopes (Norris *et al.*, 1981), and the administration of radiotherapy and chemotherapy to the CNS (Bloom, 1982). The primary concerns for patients with medulloblastoma are the risk of tumour recurrence in the posterior fossa and/or the development of supratentorial, spinal cord or systemic metastases.

Delong and Adams (1975) predicted the 'period of risk' of recurrence to be 9 months and a 5-year survival without recurrence to occur in one-third of these patients. Russell and Rubinstein (1989) claimed that recurrent medulloblastoma was most likely to appear within 2 years of initial treatment. The incidence of tumour recurrence has been estimated at 10–15 per cent (Jereb *et al.*, 1982; Park *et al.*, 1983); however, Enzmann *et al.* (1978) and Lee *et al.* (1985) reported tumour recurrence in 41 per cent (12 of 29 patients) and 56 per cent (20 of 36 children) respectively of the medulloblastoma cases described. The incidence of subarachnoid seeding and arachnoid invasion was 64 per cent and 100 per cent respectively of the cases examined by McComb *et al.* (1981), and Tomita and McLone (1983). At present, research indicates that death is the inevitable outcome when tumour recurrence or diffuse metastatic spread occurs (Laurent *et al.*, 1985; Perun *et al.*, 1987).

Other factors which appear to influence the prognosis of children with medulloblastoma include: the extent of surgical resection of the tumour with total removal resulting in a more favourable outlook than subtotal or partial resection or biopsy (Norris *et al.*, 1981; Park *et al.*, 1983; Raimondi and Tomita, 1979; Rivera-Luna *et al.*, 1987; Russell and Rubinstein, 1989), the amount of radiation administered (according to Russell and Rubinstein (1989) a dose of at least 5000 rads is required if treatment is to be effective), and the inclusion of chemotherapy in the treatment protocol. Rivera-Luna *et al.* (1987) compared 30 children who had experienced surgery and irradiation as treatment for medulloblastoma with 35 who underwent surgery, irradiation and chemotherapy. Remission rates were 34.6 per cent from 4 to 268 months (median 29.3 months) for the surgery-radiotherapy group, and 71.4 per cent from 3 to 60 months (median 21 months) for the surgery-radiotherapy-chemotherapy group. Thus the addition of chemotherapy to the treatment protocol appeared to aid remission in the patients studied by Rivera-Luna *et al.* (1987).

Park *et al.* (1983) related survival to age and sex, concluding that children over 5 years of age had a better prognosis than those 5 years of age or less. The 5-year survival rates of the 82 male and 47 female children reviewed by these authors were 53 per cent and 47 per cent respectively. In contrast, a better prognosis for females was noted by Raimondi and Tomita (1979).

Tumour extension to the brainstem was also considered to be a prognostic factor by Park *et al.* (1983). The 5-year survival rate of 42 patients with brainstem involvement was 34 per cent, whereas it was 54 per cent for the 86 patients whose brainstem remained intact.

Finally, the occurrence of extraneural metastases subsequent to medulloblastoma imply a poor prognosis. Metastatic deposits are most frequently diagnosed in the lymph nodes and the bones (Campbell *et al.*, 1984; Russell and Rubinstein, 1989).

While medulloblastomas have a less favourable prognosis than astrocytomas, advances in management techniques are improving the long-term outlook of medulloblastoma patients. Tumour recurrence and metastatic spread can occur, however, despite surgery, radiotherapy and chemotherapy, and generally indicate a poor prognosis for long-term survival.

Ependymoma

An ependymoma is a slow growing, predominantly benign neoplasm which usually arises in close relationship to the ventricles. The fourth ventricle is the most common site (Russell and Rubinstein, 1989); however, supratentorial ependymomas are also possible. The ventricles are lined with a membrane composed of ependymal cells (ependyma), hence the distinct location of this tumour type. Because of the high incidence of recurrence ependymomas have a poor prognosis (Delong and Adams, 1975; Naidich and Zimmerman, 1984; Kirsch *et al.*, 1980).

Age at onset

The peak incidence of childhood ependymoma has been reported to occur between either 3 and 7 years of age (Delong and Adams, 1975), or 1 and 5 years of age (Naidich and Zimmerman, 1984).

Male : female ratio

A higher incidence of ependymoma was reported in male children by Naidich and Zimmerman (1984). West *et al.* (1985), however, observed more females in a group of 25 patients with ependymoma.

Clinical symptoms

Generally, symptoms cannot be distinguished from astrocytoma (Delong and Adams, 1975; Naidich and Zimmerman, 1984; Kirsch *et al.*, 1980); however, since the tumour blocks the flow of cerebrospinal fluid before invading the cerebellum the initial symptoms are those associated with increased intracranial pressure rather than cerebellar deficits.

Medical prognosis

Recurrence of the tumour develops in approximately 30 per cent of the patients and is usually followed by death within a few months (Delong and Adams, 1975; Pierre-Kahn *et al.*, 1983; Ross and Rubinstein, 1989). If tumour recurrence does occur it is usually identified within 4 years of the initial diagnosis (Salazar *et al.*, 1983).

A 5-year survival rate of 39 per cent was reported by Naidich and Zimmerman (1984); however, far more favourable survival rates were determined by Salazar *et al.* (1983), and Ross and Rubinstein (1989). Fifty-one adults and children treated with surgery and radiotherapy for either infratentorial (31 patients) or supratentorial (20 patients) ependymoma (17 patients had grade 1 and 2 ependymomas, while 34 had grade 3 and 4 tumours) were reviewed by Salazar *et al.* (1983). The 10-year survival rates calculated were 75 per cent for low grade and 67 per cent for high grade ependymomas. Similarly, Ross and Rubinstein (1989) described 15 patients with malignant ependymomas (10 were situated in the posterior fossa) and found 10 patients (67 per cent) to be alive from 15 months to 14 years after surgery.

Salazar *et al.* (1983) also considered prognostic factors which may influence the survival of patients with ependymoma. A significant difference in median survival times was found for children less than 12 years of age (37 months) at the time of diagnosis and patients older than 12 years at diagnosis (18 months). In contrast, West *et al.* (1985) found that adults had a longer median survival time (52 months) than children 15 years of age or less (28.5 months). Neither tumour position above or below the tentorium, nor the extent of surgical excision significantly influenced survival in the patients studied by Salazar *et al.* (1983). The extent of radiation treatment was also correlated with survival. Patients treated with whole-brain irradiation for low grade tumours and craniospinal irradiation for high grade tumours had significantly longer survival times than those treated with partial brain irradiation.

Management of Posterior Fossa Tumours

The management of a child with a posterior fossa tumour begins when the child presents at a doctor's surgery or at a hospital casualty department suffering a combination of the clinical signs and symptoms discussed in the previous sections. A neurological examination is performed and, if warranted, the child is referred for further diagnostic examinations such as CT or magnetic resonance imaging (MRI). It is likely that the technique of choice will depend on the availability of equipment; however, the advantages of one technique over another may be a consideration in the diagnostic process. CT is more widely available, less expensive, quicker to perform, more sensitive in the detection of calcium and cysts, and allows the use of an intravenous contrast agent which enhances scan resolution. MRI enhances resolution in the CNS regions that are surrounded by bone, allows easy manipulation of the image plane, and avoids the use of ionizing irradiation and invasive intravenous contrast agents (Kadota *et al.*, 1989; Packer *et al.*, 1985).

If a positive diagnosis is made, the child is usually admitted to hospital immediately. The course of action that follows varies according to the exact location and spread of the tumour, and the age and clinical status of the child.

The majority of children with posterior fossa tumour experience hydrocephalus due to ventricular and CSF pathway obstruction. This symptom is alleviated by the surgical insertion of a shunting system. The most common shunt utilized is a ventriculoperitoneal shunt which drains fluid from the lateral ventricles into the peritoneal cavity. The shunting procedure is usually performed before surgical excision of the tumour; however, in some cases shunting may not be required until after the tumour has been resected.

Once the child has stabilized following the insertion of a shunt, a craniotomy is performed. The neurosurgeon gains access to the posterior fossa through the occipital region of the cranium. Macroscopically, tumour removal is judged as total, subtotal (at least 80 per cent of the tumour is excised), or partial. If the tumour is inaccessible, only a biopsy is taken to allow a diagnosis to be made. The extent of tumour excision depends on the neurological deficits that are likely to result from aggressive surgical resection.

The tumour tissue which was removed at surgery is analyzed and a histological diagnosis is made. Subsequent treatment depends largely on the pathologist's report and the extent of tumour resection. Most children receive whole-brain and/or spinal irradiation with an extra boost to the tumour site. Children with low grade astrocytomas are often spared craniospinal irradiation, a factor which may lead to a lower incidence of neuropsychological sequelae, including language disorders, in the long-term (see Ch. 9). A typical course of radiotherapy may consist of a total irradiation dose of 5000–6000 rads which is administered in daily fractions of 180 rads until the total dose is reached. A course of radiotherapy takes approximately 6 weeks to complete and is a gruelling experience for both the child and his/her family. The child often feels tired, irritable and nauseous while the family is required to spend many hours each week accompanying the child to the radiotherapy clinic.

Children with highly malignant tumours may also receive chemotherapy. While postoperative chemotherapy is not administered as routinely as radiotherapy, it has been suggested that when added to a regimen of surgical excision and CNS irradiation, or when implemented in cases of recurrent tumour, chemotherapy will prolong survival time (Horowitz *et al.*, 1988; van Eys *et al.*, 1988). Chemotherapy protocols can vary widely in drug selection, dosages and timing. Both chemotherapy and radiotherapy courses and the complications which may be associated with such treatments are discussed in detail in Chapter 9.

As discussed previously, many patients experience tumour recurrence despite aggressive tumour management at initial diagnosis. Depending on the site and growth characteristics of the recurrent tumour, these patients undergo reoperation, radiotherapy and/or chemotherapy. In some cases, the additional treatment is described as palliative rather than curative, with the ultimate aim being the alleviation of symptoms and an extension of the expected survival time.

Speech and Language Deficits in Posterior Fossa Tumours

Speech Deficits Associated with Posterior Fossa Tumours

It is evident from the above discussion that most childhood tumours are located in the posterior fossa (Farwell *et al.*, 1977; Matson, 1956; Naidich and Zimmerman, 1984; Segall *et al.*, 1985). This being the case, it could be expected that the most common type of speech disorder seen in association with childhood brain tumours would be an ataxic dysarthria.

Ataxic dysarthria

The first attempt to provide uniform descriptions of the dysarthrias is attributed to

Darley *et al.* (1969). These authors considered 212 adult subjects who had either pseudobulbar palsy, bulbar palsy, amyotrophic lateral sclerosis, cerebellar lesions, parkinsonism, dystonia or choreathetosis. The speech of these subjects was rated on 38 dimensions which covered the characteristics of pitch, loudness, vocal quality, respiration, prosody, articulation and overall impressions. The ten most frequent characteristics of the speech of subjects with cerebellar disorders are listed in Table 8.1.

While imprecise consonants was the most prominent feature recorded, Brown *et al.* (1970) claimed it was of little diagnostic value as any type of dysarthria could be expected to involve the imprecise production of consonants. Irregular articulatory breakdown, characterized by the sudden, inconsistent collapse of one or more syllables, was considered to be indicative of ataxic dysarthria; however, patients with dystonia and chorea also exhibited this feature. Excess and equal stress or 'scanning' speech was highly suggestive of ataxic dysarthria, while distorted vowels, harsh voice, prolonged phonemes, prolonged intervals and monopitch were frequently absent in the mild dysarthric patients.

Kent and Netsell (1975) studied a 59-year-old ataxic dysarthric using cine-radiographic and spectrographic techniques. Both their physiological and acoustic observations were compatible with the perceptual descriptions of Darley *et al.* (1969) with slow rate, excess and equal stress patterns and imprecise or distorted vowel and consonant productions being prominent on the spectrographs obtained. The cineradiographs demonstrated the occurrence of abnormally small adjustments of the tongue between the anterior and posterior positions required for vowel productions. Acquired dysarthria in adults with cerebellar lesions does therefore have a theoretical base from which the speech of adults can be predicted and described.

A number of authors have linked the presence of ataxic dysarthria in children with the presence of mass lesions in the posterior fossa (Ammirati *et al.*, 1989; Brown, 1985; Hudson *et al.*, 1989; Rekate *et al.*, 1985; Volcan *et al.*, 1986). Rekate *et al.* (1985) noted the presence of dysarthria associated with cerebellar tumours. They reviewed six

Table 8.1 Ten most deviant speech dimensions shown by subjects with cerebellar disorders

1. Imprecise consonants
2. Excess and equal stress
3. Irregular articulatory breakdown
4. Distorted vowels
5. Harsh voice
6. Phonemes prolonged
7. Intervals prolonged
8. Monopitch
9. Monoloudness
10. Slow rate

From Darley *et al.* (1969).

children between 2 and 11 years of age who had experienced acute bilateral damage to large areas of both cerebellar hemispheres. This sample included four children with medulloblastoma, one with astrocytoma and one with ependymoma. All the children were mute for 1–3 months following surgery and were severely dysarthric during recovery.

Only two of the six cases were described in detail by Rekate and co-workers. An 8-year-old girl underwent total removal of a medulloblastoma which was situated in the vermis. By 3 months after surgery, her expressive language had fully recovered although a slow, monotonous speech pattern persisted. Two and a half years later, normal academic achievement and a mild residual cerebellar dysarthria were noted. A 6-year-old boy with an astrocytoma involving the vermis and left cerebellar hemisphere was also described. He began speaking 2 weeks after surgery, demonstrating 'characteristic cerebellar dysarthria' which made him difficult to understand. Six months later his speech was described as normal.

Volcan *et al.* (1986) described another case of muteness immediately preceding dysarthria subsequent to removal of a posterior fossa tumour. They described an 8-year-old girl who had a medulloblastoma removed from the fourth ventricle which resulted in a mild right paresis, truncal ataxia, signs of right cerebellar dysfunction and muteness. Within 2 weeks she had regained monosyllabic speech but had a monotonous tone and was dysarthric. Vigorous work by her mother, a speech pathologist, preceded a marked improvement. Twelve months after surgery, a mild dysarthria was still present.

Similarly, Ammirati *et al.* (1989) described the onset of mutism in a 14-year-old boy 24 hours after the complete excision of a vermian grade 1 astrocytoma. Cranial nerve palsies, long tract signs, or dysphagia were not detected. The patient was able to pronounce two-syllable words 3 weeks after surgery, and 5 weeks after surgery was dysarthric but able to produce two- and three-word utterances. At follow-up 4 months after surgery, he exhibited a mild residual dysarthria and minimal gait ataxia. The nature of the dysarthria observed was not described. Both Rekate *et al.* (1985) and Ammirati *et al.* (1989) postulated that the mutism may have been related to bilateral involvement of the dentate nuclei and the subsequent resolution of dysarthric speech may represent a recovering cerebellar mechanism.

Although, as indicated above, a number of authors have noted the presence of dysarthria in association with tumours involving the posterior cranial fossa, the study by Hudson *et al.* (1989) is the only one reported to date that has provided a detailed description of the characteristics of the speech disorders resulting from surgical removal of posterior fossa tumours. Using the Frenchay Dysarthria Assessment (Enderby, 1983) and a perceptual analysis of connected speech, two of six children evaluated were described as dysarthric. The first exhibited a mixed ataxic-flaccid dysarthria characterized by lip, tongue and laryngeal incoordination, as well as asymmetry and restricted lip, jaw and tongue movements associated with a left facial palsy. Of the ten ataxic dysarthric characteristics identified by Darley *et al.* (1969), imprecise consonants, excess and equal stress, irregular articulatory breakdowns, prolonged phonemes and slow rate were present. A lack of volume control was also noted. Overall, this subject was largely unintelligible.

Another subject described by Hudson *et al.* (1989) demonstrated six features characteristic of ataxic dysarthria: imprecise consonants, excess and equal stress, harsh voice, prolonged phonemes, prolonged intervals and slow rate. The presence of pitch breaks, variable pitch, a lack of volume control, and explosive onsets was also reported. Although a third subject exhibited a reduced range and speed of lip and tongue movements he was not considered to be dysarthric.

In addition to the dysarthric features reported, Hudson *et al.* (1989) noted the retention of immature speech patterns in two subjects aged 6 years 2 months and 8 years 10 months at the time of assessment. The phonological processes recorded included stopping, post-vocalic devoicing, syllable reduction and progressive assimilation. The underlying basis for the observed developmental speech disorders can only be speculated upon at this stage; however, it is possible that the medical and emotional trauma experienced by these two children when aged 3 years 9 months and 2 years 1 month, respectively, may have interrupted the normal developmental pattern of speech acquisition.

Although a limited number of studies involving small subject numbers have reported some of the characteristics of acquired childhood neurological speech disorders, details of the speech disorders shown by children following removal of posterior fossa tumours remain largely unknown. Characteristics of ataxic dysarthria, as determined by Darley *et al.* (1969) for an adult population, have been identified in children treated for posterior fossa tumour. Additional features of dysarthria have also been described. Developmental speech errors have been recorded in two patients treated during the period of rapid speech and language acquisition.

In view of the high proportion of childhood tumours which involve the posterior cranial fossa, further research in this area needs to be carried out using the characteristics of specific dysarthria syndromes, in particular ataxic dysarthria, specified in the adult literature as a guideline for the formulation of hypotheses.

Language and Posterior Fossa Tumours

Although the posterior fossa site of the majority of childhood tumours does not lead to the prediction of an associated language deficit, there are a number of features occurring secondary to posterior fossa tumours which could possibly lead to the occurrence of language problems.

Hydrocephalus usually accompanies posterior fossa tumours because in many cases these tumours either emerge from or invade the fourth ventricle, thereby obstructing the flow of CSF. Subsequent dilation of the lateral ventricles may result in compression of the cerebral cortex. The mass effect of the tumour itself may also impede the CSF flow as well as contribute to tissue destruction and cortical compression. The invasion and compression of cerebral tissue may also result in vascular changes which could be related to dysfunction in the central speech and language centres. In addition, radiotherapy administered after surgical removal of posterior fossa tumours in order to prevent tumour spread or recurrence, has been reported to cause aphasia in some adults and intellectual deficits in some children (Bamford *et al.*, 1976; Broadbent *et al.*, 1981; Burns and Boyle, 1984; Danoff *et al.*, 1982; Duffner *et al.*, 1983; Kun *et al.*, 1983; Silverman *et al.*, 1984). LeBaron *et al.* (1988), however, reported major academic, motor, sensory, cognitive and emotional disturbance in more than 50 per cent of the 15 cerebellar tumour patients reviewed irrespective of the inclusion of radiotherapy in the treatment protocol. The apparent cortical involvement prompted LeBaron and co-workers to stress the need for further research into this area before any associated neuropsychological deficits can be attributed to the effects of CNS prophylaxis alone. The reader is referred to Chapter 9 for a detailed review of the speech, language and intellectual deficits that have been associated with CNS prophylaxis.

Carrow-Woolfolk and Lynch (1982) listed traumatic injury, brain tumours and epilepsy as the three primary causes of acquired aphasia. Accordingly, children with tumours have been included in samples of acquired aphasics (Alajouanine and Lhermitte, 1965; Carrow-Woolfolk and Lynch, 1982; Cooper and Flowers, 1987; Hécean, 1976; Miller *et al.*, 1984; Van Dongen *et al.*, 1985); however, the majority of studies do not differentiate between various causes of acquired language disorders, nor do they describe tumour sites or treatments.

Alajouanine and Lhermitte (1965) studied 32 children with cerebral lesions between 6 and 15 years of age. Two of these children had undergone surgery for astrocytoma removal; however, the sites of the tumours were not provided. While a posterior fossa location is more common in children, astrocytomas can also originate in the cerebral hemispheres. Alajouanine and Lhermitte (1965) reported that the reduction of expressive activities (oral, written and gesture) was the most prominent feature of the acquired language disorders exhibited by the subject group.

This reduction of expression was noted in all 32 children and was not related to the presence of dysarthria. No or limited oral expression was also reported in two of the other tumour studies previously discussed (Rekate *et al.*, 1985; Volcan *et al.*, 1986). However, in the latter studies the reduction in expression could have been caused by the presence of mutism and/or dysarthria and consequently a language disturbance may or may not have existed. Alajouanine and Lhermitte (1965) noted simplified rather than erroneous syntax, and severe reading and writing disturbances. The aphasic characteristics seen in adults such as logorrhea, phonemic or semantic paraphias, verbal stereotypes and perseverations were not detected in the cases of acquired aphasia studied. The general pattern of simplified syntax, severe reading and writing disturbances and reduced oral expression is commonly reported in the literature with the addition of comprehension and word-finding difficulties in some cases (Carrow-Woolfolk and Lynch, 1982; Satz and Bullard-Bates, 1981; Van Dongen *et al.*, 1985).

While several authors have attempted to specify a common set of characteristics of acquired childhood aphasia (see Ch.1) Cooper and Flowers (1987), in a study of children with aphasia resulting from different causes, were unable to identify one particular language deficit or a cluster of deficits as common to their group of brain-injured children. Fifteen children with histories of closed head injury, stroke, encephalitis or brain tumour (one patient showed a posterior fossa mass on CT) were assessed between 1 and 10 years post-onset using a battery of language and academic tests. The subjects performed significantly below a group of non-brain-injured controls in the areas of word, sentence and paragraph comprehension; naming; oral production of complex syntactic constructions; and word fluency. Within the subject group, language deficits ranged from no or only mild impairment to significant language deficits. Two of the 15 subjects were receiving academic assistance of some kind. In particular, the child who had been treated for posterior fossa tumour when 10, had, when 6 years old, demonstrated aphasia, reduced receptive skills and monosyllabic verbalizations at diagnosis. Twelve months later, the child was enrolled in full-time special education and was receiving speech therapy, occupational therapy and physiotherapy. On assessment, particular difficulties were noted on sentence formulation and naming tasks. Unfortunately, details of the medical management of this case were not provided. In his sample of 26 children with cortical lesions Hécaen (1976) also included two cases of tumour. It was found that in one of these cases, the presence of a tumour in the left cerebral hemisphere resulted in muteness lasting 2 months, and articulation, reading and writing disorders from which there was no change.

To date, the only study which has systematically addressed the speech and language abilities of children treated for posterior fossa tumours was reported by Hudson *et al.* (1989). This study differed from those discussed previously in that the group of six children all had a posterior fossa tumour and were investigated using a battery of language assessments. The subjects showed language abilities that ranged from normal to severely impaired, a language impairment being evidenced in four of the six children studied. Subject 1, a 6-year-old boy who was assessed 2 years 5 months after surgery, performed below the normal range in the areas of expressive semantics, receptive syntax and expressive syntax. At the time of assessment, he was repeating pre-school as his teacher believed he would be unable to cope with Grade 1. Subject 2 demonstrated a severe language impairment with all of the language abilities assessed falling well below the normal range. Subject 2 was assessed 6 years 1 month after surgery at 8 years 8 months of age. At this time, he was enrolled in Grade 1 at a small country school. The third subject (Subject 3) underwent a language evaluation 6 years 9 months after surgical removal of a posterior fossa tumour. He was 8 years 10 months of age at the time of assessment. The only language deficit recorded in this case was a word-retrieval problem. Finally, a 15 year 4 month-old male who was treated for posterior fossa tumour when 13 years of age demonstrated reading difficulties. Two further children (Subjects 4 and 6) performed within normal limits on all the language tests administered. It is notable that the four children with evidence of language deficits had received CNS prophylaxis after surgery, while Subjects 4 and 6 underwent tumour resection only.

Overall, the linguistic problems identified by Hudson *et al.* (1989) in children treated for posterior fossa tumours included deficits in the areas of expressive vocabulary and word finding, receptive syntax, expressive syntax and reading. A characteristic pattern of non-fluent or fluent acquired aphasia was not determined by Hudson *et al.* (1989), suggesting that the generalizations which have been made regarding the anticipated features of childhood aphasia (see Ch.1) may not apply to children suffering posterior fossa tumours. While the site of lesion was uniform in the subject group, factors which could have influenced the language abilities observed included age at onset, tumour type, extent of surgical excision, the insertion of ventriculoperitoneal shunts and the administration of radiotherapy and/or chemotherapy. Research utilizing a larger subject group is necessary before the many variables associated with posterior fossa tumour management can be analyzed.

In summary, symptoms of acquired childhood aphasia include simplified syntax, severe reading and writing disturbances, mutism, word-finding difficulties, comprehension difficulties at the word, sentence and paragraph levels, and articulation errors. Traditionally, childhood aphasia has been considered non-fluent; however, the presence of paraphasias, neologisms and logorrhea in the form of a fluent aphasia has also been observed (see Ch.1). Such generalizations in cases of acquired language deficits have not been supported by Hudson *et al.* (1989) who failed to recognize characteristic patterns of deficit in a group of children treated for posterior fossa tumours. Their findings suggested that while children with posterior fossa tumours may exhibit a language impairment, it is unlikely that the language deficits observed will fall into one characteristic pattern such as the non-fluent aphasia said to be shown by brain-injured children in a number of earlier studies (see Ch. 1). Exact lesion sites are rarely referred to in the literature making any predictions about the effects of posterior fossa tumour removal on language functions difficult.

Prognosis for Recovery of Speech/Language Function

Overall, improvement in aphasic children is considered to be more rapid and complete than in adults. Alajouanine and Lhermitte (1965) reported recovery in two-thirds of their children when reassessed at least 12 months after injury. While Carrow-Woolfolk and Lynch (1982) observed that children under 10 years of age have a fair chance of reacquiring verbal skills within 1 year, Alajouanine and Lhermitte (1965) did not find a significant difference in the speed of recovery between children less than 10 years of age and children 10 or more years of age. The recovery of aphasia has been related to the cause, the site, the extent and the reversibility of the cerebral lesion (Alajounanine and Lhermitte, 1965; Van Dongen and Loonen, 1977) as well as to the age at injury (Satz and Bullard-Bates, 1981).

While it has been reported that younger children with acquired aphasia have a more favourable prognosis than older children (Carrow-Woolfolk and Lynch, 1982), it is possible that the reverse is true in children who experience surgery and CNS prophylaxis for the treatment of brain tumour. There is a need for prospective studies documenting the speech and language recovery of brain tumour patients; however, studies of intellectual functioning have suggested that children with tumours who are less than 6 years of age at diagnosis and treatment have a greater risk of intellectual deterioration than those older than 6 years (Danoff *et al.*, 1982; Mulhern and Kun, 1985). Whether or not a deterioration in language abilities parallels the reported decline in intellectual functioning has not as yet been determined.

Implications for Speech and Language Management

From the information available to date, it is clear that all aspects of speech and language functioning in children treated for brain tumours need to be assessed. At this stage, no characteristic language patterns have been identified to give the clinician a starting point for patient management, or to alert the clinician to specific areas that are more likely to require in-depth evaluation in tumour cases. Following a comprehensive language assessment, an individualized therapy programme can be devised. Therapy for this population can never be prescriptive as it is essential the clinician evaluates each child's language abilities in the context of the tumour treatment being administered, the presence of other complicating factors such as hydrocephalus and ventriculoperitoneal shunts, the presence of any intellectual deterioration, the educational status of the child, the involvement of other medical and educational services and the emotional state of the child and his/her family.

The information available on the speech of brain tumour patients suggests that the clinician needs to consider both developmental and acquired disorders when assessing these children. Depending on the therapist's initial clinical impressions, either a dysarthria assessment (Hudson *et al.*, 1989) successfully utilized the Frenchay Dysarthria Assessment, a test designed for adults, in the assessment of children treated for posterior fossa tumours) or an articulation/phonological assessment should be administered. In addition, the occurrence of mutism after surgery has been documented and indicates a need for speech therapy intervention. Like language therapy, speech therapy requires individualized programming depending on the nature of the child's speech and the child's medical, educational and intellectual skills.

Finally, suggestions that neurological deterioration can occur from months to years after the completion of treatment for brain tumours (Kun *et al.*, 1983; Mulhern and Kun, 1985; Silverman *et al.*, 1984) implies a need to obtain initial baseline measurements and to review children at 6- or 12-monthly intervals for several years, whether or not speech therapy was recommended subsequent to the initial assessment. Thus, speech/language pathologists should take an active role in the long-term management of children treated for brain tumours, even if intervention is not initially warranted or has been discontinued.

References

ALAJOUANINE, T. H. and LHERMITTE, F. (1965) 'Acquired aphasia in children', *Brain*, **88**, pp. 653–62.

AMMIRATI, M., MIRZAI, S. and SAMII, M. (1989) 'Transient mutism following removal of a cerebellar tumour: A case report and review of the literature', *Child's Nervous System*, **5**, pp. 12–14.

ARON, B. S. (1971) 'Medulloblastoma in children: Twenty-two years' experience with radiation therapy', *American Journal of Diseases of Childhood*, **121**, pp. 314–17.

AUER, R. N., RICE, G. P. A., HINTON, G. F., AMACHER, A. L. and GILBERT, J. J. (1981) 'Cerebellar astrocytoma with benign histology and malignant clinical course', *Journal of Neurosurgery*, **54**, p. 128.

BAMFORD, F. N., JONES, P. M., PEARSON, D., RIBEIRO, G. G., SHALET, S. M. and BEARDWELL, C. G. (1976) 'Residual disabilities in children treated for intracranial space-occupying lesion', *Cancer*, **37**, pp. 1149–51.

BERNELL, W. R., KEPES, J. J. and SEITZ, E. P. (1972) 'Late malignant recurrence of childhood cerebellar astrocytoma: Report of 2 cases', *Journal of Neurosurgery*, **37**, pp. 470–4.

BLOOM, H. J. G. (1982) 'Medulloblastoma in children: Increasing survival rates and further prospects', *International Journal of Radiation, Oncology, Biology, Physics*, **8**, pp. 2023–7.

BROADBENT, V. A., BARNES, N. D. and WHEELER, T. K. (1981) 'Medulloblastoma in childhood: Long-term results of treatment', *Cancer*, **48**, pp. 26–30.

BROWN, J. K. (1985) 'Dysarthria in children: neurologic perspective', in Darby, J.K. (Ed.) *Speech and Language Evaluation in Neurology: Childhood Disorders*, Orlando, Grune and Stratton, pp. 133–84.

BROWN, J. R., DARLEY, F. L. and ARONSON, A. E. (1970) 'Ataxic dysarthria', *International Journal of Neurology*, **7**, pp. 302–18.

BURNS, M. S. and BOYLE, M. (1984) 'Aphasia after successful radiation treatment: A report of two cases', *Journal of Speech and Hearing Disorders*, **94**, pp. 107–11.

CAMPBELL, A. N., CHAN, H. S. L., BECKER, L. E., DANEMAN, A., PARK, T. S. and HOFFMAN, H. J. (1984) 'Extracranial metastases in childhood primary intracranial tumours. A report of 21 cases and review of the literature', *Cancer*, **53**, p. 974.

CARROW-WOOLFOLK, E. and LYNCH, J. (1982) *An Integrated Approach to Language Disorders in Children*, Orlando, Grune & Stratton, Ch. 15.

COOPER, J. A. and FLOWERS, C. R. (1987) 'Children with a history of acquired aphasia: Residual language and academic impairments', *Journal of Speech and Hearing Disorders*, **52**, pp. 251–62.

DANOFF, B. R., CHOWCHOCK, S., MARQUETTE, C., MULGREW, L. and KRAMER, S. (1982) 'Assessment of the long-term effects of primary radiation therapy for brain-tumours in children', *Cancer*, **49**, pp. 1580–6.

DARLEY, F. L., ARONSON, A. E. and BROWN, J. R. (1969) 'Differential diagnostic patterns of dysarthria', *Journal of Speech and Hearing Disorders*, **12**, pp. 246–69.

DAVIS, C. H. and JOGLEKAR, V. M. (1981) 'Cerebellar astrocytomas in children and young adults', *Journal of Neurology, Neurosurgery and Psychiatry*, **44**, pp. 820–8.

DELONG, G. R. and ADAMS, R. D. (1975) 'Clinical aspects of tumours of the posterior fossa in childhood', in Vinken P. J., and Bruijn, G. W. (Eds) *Handbook of Clinical Neurology, Vol.18: Tumours of the Brain and Skull*, Part III, Amsterdam, North Holland, pp. 387–411.

DEUTSCH, M. and REIGEL, D. H. (1980) 'The value of myelography in the management of childhood medulloblastoma', *Cancer*, **45**, pp. 2194–7.

DUFFNER, P. K., COHEN, M. E. and THOMAS. P. R. M. (1983) 'Late effects of treatment on the intelligence of children with posterior fossa tumours', *Cancer*, **51**, pp. 233–7.

ENDERBY, P. M. (1983) *Frenchay Dysarthria Assessment*, San Diego, College-Hill Press.

ENZMANN, D. R., NORMAN, D., LEVIN, V., WILSON, C. and NEWTON, T. H. (1978) 'Computed tomography in the follow-up of medulloblastomas and ependymomas', *Radiology*, **128**, pp. 57–63.

FARWELL, J. R., DOHRMANN, G. J. and FLANNERY, J T. (1977) 'Central nervous system tumours in children', *Cancer*, **40**, pp. 3123–32.

GEISSINGER, J. D. and BUCY, P. C. (1971) 'Astrocytomas of the cerebellum in children', *Archives of Neurology*, **24**, pp. 125–35.

GJERRIS, F. (1978) 'Clinical aspects and long-term prognosis of infratentorial intracranial tumours in infancy and childhood', *Acta Neurologica Scandinavica*, **57**, pp. 31–52.

GJERRIS, F. and KLINKEN, L. (1978) 'Long-term prognosis in children with benign cerebellar astrocytoma', *Journal of Neurosurgery*, **49**, pp. 179–84.

GOL, A. (1963) 'Cerebellar astrocytomas in children', *American Journal of Diseases of Children*, **106**, pp. 21–4.

GOL, A. and McKISSOCK, W. (1959) 'The cerebellar astrocytomas: A report on 98 verified cases', *Journal of Neurosurgery*, **16**, pp. 287–96.

HÉCAEN, H. (1976) 'Acquired aphasia in children and the oncogenesis of hemispheric functional specialization', *Brain and Language*, **3**, pp. 114–34.

HIRSCH, J. F., ROSE, C. S., PIERRE-KAHN, A., PFISTER, A. and HOPPE-HIRSCH, E. (1989) 'Benign astrocytic and oligodendrocytic tumours of the cerebral hemispheres in children', *Journal of Neurosurgery*, **70**, pp. 568–72.

HOOPER, R. (1975) 'Intracranial tumours in childhood', *Child's Brain*, **1**, pp. 136–40.

HOROWITZ, M. E., MULHERN, R. K., KUN, L. E., KOVNAR, E., SANFORD, R. A., SIMMONS, J., HAYES, A. and JENKINS, J. J. (1988) 'Brain tumours in the very young child', *Cancer*, **61**, pp. 428–34.

HOSHINO, T., RODRIGUEZ, L. A., CHO, K. G., LEE, K. S., WILSON, C. B., EDWARDS, M. S. B., LEVIN, V. A. and DAVIS, R. L. (1988) 'Prognostic implications of the proliferative potential of low-grade astrocytomas', *Journal of Neurosurgery*, **69**, pp. 839–42.

HUDSON, L. J., MURDOCH, B. E. and OZANNE, A. E. (1989) 'Posterior fossa tumours in childhood: Associated speech and language disorders post-surgery', *Aphasiology*, **3**, pp. 1–18.

ILGREN, E. B. and STILLER, C. A. (1986) 'Cerebellar astrocytomas: Therapeutic management', *Acta Neurochirugia* (Wien), **81**, pp. 11–26.

JEREB, B., REID, A. and AHUJA, R. K. (1982) 'Patterns of failure in patients with medulloblastoma', *Cancer*, **50**, pp. 2941–7.

JOOMA, R. and KENDALL, B. E. (1982) 'Intracranial tumours in the first year of life', *Neuroradiology*, **23**, pp. 267–74.

KADOTA, R. P., ALLEN, J. B., HARTMAN, G. A. and SPRUCE, W. E. (1989) 'Brain tumours in children', *Journal of Pediatrics*, **114**, pp. 511–19.

KENT, R. and NETSELL, R. (1975) 'A case study of an ataxic dysarthric: Cineradiographic and spectrographic observations', *Journal of Speech and Hearing Disorders*, **40**, pp. 115–34.

KIRSCH, W. M., MASFERRER, R., KIM, Y. D., KRAUTH, L. E., NORENBERG, M. and SCHROEDER, M. (1980) 'Intracranial tumours: Their pathology, specific properties and prospects for future control', in Rosenberg, R. N. (Ed.) *Neurology*, New York, Grune & Stratton.

KLEIN, D. M. and MCCULLOUGH, D. C. (1985) 'Surgical staging of cerebellar astrocytomas in childhood', *Cancer*, **56**, pp. 1810–11.

KLEINMAN, G. M., SCHOENE, W. C., WALSHE, T. M. and RICHARDSON, E. P. (1978) 'Malignant transformation in benign cerebellar astrocytoma', *Journal of Neurosurgery*, **49**, pp. 111–18.

KOH, S. J., BROWN, R. E. and SIMMONS, J. C. H. (1985) 'Glioblastoma in children', *Pediatric Pathology*, **4**, pp. 67–79.

KUN, L. E., MULHERN, R. K. and CRISCO, J. J. (1983) 'Quality of life in children treated for brain tumours', *Journal of Neurosurgery*, **58**, pp. 1–6.

LAURENT, J. P., CHANG, C. H. and COHEN, M. E. (1985) 'A classification for primitive neuroectodermal tumours (medulloblastoma) of the posterior fossa', *Cancer*, **56**, pp. 1807–9.

LAWS, E. R., BERGSTRALH, E. J. and TAYLOR, W. F. (1987) 'Cerebellar astrocytoma in children', *Progress in Experimental Tumour Research*, **30**, pp. 122–7.

LEBARON, S., ZELTZER, P. M., ZELTZER, L. K., SCOTT, S. E. and MARLIN, A. E. (1988) 'Assessment of quality of survival in children with medulloblastoma and cerebellar astrocytoma', *Cancer*, **62**, pp. 1215–22.

LEE, Y. Y., GLASS, J. P., VAN EYS, J. and WALLACE, S. (1985) 'Medulloblastoma in infants and children: Computed tomographic follow-up after treatment', *Radiology*, **154**, pp. 677–82.

LEE, Y. Y., VAN TASSEL, P., BRUNER, J. M., MOSER, R. P. and SHARE, J. C. (1989) 'Juvenile pilocytic astrocytomas: CT and MR characteristics', *American Journal of Neuroradiology*, **10**, pp. 363–70.

MABON, R. F., SVIEN, H. J., ADSON, A. W. and KERNOHAN, J. W. (1950) 'Astrocytomas of the cerebellum', *Archives of Neurology and Psychiatry*, **64**, pp. 75–88.

McCOMB, J. G., DAVIS, R. L. and ISAACS, H. (1981) 'Extraneural metastatic medulloblastoma during childhood', *Neurosurgery*, **9**, pp. 548–51.

MATSON, D. D. (1956) 'Cerebellar astrocytoma in childhood', *Pediatrics*, **18**, pp. 150–8.

MILLER, J. F., CAMPBELL, T. F., CHAPMAN, R. S. and WEISMER, S. E. (1984) 'Language behaviour in acquired childhood aphasia', in Holland A. (Ed.) *Language Disorders in Children*, Baltimore, College-Hill Press.

MULHERN, R. K. and KUN, L. E. (1985) 'Neuropsychologic function in children with brain tumours: III. Interval changes in the six months following treatment', *Medical and Pediatric Oncology*, **13**, pp. 318–24.

NAIDICH, T. P. and ZIMMERMAN, R. A. (1984) 'Primary brain tumours in children', *Seminars in Roentgenology*, **19**, pp. 100–14.

NORRIS, D. G., BRUCE, D. A., BYRD, R. L., SCHUT, L., LITTMAN, P., BILANIUK, L. T., ZIMMERMAN, R. A. and CAPP, R. (1981) 'Improved relapse-free survival in medulloblastoma utilizing modern techniques', *Neurosurgery*, **9**, pp. 661–3.

PACKER, R. J., BATNITZKY, S. and COHEN, M. E. (1985) 'Magnetic resonance imaging in the evaluation of intracranial tumours of childhood', *Cancer*, **56**, pp. 1767–72.

PARK, T. S., HOFFMAN, H. J., HENDRICK, E. B., HUMPHREYS, R. P. and BECKER, L. E. (1983) 'Medulloblastoma: Clinical presentation and management', *Journal of Neurosurgery*, **58**, pp. 543–52.

PARKIN, D. M., STILLER, C. A., DRAPER, G. J. and BIEBER, C. A. (1988) 'The international incidence of childhood cancer', *International Journal of Cancer*, **42**, pp. 511–20.

PERUN, J., CARCAVILLA, L., EIRAS, J., ALBERDI, J., PISON, J. and ARANA, T. (1987) 'Medulloblastomas: A review of 11 cases', *Child's Nervous System*, **3**, pp. 361–3.

PIERRE-KAHN, A., HIRSCH, J. F., ROUX, F. X., RENIER, D. and SAINTE-ROSE, C. (1983) 'Intracranial ependymomas in childhood. Survival and Functional Results of 47 cases', *Child's Brain*, **10**, pp. 145–56.

RAIMONDI, A. J. and TOMITA, T. (1979) 'Medulloblastoma in childhood: Comparative results of partial and total resection', *Child's Brain*, **5**, pp. 310–28.

REKATE, H. L., GRUBB, R. L., ARAM, D. M., HAHN, J. F. and RATCHESON, R. A. (1985) 'Muteness of cerebellar origin', *Archives of Neurology*, **42**, pp. 697–8.

RIVERA-LUNA, R., RUEDA-FRANCO, F., LANCHE-GUEVARA, M. T. and MARTINEZ-BUERRA, G. (1987) 'Multidisciplinary treatment of medulloblastomas in childhood', *Child's Nervous System*, **3**, pp. 228–31.

ROSS, G. W. and RUBINSTEIN, L. J. (1989) 'Lack of histopathological correlation of malignant ependymomas with postoperative survival', *Journal of Neurosurgery*, **70**, pp. 31–6.

RUSSELL, D. S. and RUBINSTEIN, L. J. (1989) *Pathology of Tumours of the Nervous System* 5th Ed., London, Edward Arnold.

SALAZAR, O. M., CASTRO-VITA, H., VAN HOUTTE, P., RUBIN, P. and AYGUN, C. (1983) 'Improved survival in cases of intracranial ependymoma after radiation therapy: Late report and recommendations', *Journal of Neurosurgery*, **59**, pp. 652–9.

SATZ, P. and BULLARD-BATES, C. (1981) 'Acquired aphasia in children', in Sarno, M. T,, (Ed.) *Acquired Aphasia*, New York, Academic Press.

SEGALL, H. D., BATNITZKY, S., ZEE, C. S., AHMADI, J., BIRD, C. R. and COHEN, M. E. (1985) 'Computed tomography in the diagnosis of intracranial neoplasms in children', *Cancer*, **56**, pp. 1748–55.

SILVERMAN, C. L., PALKES, H., TALENT, B., KOVNAR, E., CLOUSE, J. W. and THOMAS, P. R. M. (1984) 'Late effects of radiotherapy on patients with cerebellar medulloblastoma', *Cancer*, **54**, pp. 825–9.

TADMOR, R., HARWOOD-NASH, D. C. F. and SAVOIARDO, M. (1980) 'Brain tumours in the first two years of life: CT diagnosis', *American Journal of Neuroradiology*, **1**, pp. 411–17.

TADMOR, R., HARWOOD-NASH, D. C., SCOTTI, G., SAVOIARDO, M., MUSGRAVE, M. A., FITZ, C. R., CHUANG, S. and MODAN, M. (1982) 'Intracranial neoplasms in children: The effect of computed tomography on age distribution', *Radiology*, **145**, pp. 371–3.

TEW, J. M., FEIBEL, J. H. and SAWAYA, R. (1984) 'Brain tumours: Clinical aspects', *Seminars in Roentgenology*, **19**, pp. 115–28.

TOKARS, R. P., SUTTON, H. G. and GRIEM, M. L. (1979) 'Cerebellar medulloblastoma: Results of a new method of radiation treatment', *Cancer*, **42**, pp. 129–36.

TOMITA, T. and MCLONE, D. G. (1983) 'Spontaneous seeding of medulloblastoma: Results of cerebrospinal fluid cytology and arachnoid biopsy from the cisterna magna', *Neurosurgery*, **12**, pp. 265–7.

USHIO, Y., ARITA, N., YOSHIMINE, T., IKEDA, T. and MOGAMI, H. (1987) 'Malignant recurrence of childhood cerebellar astrocytoma: Case report', *Neurosurgery*, **21**, pp. 251–5.

VAN DONGEN, H. R. and LOONEN, M. C. B. (1977) 'Factors related to prognosis of acquired aphasia in children', *Cortex*, **13**, pp. 131–6.

VAN DONGEN, H. R., LOONEN, C. B. and VAN DONGEN, K. J. (1985) 'Anatomical basis for acquired fluent aphasia in children', *Annals of Neurology*, **17**, pp. 306–9.

VAN EYS, J., BARAM, T. Z., CANGIR, A., BRUNER, J. M. and MARTINEZ-PRIETO, J. (1988) 'Salvage chemotherapy for recurrent primary brain tumours in children', *Journal of Pediatrics*, **113**, pp. 601–6.

VOLCAN, I., COLE, G. P. and JOHNSTON, L. (1986) 'A case of muteness of cerebellar origin', *(Letter to the editor). Archives of Neurology*, **43**, pp. 313–14.

WALLNER, K. E., GONZALES, M. F., EDWARDS, M. S., WARA, W. M. and SHELINE, G. E. (1988) 'Treatment results of juvenile pilocytic astrocytoma', *Journal of Neurosurgery*, **69**, pp. 171–6.

WEST, C. R., BRUCE, D. A. and DUFFNER, P. K. (1985) 'Ependymomas: Factors in clinical and diagnostic staging', *Cancer*, **56**, pp. 1812–16.

Chapter 9

Effect of CNS Prophylaxis on Speech and Language Function in Children

Lisa J. Hudson, Deborah L. Buttsworth and Bruce E. Murdoch

Introduction

Modern medicine has brought new knowledge to the complex task of treating the various forms of childhood cancer. In addition to radical surgery, the current treatment of childhood cancers usually involves the use of techniques such as radiotherapy and chemotherapy, both of which may cause structural and functional changes in the central nervous system (CNS). These structural and functional changes, in turn, may cause a reduction in overall intellectual and cognitive function, including language. It is important, therefore, that speech/language pathologists are aware of the possible implications of treatment involving either radiotherapy and/or chemotherapy on the speech/language abilities of children with cancerous conditions.

Radiotherapy

An Introduction to Radiotherapy

Radiotherapy is the treatment of disease using ionizing radiation. The use of radiation as a treatment modality was first attempted in the late nineteenth century and followed closely on the discovery near the end of last century of X-rays by Roentgen, radioactivity by Becquerel and radium by the Curies (Kaplan, 1975). During the treatment process, tissues containing neoplastic cells are exposed to a beam of radiation. Because cancer cells are particularly sensitive to radiation, their rapid multiplication is controlled, and ultimately, the abnormal cells are destroyed while the surrounding normal tissue remains relatively intact. Much research, however, has been aimed at determining the maximum amount of radiation that can be delivered before damage to normal tissue is induced (Marks *et al.*, 1981; Marks and Wong, 1985). Despite advances in research, however, damage to normal tissue as a result of irradiation is still frequently reported.

The present section will consider the use and effects of radiation in cases of CNS cancers. The effects of irradiation to be considered will mainly include those classified as 'late-delayed' reactions. Such reactions appear from several months to years after the completion of radiotherapy and tend to be progressive and more permanent in nature than either acute reactions or 'early-delayed' reactions. Acute reactions are symptoms occurring during the course of radiotherapy, while 'early-delayed' reactions appear from a few weeks to a few months after irradiation and are usually transient.

As part of a course of radiotherapy, radiation can be administered to any body part containing either benign or malignant neoplastic cells. The amount of radiation used varies depending on the nature of the neoplasm. Radiation doses are measured in rads (radiation absorbed dose) which is a unit of measurement representing the absorbed dose of ionizing radiation.

Patients receiving CNS irradiation include those with benign or malignant neoplasms in the brain and/or spinal cord. Patients with CNS tumours usually receive a total radiation dose of 5000–6000 rads, usually in daily fractions of 180–200 rads until the total dose is reached. A typical course of radiotherapy takes 5–6 weeks to complete.

CNS radiotherapy is also required by patients who have leukaemia or lymphoma. The administration of radiation in such cases is to prevent the spread of cancer cells to the CNS and is targeted at the brain and spinal cord to a total dose of 1800–2400 rads which is less than the total dose given to tumour patients. Again, the total dose is given in daily fractions of 180–200 rads.

Sites and Types of Radiation-Induced CNS Damage

Evidence is accumulating which suggests that although radiotherapy is necessary for the survival of children with cancerous conditions, it has some long-term negative effects on brain structure and function. Radiation-related lesions have been detected in both the grey and white matter of the cerebrum and cerebellum.

White matter damage occurring subsequent to radiotherapy

The white matter damage detected in patients who have received radiotherapy to the CNS has primarily involved necrosis and calcification. Necrosis refers to changes in the neural tissue which are indicative of cell death. Calcification involves the deposition of calcium salts in a tissue, while dystrophic calcification is the deposition of calcium in abnormal tissue (e.g. scar tissue) without an abnormality of blood calcium.

Damage to cerebral white matter following cranial irradiation has been reported to occur in both children and adults while grey matter regions are more likely to remain intact. White matter changes can be detected from 5 months to 5 years after the completion of radiotherapy. Doses of radiation which have been associated with alterations in white matter have reportedly ranged from 2340 to 6000 rads. No specific dose level, however, has been suggested to increase the risk of white matter calcification or necrosis. Contrary to expectations, Marks *et al*. (1981) observed that white matter necrosis did not always occur in the region that received the highest radiation dose. Davis *et al*. (1986) attempted to link radiation dose and resultant damage and found that children with white matter abnormalities had received between 2600 and 5000 rads while those with calcification had received between 3500 and 5500 rads, thereby suggesting that calcification is induced by slightly higher doses of radiation than other white matter abnormalities.

Both specific and diffuse white matter damage has been reported subsequent to radiotherapy. Marks *et al*. (1981) described pathologically-proven radionecrosis in seven adults. Reported sites of damage included the white matter of the right hemisphere, the white matter adjacent to the original tumour site, the white matter of both temporal lobes, the white matter of the occipital hemisphere opposite the original tumour and in the original tumour bed.

A 14-year-old male with internal capsule calcification following radiotherapy was reported by Lichtor *et al*. (1984). Twelve years after completion of irradiation, a large calcified mass in the right internal capsule and an area of increased density in the genu of the left internal capsule were identified by computed tomography (CT). Another 14-year-old boy examined by Yamashita *et al*. (1980) 9 months after cranial irradiation demonstrated lesions within the deep white matter of both cerebral hemispheres. Grey matter damage was also diagnosed in this patient, with bilateral abnormalities being detected in the basal ganglia and cerebral peduncles. In addition to specific lesions, diffuse white matter damage following radiotherapy has also been reported by several investigators (Davis *et al*., 1986; Dooms *et al*., 1986).

While white matter abnormalities have been identified by some investigators in children who have experienced cranial irradiation, Tsuruda *et al*. (1987) failed to detect any lesions in 11 patients less than 20 years of age. These authors reviewed 95 patients who had received radiotherapy for CNS tumours. Magnetic resonance images (MRI) were viewed retrospectively and graded according to the changes involving white matter. Thirty-six of the 84 patients more than 20 years of age had symmetrical white matter lesions remote from either the tumour or operative site. Relative sparing of the brainstem, cerebellum, internal capsules and basal ganglia was noted in these cases. The severity of white matter damage increased with age at treatment. Tsuruda *et al*. (1987) were unable to explain the absence of radiation-related damage in younger patients. The authors proposed that the follow-up interval used by them of less than 2 years for the younger patients may have preceded the appearance of any long-term changes. The older patients were assessed up to 71 months after the completion of irradiation. It was also suggested that a higher percentage (45 per cent) of posterior fossa tumours in the younger group may have biased the results. The significance of posterior fossa tumours in the consideration of white matter changes was not explained by the authors.

Grey matter damage occurring subsequent to radiotherapy

Although the presence of white matter damage subsequent to radiotherapy has been discussed frequently throughout the literature, grey matter calcification has also been acknowledged as a consequence of radiation treatment. As indicated above, irradiation induced damage involving both grey and white matter lesions was observed bilaterally in the basal ganglia, the cerebral peduncles and in the deep white matter of both cerebral hemispheres by Yamashita *et al.* (1980).

Basal ganglia calcification has frequently been cited as a consequence of childhood cranial irradiation. Lee and Suh (1977) described two children who were irradiated when 2 years of age. Both evidenced extensive bilateral calcifications in the basal ganglia at intervals of 10 and 14 years after radiotherapy. One child also had calcification of the thalamus, and the other had calcification of the cerebral cortex. Similarly, Pearson *et al.* (1983) identified basal ganglia calcification in three children who were also treated when less than 5 years of age. In addition, calcification in the frontal and parietal lobes was also observed. Two older children studied by Pearson *et al.* (1983), 9 and 11 years of age when irradiated, demonstrated slight dilation of the lateral ventricles but no areas of calcification. Fourteen of the 49 children examined by Davis *et al.* (1986) had evidence of grey matter calcification. Lesions were most frequently noted at the junctions of grey and white matter, and in the basal ganglia and cerebellum.

Pontine calcification has also been reported following cranial irradiation. The CT scans of two children studied by Price *et al.* (1988) showed the presence of pontine calcification 9 months and 23 months after irradiation. Basal ganglia calcifications and cortical atrophy were also evident. One patient (patient 2) had a repeat CT scan 9 months after the initial scan which showed additional areas of calcification to be present, thereby suggesting that calcification occurring subsequent to irradiation may be progressive in nature.

Atrophy occurring subsequent to radiotherapy

Generalized cerebral and cerebellar atrophy have been identified in recipients of cranial irradiation. Davis *et al.* (1986) diagnosed generalized atrophy in 25 of the 49 children examined. Cerebral atrophy was also identified in four of the nine patients studied by Curnes *et al.* (1986), and in both children reported by Price *et al.* (1988). Finally, cerebellar atrophy was found in a 15-year-old male described by Lichtor *et al.* (1984).

Cerebrovascular changes occurring subsequent to radiotherapy

Cerebrovascular disease has also been linked to CNS irradiation. Several researchers have used arteriography to show changes to the cerebrovascular system following irradiation. Four children described by Painter *et al.* (1975) experienced cerebrovascular damage including narrowing of the left internal carotid artery and the left ophthalmic artery, displacement of both the left anterior choroidal and posterior communicating arteries, stenosis of the right anterior and middle cerebral arteries, an elevated left middle cerebral artery, a stretched left anterior choroidal artery and severe atherosclerosis throughout the vertebrobasilar system.

Mechanisms of Central Nervous System Damage Following Radiotherapy

While specific sites and types of CNS damage have been identified in patients who undergo cranial irradiation, the exact mechanism of change is currently unknown. Overall, six hypotheses have been proposed in order to explain the actual effect of radiation on nervous tissue; however, at this stage no one theory has been agreed upon. The proposed hypotheses include:

1   Radiation damage is primarily an injury to nervous tissue (Di Lorenzo *et al.*, 1978).

2   Radiation adversely affects the rapid phase of myelination that occurs early in childhood (Davis *et al.*, 1986). Davis and co-workers studied the CNS changes that occurred in 49 children given radiotherapy for brain tumours. The white matter abnormalities and the focal calcification observed, in association with the fact that damage predominantly occurred in children less than 3 years of age, formed the basis for their hypothesis.

3   Radiation causes a transient abnormality in the biochemical mechanisms that maintain myelin (Nightingale *et al.*, 1982). The failure of the nervous system to maintain myelin serves to explain the transient early-delayed reactions observed in recipients of cranial irradiation. This theory differs from that proposed by Davis *et al.* (1986) which deals with the more permanent interruption to myelination.

4   Radiation damage occurs secondary to vascular changes (Curnes *et al.*, 1986; De Reuck and vander Eecken, 1975).
    Curnes *et al.* (1986) proposed that demyelination occurs secondary to vascular changes. After using MRI to study nine patients with histories of radiotherapy, these investigators produced the following evidence to support their theory:

i   A long interval preceded the onset of symptoms.

ii   Fibrinoid changes occurred in the arteriolar walls in the affected area.

iii The most severe changes in the white matter occurred in deep locations adjacent to the ventricle where the blood supply is most tenuous.

iv A high correlation between the severity of vascular change and the severity of demyelination was determined.

De Reuck and vander Eecken (1975) also argued for a vascular change in cases of radiation necrosis and demyelination. Thirteen autopsies were performed by these investigators on subjects with suspected radiation-related damage. Focal necrosis of the brainstem and of the cerebral hemispheres corresponded to the vascular territories of deep-perforating arteries. Diffuse necrosis and demyelination was predominant in the periventricular regions with sparing of the cortex and subcortical white matter. The periventricular lesions corresponded to the periventricular arterial border-zones. Arterial border-zones are highly susceptible to generalized disturbances of the cerebral blood flow. The sparing of the cerebral cortex and subcortical white matter was explained by the rich vascular supply of these structures due to leptomeningeal anastomoses.

Evidence linking cerebrovascular disease with radiotherapy was also supplied by Kearsley (1983). Kearsley reported late cerebellar disease in two patients with histories of radiotherapy. A 47-year-old man was given 6600 rads over 42 days to a carcinoma of the left vocal cord. Seventeen years later the patient experienced episodic right-sided monocular visual blurring. Angiography revealed an embolus in the superior temporal branch of the retinal artery and irregular narrowing of the right common carotid artery at the level of the larynx. On the left side similar, but less severe, changes were noted. The second case described by Kearsley (1983) was a 47-year-old female who underwent a mastectomy. Nineteen years after irradiation she experienced episodic tingling on the left side and slurred speech. An atherosclerotic plaque at the origin of the right internal carotid artery was demonstrated by angiography.

Kearsley (1983) also presented an extensive literature review summarizing 35 cases of cerebrovascular disease following radiotherapy. Thirteen of the 35 patients described were children 12 years of age or younger. Damage to the cerebrovascular system included stenosis or occlusion of the internal carotid artery, the middle cerebral artery, the common carotid artery, the anterior cerebral artery, or the vertebrobasilar artery. Changes were limited to the area irradiated and common presentations included headaches, aphasia and sudden hemiparesis or hemiplegia. Kearsley (1983) also noted the absence of reports of late cerebrovascular changes in children irradiated for acute lymphocytic leukaemia and suggested that the lower doses of irradiation (2000–4000 rads) administered to leukaemic patients may account for this observation.

Wright and Bresnan (1976), however, provided evidence to suggest that even small amounts of radiation administered to young children can produce occlusion of the large cerebral blood vessels. The child studied by Wright and Bresnan was only a few weeks old when she received 1000 rads over a 2-month period to a haemangioma involving the left orbit. When 6 years of age she experienced two episodes of slow, slurred speech, confusion to questions, and a right hemiparesis without facial involvement. The symptoms cleared within 1 hour. Angiography showed a hypoplastic left carotid artery with occlusion of both the anterior and middle cerebral arteries. The authors attributed the transient symptoms to a transient low flow state in the affected areas of the brain.

The endothelial cell was considered to be the primary site of radiation damage by Martins *et al.* (1977). These investigators favoured the theory that damage to the cells lining the blood vessels leads to abnormal vascular permeability. This, in turn, allows the accumulation of plasma proteins in the vessel walls, which results in thickening and hyalinization of the vessels. Acute fibrinoid necrosis follows with possible rupturing of the blood vessels leading to oedema, necrosis and haemorrhages which present clinically as a cerebral mass effect.

5   Radiation damage represents an immune reaction. Irradiation promotes the synthesis of proteins with antigenic properties which could then trigger a progressive allergic reaction in the host (Di Lorenzo *et al.*, 1978). After reviewing the literature and studying two children with grey matter calcification, Lee and Suh (1977) claimed that an autoimmune reaction or hypersensitivity to radiation causes both vascular damage and demyelination. Grey matter calcification then develops as a result of the primary damage incurred.

6   White matter changes which follow irradiation represent the normal ageing process but at an accelerated rate (Tsuruda *et al.* 1987). Tsuruda and co-workers reviewed 95 patients who had received radiotherapy for a wide variety of CNS tumours. The MR images of the irradiated patients were compared with those of 180 age-matched controls. The controls had no history of radiotherapy but had experienced benign or malignant intracranial lesions. Morphologically, the deep white matter changes in both groups had similar MR images. Both groups showed an increase in changes with age, but these occurred at a greater rate in the irradiated group.

Speech, Language, Neurological and Behavioural Effects of Radiotherapy

Studies investigating the detrimental effects of CNS irradiation have largely been carried out on subjects treated for CNS tumours. In that tumours cause complications such as exerting mass effect on surrounding tissues, many investigators have found it difficult to isolate radiotherapy as the sole cause of associated language, neuropsychological and behavioural disturbances. Despite this difficulty, however, radiotherapy has frequently been implicated as the causal factor when recipients develop intellectual, behavioural, speech and/or language deficits or when structural changes in the CNS are detected in patients subsequent to treatment for cancer.

Dysarthria occurring subsequent to radiotherapy

Facial paresis and dysarthria have been reported to occur in both children and adults who underwent irradiation for intracranial tumours. For example, two of the four subjects examined by Painter *et al.* (1975) showed facial paresis or dysarthria. All four subjects underwent cranial irradiation as children and, at the time of assessment, demonstrated evidence of cerebrovascular damage. A 29-year-old man described by Painter *et al.* (1975) demonstrated dysarthria, a flaccid right hemiparesis and difficulty with respiration 24 years after undergoing partial resection of a cerebellar medulloblastoma and receiving a total dose of 4800 rads to the posterior fossa and 3600 rads to the spine. The patient subsequently died and autopsy revealed severe atherosclerosis of the vertebrobasilar system, areas of encephalomalacia in the pons and medulla, and partial occlusion of the fourth ventricle by collagenous material. Painter *et al.* (1975) also reported the case of a young girl who received 2500 rads of radiation following removal of an optic chiasm tumour when she was 8 months of age. An additional 3500 rads was administered over 4 weeks when the child was 3 years 8 months of age. At 8 years of age she had a right supranuclear facial paresis, a spastic right hemiparesis, bilateral optic atrophy and horizontal nystagmus.

Facial weakness was also identified in four of the 30 long-term survivors of childhood brain tumours examined by Bamford *et al.* (1976). An additional subject demonstrated dysphagia associated with a palatal weakness.

One of the six adults considered by Martins *et al.* (1977) exhibited a marked dysarthria. A 54-year-old woman developed dysarthric speech 16 months after 6885 rads of radiotherapy to the suprasellar region. Based on the findings of CT scans and the clinical presentation, radionecrosis in the frontal lobes was diagnosed. Other symptoms included an unsteady gait, confusion, memory loss, headaches, lethargy and progressive dementia.

A 54-year-old woman who developed dysarthria subsequent to cranial irradiation was also described by Marks *et al.* (1981). The patient had a left temporal lobe ganglioneuroma removed, followed by 6500 rads of radiation given in 35 fractions over 52 days. Fourteen months later, receptive and expressive dysphasia, slurred speech, poor concentration and confusion developed.

Mild dysarthria was also associated with radiation damage by Nightingale *et al.* (1982). A 37-year-old woman underwent a mastoidectomy and subtotal excision of a left glomus jugulare tumour. Surgery was followed by irradiation involving 5200 rads to the tumour and 1950 rads to the brainstem. Seven weeks after the completion of radiotherapy, a mild dysarthria involving weakness of the left side of the mouth developed. Incoordination of the left arm and deafness of the left ear were also experienced at this time. Six months post-onset, a mild dysarthria and mild truncal ataxia remained. This case was described as having early-delayed radiation rhombencephalopathy which occurred within a few months of irradiation treatment.

Language disturbances subsequent to radiotherapy

There is a paucity of literature dealing specifically with language disturbances following cranial irradiation. Most studies have derived the language status of irradiated patients from the results of neuropsychological assessments rather than using tests designed to evaluate the various aspects of language functioning. Other studies have failed to indicate the means by which a language deficit or an aphasia were diagnosed. Despite the limitations of the available literature, it is apparent that language deficits subsequent to radiotherapy can occur in both children and adults.

Painter *et al.* (1975) identified 2 years after radiotherapy a right hemiparesis and an aphasia in a 9-year-old girl. The aphasia was characterized by anomia and an inability to follow simple commands. Arteriography suggested the presence of an avascular mass in the left posterior temporal lobe.

Aphasia was also identified in one of the six adults studied by Martins *et al.* (1977). A 44-year-old man experienced fluent dysphasia, headaches and seizures 10 months after 5000 rads of radiotherapy to the left temporal bone for a glomus jugulare tumour. Necrosis of the left inferior temporal gyrus was diagnosed. Twelve months later mild dysnomia and a 'minimal organic mental syndrome' remained.

Receptive and expressive aphasia were listed as symptoms of radionecrosis by Marks *et al.* (1981). A 22-year-old man was irradiated after resection of a cystic low grade astrocytoma from the left parieto-occipital region. He received 6500 rads in 30 fractions over 46 days. Increasing aphasia and seizures were experienced 18 months after irradiation by this patient. Marks *et al.* (1981) also reported the case of a 54-year-old woman with receptive and expressive aphasia following removal of a left temporal lobe ganglioneuroma and a dose of 6500 rads of radiation given in 35 fractions over 52 days.

Radiotherapy has been identified as a possible cause of linguistic deficits in children treated for brain tumours (Hudson *et al.*, 1989). Hudson *et al.* (1989) reported that the patients treated with radiotherapy (*n* = 4) following surgery for posterior fossa tumours presented with language difficulties. In particular, receptive and expressive syntax, expressive semantics, word finding difficulties and reading comprehension deficits were reported. Two children who did not receive cranial irradiation had language abilities within normal limits on assessment (Hudson *et al.*, 1989).

Two adults described by Burns and Boyle (1984) underwent speech pathology assessments following the onset of aphasia 4.5 and 1.5 years after radiotherapy for a left frontal and a temporal astrocytoma. Patient 1, a 45-year-old man, demonstrated a severe Broca's aphasia with oral-buccal apraxia and apraxia of speech. Initially, the prognosis was poor; however, rapid spontaneous improvement resulted in a normal performance on verbal and written language tasks just $2\frac{1}{2}$ weeks post-onset of aphasia. Patient 2, a 40-year-old man, presented with severe receptive and expressive language deficits 1.5 years after the completion of CNS irradiation. Speech therapy was initiated and, 1.5 years after the onset of aphasia, residual deficits included a moderate reduction in the comprehension of complex ideational material, a mild to moderate anomia and mild reading and moderate writing deficits.

While expressive and receptive language disturbances may not be an inevitable outcome of cranial irradiation, the occurrence of language deficits has been linked with radiation treatment. Patterns of dysfunction have not yet been determined. Reports in the literature suggest, however, that language deficits can appear several years after the completion of radiotherapy. Spontaneous recovery can be complete, partial or very limited. Thus, the information available suggests that speech pathologists have a role in monitoring, diagnosing and treating patients at risk for post-radiation neurological disease.

Intellectual deficits associated with radiotherapy

To date, the long-term abilities of children who have received irradiation have only primarily captured the interest of neuropsychologists. As a result, much of the research in this area has involved obtaining intelligence quotients (IQ) of children who have experienced radiotherapy. Many authors have reported evidence of either below average IQ scores in irradiated populations, or IQ scores that are within normal limits but fall below the score achieved by the control group/s used.

The long-term intellectual abilities and general neurological status of subjects administered radiotherapy as part of the treatment of paediatric brain tumours were studied by Danoff *et al.* (1982). Sixteen of the 38 subjects had no neurological or psychological disabilities, 18 were considered to have mild handicaps, three had major disabilities but were capable of self-care, and one was incapable of self-care. When the IQs were considered, six of the 36 subjects tested (17 per cent) had IQ scores of less than 69, three (8 per cent) were classified as border-line with scores of 70–9, seven (20 per cent) had scores between 80 and 89, and 20 (55 per cent) were found to be normal or above normal.

Danoff *et al.* (1982) acknowledged that variables other than radiotherapy may have influenced intelligence in the cases studied. The analysis of two variables led to the conclusion that the presence or absence of hydrocephalus did not influence IQ, while tumour extension to the hypothalamus did result in an increased incidence of intellectual handicap. The authors also stated that while the majority of subjects were functioning with minimal disability, their performance may be inferior when compared with a control group of children who have non-intracranial malignancies.

In an attempt to detect minimal intellectual impairments in children following radiotherapy, Silverman *et al.* (1984) compared the IQs of nine long-term survivors of cerebellar medulloblastoma with those of their non-irradiated siblings. The full scale IQ score of each subject was found to be significantly below his/her non-irradiated sibling. All siblings scored at least 11 points higher on the Weschsler Performance Scale than the irradiated patients. While the differences in Verbal Scale scores were less dramatic, they too were statistically significant. In addition, it was found that the greater differences between patient and sibling IQ scores occurred when the patient was assessed 5 or more years after therapy. Educational Quotients were also obtained, the patient group scoring 12–17 points below their siblings. Silverman *et al.* (1984: 829) concluded that the reduced performance IQ scores reflected a 'decreased ability to assimilate new information and apply it to unfamiliar situations'. The trend towards a more reduced IQ as time after therapy lengthened was attributed to either the cumulative effect of learning disabilities or a compounding of the difficulty of learning new concepts and using abstract reasoning.

Impaired intelligence was also detected in three of the four survivors of medulloblastoma assessed by Pearson *et al.* (1983). The children were assessed from 6 to 13 years after treatment. The intelligence tests resulted in IQ scores of 77, 71, 66 and 91. The child with an IQ of 91 was the oldest (11 years of age) at diagnosis and had undergone total removal of the medulloblastoma.

Several studies have identified intellectual disabilities in children who have been treated for brain tumours without using standardized intelligence tests. Such tests have used academic achievement, educational placement and performance on selected subtests of an intelligence scale in order to diagnose intellectual impairment. Minimal intellectual impairments, however, are likely to be overlooked when such subjective judgements are made.

Bamford *et al.* (1976) labelled 30 subjects as either superior, average, educationally subnormal or severely subnormal on the basis of educational attainment and performance on selected subtests of the Revised Stanford–Binet Scale. Three subjects (10 per cent) were classified as being superior, 10 (33 per cent) were average, 4 (13 per cent) were below average and were receiving remedial assistance within a normal school setting, while 11 (37 per cent) were described as educationally subnormal, and 2 (7 per cent) were severely subnormal. Bamford and co-workers suggested that while the direct effect of the tumour and the accompanying increase in intracranial pressure can account for any visual and motor handicaps experienced by the subjects, it is unlikely that such factors could cause long-term reductions in intelligence. Hence, radiotherapy was implicated as the most likely cause. In addition, Bamford *et al.* (1976) proposed that a lack of adequate rehabilitation following treatment for intracranial masses may actually lead to a preventable disability.

Broadbent *et al.* (1981) reported 'frank mental retardation' in three of the eight irradiated children examined. This broad diagnosis, however, was based on subjective observations and whether or not the child was attending a special school. As a result, children with more subtle intellectual deficits may have been overlooked. The youngest patient, treated when 1.1 years of age, was ataxic and had a visual field defect. When 2.9 years of age, his general abilities were approximately 6 months delayed. Another patient, treated at 1.7 years of age, was intellectually handicapped and attending a special school. The third patient was 12 years old when treated. He demonstrated considerable intellectual deterioration and from being a grammar school candidate, became virtually unemployable. While acknowledging that it is difficult to interpret the relative contributions of hydrocephalus and other aspects of the treatment, Broadbent *et al.* (1981) believed that the results indicated the need to reconsider the radiotherapy regimens for younger children.

Ninety-one childhood cases of primary brain tumours treated with irradiation were reviewed by Deutsch (1982). All children were younger than 5 years of age at diagnosis. At the 5-year survival stage at least 14 of the 19 known to be disease-free had learning disabilities. Of these, two were severely intellectually handicapped and had been placed in institutions. The other 12, however, attended regular schools.

While the studies described above used children treated for brain tumours as the subject group, Copeland *et al.* (1985) studied the neuropsychological sequelae of children who required radiotherapy in the treatment of leukaemia or lymphoma. Three groups of children who had survived childhood cancer for at least 5 years were considered. Group 1 included 24 children with either leukaemia or lymphoma who had received chemotherapy including intrathecal medication but no CNS irradiation. The 25 children in group 2 also had leukaemia or lymphoma, but were given both chemotherapy and radiotherapy (2400 rads over a 16-day period). Group 3 consisted of a control group of patients with solid tumours and Hodgkin's disease. The control group had been treated with chemotherapy, surgery, and, in some cases, irradiation to sites remote from the head and neck. As all groups received chemotherapy, radiotherapy was the variable being examined.

The irradiated leukaemia/lymphoma group (group 2) performed significantly below groups 1 and 3 in the areas of arithmetic, block design, coding, written spelling, visuomotor integration, spatial memory and fine motor skills. These deficits resulted in a reduction of full scale IQ for group 2. It was concluded that radiation primarily affects non-language skills and language skills remain intact. However, it is important to note that the language tests given included the Peabody Picture Vocabulary Test

(PPVT), a rapid automatized naming test, and word fluency test. These short assessments only permit the examination of semantic abilities. The status of a patient's expressive syntax, receptive syntax, pragmatics or morphology therefore cannot be assumed on the basis of the three semantic assessments used by Copeland *et al.* (1985).

The reported incidences of intellectual impairment subsequent to cranial irradiation range from 25 per cent to 60 per cent. Variables which may influence the incidences reported are discussed later in this chapter. The risk of experiencing below average intelligence as a result of radiotherapy has been reported throughout the literature. However, it is important that professionals and parents are also aware that, while a child's IQ may fall within the average range, it may actually be significantly below the child's pre-treatment ability. Rehabilitation following treatment for childhood cancers should, therefore, take this possibility into consideration.

Motor deficits occurring subsequent to radiotherapy

Motor deficits have been reported to appear in some patients following radiotherapy. Ataxia, unsteady gait and limb incoordination following radiotherapy are frequently reported throughout the literature irrespective of the site of the original tumour (Bamford *et al.*, 1976; Broadbent *et al.*, 1981; Martins *et al.*, 1977; Nightingale *et al.*, 1982; Pearson *et al.*, 1983; Silverman *et al.*, 1984). In addition, Copeland *et al.* (1985) studied children with leukaemia or lymphoma and found that the 25 children in the irradiated leukaemia/lymphoma group demonstrated fine motor abilities which were significantly below those demonstrated by the non-irradiated leukaemia/lymphoma group and a group of children with solid tumours or Hodgkin's disease. This observation was made in the absence of the complicating factors often associated with tumours, giving further support to the reported link between motor deficits and radiotherapy.

Spastic and flaccid hemiplegias of either the left or right sides of the body have also been reported in patients who have completed courses of radiotherapy (Bamford *et al.*, 1976; Marks *et al.*, 1981; Painter *et al.*, 1975). Bamford *et al.* (1976) also noted the presence of cranial nerve palsies in 12 (40 per cent) of the 30 patients reviewed by them at least 5 years after treatment for intracranial space-occupying lesions. Nerve palsies were the cause of squint in seven patients and facial weakness in four. Dysphagia due to a palatal weakness was present in one patient.

Thus it appears that motor deficits can occur as a direct result of the radiotherapy administered in the treatment of cerebral tumours, leukaemia or lymphoma.

Sensory deficits occurring subsequent to radiotherapy

Both visual and hearing impairments have been associated with radiotherapy given for the treatment of brain tumours. Painter *et al.* (1975) described an 8-year-old girl who developed bilateral optic atrophy and horizontal nystagmus 4 years 4 months after completing radiotherapy for a glioma of the optic chiasm.

Of the 30 long-term survivors of brain tumours reviewed by Bamford *et al.* (1976), 11 had correctable defects of acuity, while three experienced severe visual handicaps. Hearing impairments were detected in two of the 30 subjects. One was described as partially deaf and the other as totally deaf.

Other neurological and neuropsychological findings

Other symptoms which have been noted in patients given radiotherapy for the treatment of brain tumours include: confusion (Marks *et al.*, 1981; Pearson *et al.*, 1983), poor concentration (Marks *et al.*, 1981; Pearson *et al.*, 1983), progressive dementia (Martins *et al.*, 1977), lethargy (Martins *et al.*, 1977), hyperactivity (Pearson *et al.*, 1983), poor school performance/learning disabilities (Deutsch, 1982; Pearson *et al.*, 1983), headaches (Martins *et al.*, 1977; Painter *et al.*, 1975) and seizures (Marks *et al.*, 1981; Martins *et al.*, 1977; Painter *et al.*, 1975).

In summary, while there is a paucity of reports describing the speech and language characteristics of children who have received cranial irradiation for the treatment of cancer, the literature available indicates that speech and language disorders do occur subsequent to radiotherapy. Clearly there is a need for research which is specifically designed to analyze subjects' communication abilities. The negative effect of radiation on intelligence has been widely reported. A risk of motor and sensory abnormalities has also been identified as a consequence of CNS irradiation.

Effect of Age at Irradiation on CNS Damage and Neuropsychological Functioning

Numerous reports in the literature indicate a trend for a greater number of younger than older children to be negatively affected by irradiation. Several studies have compared the CNS status and/or the neuropsychological functioning of younger and older children after therapy. The ages used, however, to differentiate between 'young' and 'old' children have included 2, 3, 5 and 11 years. The use of varying age ranges throughout the literature suggests that a specific age below which damage is most likely to occur is difficult to determine.

Effect of age at irradiation on CNS damage

Davis *et al* (1986) reviewed 49 children with histories of intracranial tumours and subsequent treatment with irradiation. Three age groups were considered: younger than 3 years of age ($n = 14$), 3–12 years of age ($n = 22$), and older than 12 years of age ($n = 13$). It was found that both focal calcification and white matter abnormalities occurred predominantly in younger children, particularly those less than 3 years of age when treated. The incidence of atrophy varied little with respect to age at time of treatment.

Five children who had survived from 6 to 13 years after being treated surgically and with radiation for medulloblastoma were studied by Pearson *et al.* (1983). Three children who were irradiated with 3000–3900 rads when less than 5 years of age demonstrated varying degrees of intracranial calcification of the basal ganglia, as well as the frontal and parietal lobes on CT scan. Poor attention spans, hyperactivity, poor school performances and IQ scores of 77, 71 and 66 were noted in the three children. The authors concluded that there appears to be a correlation between age at treatment and the presence and extent of intracranial calcification.

In contrast, as discussed earlier, Tsuruda *et al.* (1987) failed to detect irradiation-related changes in patients less than 20 years of age. Tsuruda *et al.* (1987) obtained MR images from 95 patients who had received radiotherapy for a wide variety of CNS tumours. Eleven of the 95 patients were less than 20 years of age. The MR images were compared with those of a control group consisting of 180 age-matched patients with no history of radiotherapy but with benign or malignant intracranial tumours. Tsuruda *et al.* (1987) were unable to explain this observation but suggested that a follow-up interval of less than 2 years and a higher percentage (45 per cent) of posterior fossa tumours may have biased the results.

Effect of age at irradiation on neuropsychological outcome

Researchers have found that 'younger' children tend to have a greater risk of developing neuropsychological deficits than children who are older at the time of cranial irradiation. A critical age of 3 years was determined by Danoff *et al.* (1982) after reviewing 38 patients who had been treated for paediatric brain tumours. An increased incidence of intellectual handicap was recorded for the patient group who had received cranial irradiation when less than 3 years of age. Bamford *et al.* (1976), however, claimed that the disabilities observed in 30 children given irradiation for the treatment of brain tumours were most severe in those children treated when less than 11 years of age. Deficits identified included visual handicaps, hearing impairments, motor abnormalities and intellectual handicaps.

All 91 cases of childhood brain tumours reviewed by Deutsch (1982) were treated with cranial irradiation when less than 5 years of age. Deutsch did not find a significant correlation between age at diagnosis and prognosis in children from birth to 5 years of age. However, there was a trend for patients over 24 months of age to do slightly better than those treated in the first two years of life.

Another two children treated when less than 2 years of age were described by Broadbent *et al.* (1981). The patients received radiotherapy for medulloblastoma when 1.1 and 1.7 years old. They demonstrated ataxia, visual field defects and intellectual handicaps. However, a third child assessed by Broadbent *et al.* (1981) was nearly 12 years of age when treated, yet experienced intellectual deterioration following radiotherapy, thereby suggesting that damage following irradiation is not confined to younger children. Likewise Copeland *et al.* (1985) concluded that radiation exerts detrimental effects on neuropsychological skills regardless of age at diagnosis. Nevertheless children younger than 5 years of age at diagnosis are more likely to have cognitive deficits.

While most authors have indicated that young children are at risk for long-term neuropsychological deficits following radiotherapy, Hodges and Smithells (1983) stressed the need to identify such deficits in older children as well. Hodges and Smithells (1983) described an 11-year-old boy who underwent partial removal of a cerebellar astrocytoma followed by 4500 rads of irradiation given in 15 fractions over 21 days. Five years after treatment, right occipital lobe calcification was detected and a gradual deterioration in mental function had occurred. The patient was enrolled in a school for the intellectually handicapped. Thus the need to monitor the educational progress of all children, regardless of age, was stressed.

While it is evident that all children should be monitored closely for several years following radiotherapy, it appears that the long-term monitoring of children less than 5 years of age at the time of treatment is particularly important. The increased risk of radiation damage for young children has not been explained. Radiation may significantly interrupt normal brain development by interfering with the rapid phase of myelination seen in childhood (Davis *et al.*, 1986). Perhaps radiation interrupts the development of normal intellectual, speech and/or language skills when administered to a young child, or perhaps the damage induced by irradiation results in a cumulative effect on the child's ability to learn. As development proceeds, the gap in performance between an irradiated child and his/her peers may widen.

Effect of Dose, Time, Fractionation and Volume Irradiated

Marks *et al.* (1981) reviewed 152 children and adults who had had primary brain tumours irradiated between 1974 and 1976. Of the 139 patients who received more than 4500 rads, seven adults had pathologically-proven radionecrosis, representing an incidence of 5 per cent. It was found that radionecrosis did not develop below radiation doses biologically equivalent to 5400 rads administered in 30 fractions over 42 days. The risk of radionecrosis could not be associated with administering the radiation over a shorter time period, giving the dose in larger fractions or irradiating a larger field. While radiation dose was important in determining risk, the degree of necrosis was not always greatest in those areas of the brain which received the highest dose.

As a result of the findings of Marks *et al.* (1981), the Mallinckrodt Institute of Radiology reduced the radiation doses administered to patients by an average of 7 per cent. Marks and Wong (1985) subsequently reported that of 198 patients irradiated between 1976 and 1981, none demonstrated evidence of cerebral radionecrosis. Further analyses were performed on a total of 337 patients who received more than 4500 rads between 1974 and 1981. Incidences of cerebral radionecrosis were calculated as being 1.5 per cent at 5500 rads of irradiation and 4 per cent at 6000 rads. While the earlier study of Marks *et al.* (1981) could not relate risk to time and fractionation of radiotherapy, Marks and Wong (1985) concluded that the risk of damage is greater when patients are given a course of radiotherapy involving shorter periods of time or larger daily fractions.

The significance of fractionation in calculating the risk of radiotherapy was stressed by Martins *et al.* (1977). After studying six cases of radionecrosis in adults treated for benign intracranial neoplasms and reviewing the available literature, Martins *et al.* (1977) suggested that the risk of radiotherapy increases when a dose of 5000–7000 rads is fractionated at greater than 200 rads per day.

The time period over which a course of radiotherapy is administered was considered by Nguyen *et al.* (1988). Thirty-nine adults were followed for at least 2 years after receiving radiotherapy for head and neck cancers. No patient had CNS involvement. Patients were given 6600–7200 rads in two series of 3300 to 3600 rads each. The two series were separated by a 2–4 week interval. Irradiation was delivered in 6–8 daily fractions of 90 rads each with the fractions being separated by 2-hour-intervals. Clearly, this programme differs from the more commonly used 180–200 rads per day regimen.

Of the 39 patients studied by Nguyen *et al.* (1988) 27 (69 per cent) had one or more late complications. Damage experienced by the patients included cervical fibrosis, mucosal necrosis, trismus, bone necrosis and recurrent laryngeal oedema. The type and frequency of late effects could not be related to the field sizes and dosimetric data, or the different regimens of irradiation. Although the CNS was not involved in these cases, the study suggests that the interval between fractions is crucial in determining the tolerance of normal tissues to irradiation as the time between fractions allows for the repair of any damage incurred.

Two courses of radiotherapy were compared by Safdari *et al.* (1985). Within 2 weeks of undergoing surgery for either primary or secondary intracranial tumours, 164 patients began radiation treatment. Group A included 118 patients who were given 280–300 rads three times a week up to a total dose of 4500–5000 rads. Two-thirds of the total dose was delivered to the whole brain and one-third to the tumour site. Group B consisted of 46 patients who received 850 rads on days 1, 3, 21 and 23 to a total dose of 3400 rads, with 1700 rads being delivered to the whole brain and 1700 rads to the tumour site. This split-regimen therapy actually corresponded to a biological equivalent dose of 200 rads per day (1000 rads per week) to a total dose of 5400 rads.

Four patients in each group had a histologically-proven radiation-induced lesion, resulting in an incidence of 3.4 per cent for Group A and 8.7 per cent for Group B. The difference between groups was not significant. However, a significant difference between groups was detected when the median time of onset was considered. Radiation-induced lesions were identified 21 months after radiotherapy in Group A and 8.5 months after the completion of radiotherapy in Group B. Thus, the rapidity of onset of radiation necrosis appeared to be related to the total dose and the fractionation of radiation.

Summary of Radiotherapy

Although CNS irradiation is vital for the survival of children with cancer, such treatment can induce detrimental changes to the structure and function of the nervous system. CNS necrosis and calcification, particularly of white matter, have been observed in children treated with radiotherapy. Cerebral atrophy and cerebrovascular damage have also been attributed to CNS irradiation. Speech, language, intellectual, motor and sensory deficits have been observed, with and without associated structural damage to the nervous system. Such observations and the fact that radiation damage can appear many years after the completion of treatment stress the need to monitor the speech, language, educational and functional abilities of children who experience CNS irradiation regardless of the child's age or the radiation dose received.

Chemotherapy

Chemotherapy is the treatment of cancerous conditions by chemical agents or drugs. Drug administration for the treatment of childhood cancer was first reported in the late 1940s when the beneficial effects of drug therapy in the treatment of patients with leukaemia were described by Farber *et al.* (1948). Although in the early years of chemotherapy cytotoxic drugs were usually administered as single agents, in more recent times, to heighten the effect of the drugs, chemotherapy has generally involved the administration of a combination of drugs (McWhirter and Masel, 1987). A list of chemical agents commonly used in the treatment of childhood cancer is shown in Table 9.1.

Table 9.1 Agents commonly used in protocols for the treatment of childhood cancer

Drug name	Abbreviation	Route of administration	Possible side effects	Administered for
Actinomycin D (dactinomycin)		IV	nausea vomiting stomatitis diarrhoea hair loss myelosuppression	Wilm's tumour sarcomas
Adriamycin (doxorubicin)		IV	nausea vomiting stomatitis hair loss myelosuppression cardiac failure if correct precautions not taken	acute leukaemias lymphomas sarcomas Wilm's tumour neuroblastomas etc
Bleomycin		IV IM S	mucositis dermatitis hair loss fever myalgia pulmonary complications	lymphomas germ cell tumours
Busulphan		Oral	myelosuppression	chronic myeloid leukaemia
CCNu (lomustine)		Oral	phlebitis nausea vomiting myelosuppression pulmonary fibrosis	lymphomas gliomas
Chlorambucil		Oral	myelosuppression nausea vomiting aspermia amenorrhoea possibly secondary primary tumours, esp. leukaemia	Hodgkin's disease histiocytosis x
Cis-platin		IV	renal tubular damage hypomagnesaemia ototoxicity leading to hearing loss severe nausea and vomiting	osteosarcoma neuroblastoma germ cell tumours
Cyclophosphamide	CTX	IV	myelosuppression hair loss haemorrhagic cystitis sterility in males	lymphomas neuroblastomas sarcomas Ewing's tumour etc

Table 9.1 Continued

Drug name	Abbreviation	Route of administration	Possible side effects	Administered for
Cytosine arabinoside	Ara-C	IT IV IM S	myelosuppression megaloblastic erythropoiesis nausea mucositis fever macular rash conjunctival inflammation	ALL non-Hodgkin's lymphoma
Daunorubicin	DNR	IV	nausea vomiting stomatitis hair loss cardiac complications	acute leukaemias
DTIC (dacerbazine)		IV	nausea vomiting myelosuppression influenza-like syndrome (occasionally)	Hodgkin's disease neuroblastoma sarcomas melanoma
5-Fluorouracil		IV	myelosuppression stomatitis diarrhoea	primary liver tumours
L-asparaginase	L-asp	IV IM	nausea vomiting abdominal pain anorexia & weight loss hypoglycaemia hypofibrinogenaemia	ALL lymphomas
Melphalan		IV Oral	myelosuppression nausea vomiting	osteosarcoma neuroblastoma
6-Mercaptopurine	6-MCP	Oral	myelosuppression cholestatic jaundice nausea vomiting anorexia	acute leukaemias
Methotrexate		IT IV IM Oral / IT only	myelosuppression oral ulceration diarrhoea hepatic fibrosis or cirrhosis pulmonary infiltrates skin rash hair loss osteoporosis nephropathy (if dose is high) arachnoiditis dementia peripheral neuropathy seizures coma	ALL osteosarcoma (high dose)
Nitrogen mustard		IV	severe nausea and vomiting myelosuppression diarrhoea thrombophlebitis	Hodgkin's disease

Table 9.1 Continued

Drug name	Abbreviation	Route of administration	Possible side effects	Administered for
Prednisone	Pred.			ALL
Procarbazine		Oral	myelosuppression nausea vomiting confusion peripheral neuropathy ataxia myalgia	lymphomas gliomas
Thioguanine		Oral	myelosuppression nausea vomiting	acute non-lymphocytic leukaemias
Vinblastine		IV	myelosuppression nausea vomiting constipation peripheral neuropathy	lymphomas germ cell tumours histiocytosis x
Vincristine	VCR	IV	peripheral neuropathy hair loss abdominal pain muscle pains constipation	acute leukaemias lymphomas sarcomas Wilm's tumour neuroblastoma
Teniposide Etoposide	VM-26 VP-26	IV	myelosuppression stomatitis hair loss fever hypotension generalized erythema and bronchospasm	acute leukaemias lymphomas gliomas

ALL = acute lymphoblastic leukaemia
IT = intrathecal, i.e. through the theca of the spinal cord into the subarachnoid space
IV = intravenous
IM = intramuscular
S = subcutaneous

For the purposes of chemotherapy, drugs are combined and administered according to highly complicated protocols determined by three principles which, according to McWhirter and Masel (1987), include:

1   Each drug should have been proven to be effective against the particular tumour concerned.
2   Each drug included should preferably have a different mode of action.
3   Ideally as little overlap as possible should exist in regard to the toxicities of the drugs included.

Chemotherapy is used in a number of different ways in the treatment of childhood cancers. In some conditions, especially where there is no disease mass (tumour) present such as in acute non-lymphoblastic leukaemia, chemotherapy may be the only form of treatment administered. In other conditions chemotherapy may be given as an initial treatment before another form of treatment such as surgery or radiotherapy. For instance, chemotherapy may be used initially to reduce the size of a large tumour to enable surgery to be carried out. Also, chemotherapy is given to induce remission in patients with acute lymphoblastic leukaemia before a course of radiotherapy.

Chemotherapy is also used in combination with another treatment method (i.e. as an adjunctive therapy) in the treatment of some childhood cancers. For example, chemotherapy and radiotherapy are often administered in combination to patients with acute lymphoblastic leukaemia to prevent the spread of cancer cells to the CNS (CNS prophylaxis). Furthermore, in those cases of childhood cancer that cannot be cured by chemotherapy, or indeed by any other form of treatment, chemotherapy is often used as a palliative therapy (i.e. a therapy aimed at alleviating the disease without curing it). For example, children with leukaemia who have suffered several relapses and are deemed not to be curable may be given chemotherapy to palliate the disorder. However, for reasons that will be discussed later in this chapter, it is important that before using drugs for this purpose the likelihood of any undesirable side-effects should be considered.

Unfortunately, despite the many positive aspects of chemotherapy in the treatment of childhood cancer, in recent years a number of researchers have documented a possible link between chemotherapy and the occurrence of long-term negative side-effects, including alterations in brain structure and function, which in turn may be associated with a reduction in overall intellectual and cognitive functioning, including language. One group of children that has been reported to exhibit negative side-effects following treatment with chemotherapy for a malignant disorder are children with acute lymphoblastic leukaemia. The effects of chemotherapy on brain structure and function in this group will now be examined to illustrate the possible implications of this type of therapy for the speech/language pathologist and neuropsychologist.

Acute Lymphoblastic Leukaemia: An Example of a Childhood Cancer Treated by Chemotherapy

Description of leukaemia

Leukaemia is a progressive, malignant disease of the blood-forming organs, marked by distorted proliferation and development of leucocytes and their precursors in the blood and bone marrow. Of the paediatric malignancies, acute leukaemias are the most common, accounting for about 30 per cent of all newly diagnosed cases (Duffner *et al.*, 1985; Neglia and Robison, 1988). Included in the several groups of leukaemia is one to which children are particularly susceptible: acute lymphoblastic leukaemia.

Acute lymphoblastic leukaemia is the most common form of leukaemia (accounting for approximately 80 per cent of leukaemias), and is associated with hyperplasia and overactivity of the lymphoid tissue, in which the majority of leucocytes (white cells) are lymphocytes or lymphoblasts. Although acute lymphoblastic leukaemia is a disease of both children and adults, it predominantly affects children, with an initial peak incidence of the disease occurring between 3 and 5 years of age. Neglia and Robison (1988) point out that this peak does not occur uniformly throughout the world, and is not present in Africa and various developing nations (Ansel and Nabemezi, 1974; Davies, 1965; Edington and Hendrikse, 1973). The incidence of acute lymphoblastic leukaemia is higher in males than females and, although the exact figures vary with the particular type, this pattern is consistent across both geographical boundaries and racial groups (Neglia and Robinson, 1988). One survey in the USA found that for children under 15 years of age the annual incidence of acute lymphoblastic leukaemia among males is 22.3 per million, whereas for females it is 15.7 per million (Young and Miller, 1975).

Treatment of acute lymphoblastic leukaemia

Treatment of leukaemia is aimed at inducing, consolidating and maintaining remission and involves the use of multiple cytotoxic drugs in complex protocols.

Induction therapy
According to Miller (1982) there are three aims to the induction of remission in acute lymphoblastic leukaemia. These are: (1) to destroy as many leukaemic cells as rapidly as possible, (2) to preserve normal haematopoietic cells, and (3) to restore haematopoiesis (production of red blood cells) as quickly as possible. Remission has been reported to occur in 85 per cent of children with acute lymphoblastic leukaemia when treated with two cytotoxic drugs (usually vincristine and prednisone) in combination (Poplack and Reaman, 1988). An even better remission rate of 95 per cent has been reported when a third agent (e.g. L-asparaginase) is added to the treatment protocol (Miller, 1982).

Treatment protocols containing four or more active agents, however, are used only in the treatment of cases with a poor prognosis because they are associated with a higher incidence of complications and toxicity during induction (Hughes *et al.*, 1975). An example of a protocol used in the treatment of acute lymphoblastic leukaemia is shown in Table 9.2.

Consolidation therapy

Children with acute lymphoblastic leukaemia are at risk of developing CNS leukaemia (Littman *et al.*, 1987). The blood-brain barrier, while protecting the CNS by monitoring the chemicals allowed to enter the CNS, does not offer adequate protection from infiltration of leukaemic cells. Moreover, systemic chemotherapy has no effect on leukaemic cells present in the CNS since the therapeutic agents cannot cross the blood-brain barrier to gain access to the invading leukaemic cells. Consequently, the CNS acts as a sanctuary site for leukaemic cells which are then able to proliferate and eventually to metastasize to the bone marrow and other peripheral sites and thereby cause a systemic relapse. Without prophylaxis to prevent overt leukaemic infiltration of the CNS, many children who survive acute lymphoblastic leukaemia develop CNS leukaemia, which is difficult to eradicate, causes considerable discomfort and is associated with a risk of further neurological complications (Chessells, 1985a; Ochs *et al.*, 1985).

The incidence of CNS leukaemia in children with acute lymphoblastic leukaemia is considerably reduced by adequate presymptomatic prophylaxis with cranial irradiation in conjunction with intrathecal methotrexate (Hustu and Aur, 1978; Kim *et al.*, 1972). In fact the risk of developing CNS leukaemia can be reduced from as high as 50–60 per cent in children receiving minimal or no prophylactic CNS treatment

Table 9.2 An example of a treatment protocol used on a child with common acute lymphocytic leukaemia in 1981

Stage of treatment	Cytotoxic drugs	Treatment regimen	
			1 8 15 22 29 36 43 50
Induction	Vincristine	$2\,mg/m^2$	
	Prednisone	$50\,mg/m^2$	
	L-Asparaginase	$10\,000\,mg/m^2$	
CNS Prophylaxis	Cranial Irradiation	$1800\,rad$	
	Intrathecal		
	Methotrexate	$12\,mg/m^2$	
	Vincristine	$2\,mg/m^2$	
Maintenance	Vincristine	$1.5\,mg/m^2$	
	Methotrexate	$30\,mg/m^2$ each week for 6 weeks) then 2 weeks	
	6-Mercaptopurine	$75\,mg/m^2$ each day for 6 weeks) off	

(Green *et al.*, 1980; Littman *et al.*, 1987; Ludwig *et al.*, 1987; Moe, 1984) to 3–10 per cent by administering prophylactic cranial irradiation and intrathecal methotrexate during early phases of therapy when no signs of CNS leukaemia are present (Chessells, 1985b; Ch'ien *et al.*, 1981; Kaleita and Al-Mateen, 1985; Littman *et al.*, 1987; Moe, 1984; Pinkel, 1979).

Although the need for CNS prophylaxis is unquestionable, evidence is accumulating which suggests that this therapy may be associated with adverse long-term sequelae (Moss *et al.*, 1981). The increase in the number of survivors of acute lymphoblastic leukaemia has led to the recognition of some important late sequelae of the disease and its treatment (McWhirter *et al.*, 1986). With improvement in survival, especially for children with the most favourable outlook, there has been a shift in emphasis, with almost as much concern shown for the late effects of treatment as for the improvement of present therapy itself (Esseltine *et al.*, 1981; Meadows *et al.*, 1981). Among the late consequences are structural neurological changes and a range of adverse late neuropsychological sequelae which are discussed later in this chapter.

Maintenance therapy

Maintenance chemotherapy is also an essential part of the treatment of children with acute lymphoblastic leukaemia. Without some form of maintenance therapy remission in most patients lasts only 1–2 months (Frei, 1965). As in the case of remission induction, most maintenance therapy programmes employ a multiple-drug regimen. The choice of drugs varies according to different risk groups. As an example, a multiple-agent regimen may involve reinforcement chemotherapy with periodic (i.e. monthly or quarterly) chemotherapy pulses. The two most frequently administered drugs in reinforcement therapy are methotrexate (administered weekly or twice weekly) and 6-mercaptopurine (daily). In addition, remission appears to be prolonged by intermittent pulses of vincristine and prednisone, with or without L-asparaginase. It must be noted, however, that pulsed chemotherapy may not be required for all patients (Fernbach *et al.*, 1975; Rivera and Mauer, 1987; Simone, 1976). As in remission induction it has been found that although multiple-drug regimens are superior to single drug treatments for the purpose of maintenance therapy, adding too many chemotherapeutic agents to the protocol merely serves to increase the toxicity and morbidity associated with the treatment without having any significant effect on remission duration or survival in most patients (Aur *et al.*, 1978; Haghbin, 1976) except perhaps for those with a very poor prognosis.

Adverse Effects of Treatment for Acute Lymphoblastic Leukaemia

Four decades ago, acute lymphoblastic leukaemia together with most other forms of cancer, was virtually always rapidly fatal (Southam *et al.*, 1951; Tivey, 1952). Over the past 20 years, therapy for childhood acute lymphoblastic leukaemia has become so effective that at least 50 per cent of patients can be expected to achieve long-term disease-free remission (Aur *et al.*, 1978; Holland and Glidewell, 1972; Jacquillat *et al.*, 1973; McCalla, 1985; Miller, 1980; Till, Hardisty and Pike, 1973). Subsequently, with such advances in treatment, acute lymphoblastic leukaemia is no longer viewed as an almost invariably fatal disease, but as a life-threatening illness, with long-term disease-free survival frequently achieved, and cure as a realistic goal (McCalla, 1985; Meadows *et al.*, 1980; Muchi *et al.*, 1987). Consequently, as a result of the improvements in treatment, a group of children have emerged who, having survived the brain insults sustained from the necessary chemo- and radiotherapy, go on to develop undesirable neurological and neuropsychological sequelae (Eiser, 1978; Ochs and Mulhern, 1988).

Structural changes in the brain

Studies using CT scans have identified a number of structural brain abnormalities in leukaemic patients who have received CNS prophylaxis. These abnormalities include: focal areas of white matter hypodensity, ventricular dilation and cerebral calcifications (Ochs *et al.*, 1980, 1986; Peylan-Ramu *et al.* 1978; Pizzo *et al.*, 1979). Microangio-pathies (calcification of cerebral blood vessels) have also been identified in patients treated with cranial radiation and intrathecal and intravenous methotrexate (Chi'en *et al.*, 1981; Price and Birdwell, 1978).

The findings of several post-mortem investigations have also suggested that chemotherapy for the treatment of leukaemia might be responsible for inducing structural changes in the brain. Smith (1975) performed autopsies on 20 patients with acute lymphoblastic leukaemia, acute myeloid leukaemia, hairy cell leukaemia or non-Hodgkin's lymphoma. Ten had received intrathecal methotrexate while ten patients were not given intrathecal therapy. Patients were between 6 months and 67 years of age at the time of diagnosis. Damage to the brain in patients given intrathecal methotrexate included the destruction of oligodendroglial cells, white matter swelling, moderate to severe astrocytosis, petechial haemorrhages, oedema and coagulative necrosis. The damage was confined to the white matter of both the cerebrum and cerebellum.

Although nine of the ten patients given intrathecal methotrexate also received up to 2400 rads of radiotherapy, Smith (1975) attributed the damage to the course of chemotherapy. She claimed that damage occurring to the brain following radiotherapy usually appears many years after the conclusion of treatment. However, Smith (1975) failed to indicate the delay between the conclusion of chemotherapy and the detection of CNS damage in the 20 patients studied. In addition, it was claimed that the lesion types observed following the irradiation of intracranial tumours differed from those experienced by patients treated with chemotherapy for leukaemia. Smith (1975) described irradiation-related damage as being more severe and involving the cerebrovascular system. While Smith recognized that the relatively low doses of irradiation used to treat patients with leukaemia might exacerbate the damage, it was concluded that methotrexate itself directly affects the oligodendrocyte.

Another case of intracranial damage following a course of intrathecal methotrexate was reported by Skullerud and Halvorsen (1978). A 2-year-old boy with acute leukaemia was given methotrexate intrathecally (6.5 mg per week for 3 weeks followed by monthly injections of 6.5 mg). Radiotherapy was not administered in this case. Twenty-four hours after completing the fifth intrathecal methotrexate treatment, the child developed progressive flaccid paresis. Mental deterioration was observed and he died 18 days after the onset of the symptoms. Autopsy revealed areas of incomplete necrosis with astrocytosis on the base of the brain and along the insula, around the foramina of Luschka, and over the superior and inferior colliculi. Similar lesions were also found over the surface of the cerebellum, particularly over the vermis. In contrast to the findings of Smith (1975), there were no lesions in the central white matter of the brain or spinal cord, or along the ependyma of the ventricles. It was concluded that methotrexate alone caused the lesions observed because methotrexate was the only drug the patient received intrathecally, and as tests showed no evidence of leukaemia within the CNS, the cancer could not have caused the damage. Skullerud and Halvorsen (1978) also noted that the most extensive tissue destruction occurred in areas which are in direct contact with the CSF and therefore with the methotrexate.

Neurological changes

Progressive dementia was observed by Pizzo *et al.* (1976) in a 6-year-old girl undergoing a course of intrathecal methotrexate without radiotherapy for relapse of meningeal leukaemia. The patient was disoriented to time and place, demonstrated a gait disturbance and experienced a significant deterioration of reading and arithmetical abilities. Intrathecal methotrexate was discontinued and during the next 6 months the symptoms disappeared completely. The authors surmised that the lack of radiotherapy in this case eliminated the possibility that alteration of the blood-brain barrier enhanced the toxicity of intrathecal methotrexate.

Meadows and Evans (1976) also attributed the neurological symptoms observed in patients treated for leukaemia to methotrexate administered to the CNS. Four of the 23 children assessed by them demonstrated severe impairments including spastic quadriplegia or paraplegia and limited responsiveness. It must be noted, however, that three of the four severely impaired children also received up to 3400 rads of irradiation.

Five of the children assessed by Meadows and Evans (1976) demonstrated mild neurological dysfunction. Two had abnormal psychological test results and three required special education. Of the five patients showing minimal neurological deficits, three were given radiotherapy. However, it was claimed that in two cases the administration of radiation followed the signs of minimal cerebral dysfunction. Five of the 23 children examined by these workers had EEG abnormalities but were clinically asymptomatic. Nine patients had no signs of neurological abnormalities. These nine patients did not receive cranial irradiation, suggesting that methotrexate should not be cited as the sole cause of CNS damage in this study.

Meadows and Evans (1976) observed that the only clinical feature common to the 14 patients with some degree of neurological impairment was the administration of methotrexate in high doses (5–10 mg/kg per month) over prolonged periods (2–7 years). While it was postulated that radiation may cause changes in the blood-brain barrier allowing methotrexate to diffuse more easily into the white matter, the authors concluded that methotrexate alone does have a direct effect on the nervous system as not all of their patients had received radiotherapy. However, in order to isolate the elements which may contribute to any long-term deficits, it was recommended that patients receive detailed neurological and psychological examinations before, and at regular intervals after, CNS prophylaxis.

Despite the claims that methotrexate has negative effects on the structure and function of the nervous system, two studies involving relatively large patient groups have failed to detect any long-term damage to the CNS. Ochs *et al.* (1980) examined 43 children with acute lymphoblastic leukaemia. Ten patients were given intrathecal methotrexate while 33 received intrathecal methotrexate in combination with intravenous methotrexate. All patients received weekly oral methotrexate. Patients were assessed using CT between 10 and 59 months (median = 29) after the completion of treatment. It was concluded that none of the 43 patients had evidence of intracerebral calcification or areas of decreased attenuation coefficient (i.e. hypodense areas) on CT scans. While mild ventricular dilation and visualization of the cortical sulci was detected in four patients, such features were also observed in control subjects.

Neuropsychological sequelae

In addition to causing structural and neurological abnormalities, a number of recent reports in the literature have indicated that CNS prophylaxis may also have detrimental effects on various neuropsychological functions. Several researchers have reported the presence of intellectual impairment in children treated for acute lymphoblastic leukaemia with cranial irradiation and chemotherapy (Duffner *et al.*, 1985; Eiser, 1978; Meadows *et al.*, 1981; Said *et al.*, 1987; Taylor *et al.*, 1987). A subtle but significant lowering of intelligence quotients (IQs) was noted in long-term survivors of acute lymphoblastic leukaemia by Duffner *et al.* (1983) and Taylor *et al.* (1987). It has been suggested that CNS prophylaxis, in the form of cranial irradiation or the combination of radiotherapy and intrathecal methotrexate, is a primary factor in the development of the reported mild neuropsychological deficits (Eiser 1978; Tamaroff *et al.*, 1982; Tebbi, 1982).

The possibility that a combination of methotrexate and cranial irradiation (2400 rads) could be responsible for intelligence deficits was also noted by Twaddle *et al.* (1983). These investigators estimated pre-treatment IQs of leukaemic patients and solid tumour patients from corrected measures of sibling IQ. A significant difference between the estimates and post-treatment IQs was found in the acute lymphoblastic leukaemia group, but not in the solid tumour group. Twaddle *et al.* (1983) noted that higher functions of intelligence were particularly affected in the leukaemic group, such as verbal associate reasoning and reasoning with abstract material.

In addition to intellectual impairment, other neuropsychological deficits following CNS prophylaxis for acute lymphoblastic leukaemia have also been reported in the literature. Memory deficits are frequently noted (e.g. Chessells, 1985a; Copeland *et al.*, 1985; Eiser, 1980; Mulhern *et al.*, 1987). Difficulty in concentration and attention problems also exist (Chessells, 1985a; Said *et al.*, 1987). Reading deficits have been found both in children with acute lymphoblastic leukaemia in complete continuous remission (Eiser, 1980) and in leukaemic children who have suffered a relapse (Mulhern *et al.*, 1987). In addition, Mulhern *et al.* (1987) reported spelling and mathematical difficulty in children with acute lymphoblastic leukaemia who had suffered a relapse.

Despite the evidence that a combination of chemotherapy and radiotherapy in the form of CNS prophylaxis may have long-term effects on various neuropsychological abilities, the effect of chemotherapy alone on these functions is less certain. Tamaroff *et al.* (1982) failed to detect neuropsychological deficits following the administration of intrathecal methotrexate. Forty-one children with acute lymphoblastic leukaemia were assessed within 1 year of completing a 36-month course of intrathecal methotrexate. Methotrexate was administered at regular intervals in a dose of $6.25 \, mg/m^2$ and was the sole agent of CNS prophylaxis. A control group of 33 children with embryonal rhabdomyosarcoma who had no central nervous disease or treatment were also studied. There was no significant difference in IQ between the two groups for children less than 8 years of age. When children older than 8 years of age were considered, the children with acute lymphoblastic leukaemia achieved IQ scores significantly greater than the children suffering from embryonal rhabdomyosarcoma. In addition, 12 of the 21 younger children were reassessed at an average of 57.4 months after the initial examination. No long-term intellectual changes were detected. The authors concluded that intrathecal methotrexate alone does not have either short-term or long-term effects on general intellectual functioning. Tamaroff *et al.* (1982) suggested that the 2400 rads of cranial radiation given to patients in other studies may be responsible for any reported deficits or perhaps radiation and methotrexate in combination produce the neurological deficits.

Language disturbances

Although considering the disruption to higher functions of intelligence noted by Twaddle *et al.* (1983) it is likely that subtle deficits in language function also occur in children treated for leukaemia, to date, little research has been focused on the linguistic abilities of this population. Higher level language problems were identified by Taylor *et al.* (1987) in children with acute lymphoblastic leukaemia following irradiation. These workers included four age-normed assessments of language (the Expressive One Word Picture Vocabulary Test, the Token Test, the Word Fluency Test and the Verbal Selective Reminding Test) in their test battery and reported that leukaemic subjects performed less well than their siblings on tasks requiring speech and accuracy (word fluency, contingency naming) and on a task requiring the ability to follow multiple element directions (Token Test). Apart from the study by Taylor *et al.* (1987) the majority of comments in the literature relating to the language abilities of acute lymphoblastic leukaemia subjects following treatment are based on neuropsychological measures rather than a comprehensive language assessment. Consequently, although a number of authors have noted that language function remains intact following CNS prophylaxis in childhood leukaemia (Brouwers *et al.*, 1985; Copeland *et al.*, 1985; Eiser, 1978, 1980), effects on language may have been missed by these researchers due to the lack of sufficiently sensitive or specifically-designed measures of language.

Jackel *et al.* (in press) investigated the language abilities of a group of 10 children treated at least 4 years previously for acute lymphoblastic leukaemia. They found that overall the linguistic deficits shown by these children were mild. As a group, however, the leukaemic subjects performed significantly worse than controls matched for age and sex on the TOAL-2, CELF, and Boston Naming Test. Individually, the leukaemic subjects varied in their performance on the language measures.

In addition to language difficulties, problems academically, especially in the areas of English and Mathematics, were reported by Jackel *et al.* in five of their leukaemia subjects. Difficulties reportedly became more noticeable as higher levels of secondary school were attempted. Academic performance has received consideration in the literature relating to acute lymphoblastic leukaemia (Copeland *et al.*, 1985; Moore *et al*, 1986; Ochs *et al.*, 1986, Taylor *et al.*, 1987; Whitt *et al.*, 1984). The Wide Range Achievement Test (WRAT) which considers reading, spelling and arithmetic has been widely used to measure academic performances of acute lymphoblastic leukaemia subjects and controls. Significantly poorer WRAT outcomes have been reported for leukaemic patients than for their siblings (Taylor *et al.*, 1987) and solid tumour controls (Copeland *et al.*, 1985; Moore *et al.*, 1986). Studies that compared WRAT results of leukaemia subjects who had received cranial irradiation with those who had received prophylaxis consisting of drug therapy only, have not identified significant differences (Copeland *et al.*, 1985; Ochs *et al.*, 1986; Whitt *et al.*, 1984).

Effect of age at diagnosis

In an attempt to identify the possible factors associated with the occurrence of neuropsychological deficits following treatment in acute lymphoblastic leukaemia in children, a number of researchers have considered the effects of age at diagnosis (Copeland et al., 1985; Eiser, 1978, 1980; Eiser and Lansdown, 1977; Jannoun, 1983; Meadows et al., 1981; Moore et al., 1986; Rowland et al., 1982; Said et al., 1987; Stehbens et al., 1983) and cranial radiation dosage (Said et al., 1987; Tamaroff et al., 1985) on the degree of neuropsychological impairment in children treated for acute lymphoblastic leukaemia.

Said et al. (1987) supported the findings of earlier workers that the severity of neuropsychological after-effects in subjects treated for acute lymphoblastic leukaemia was related to their age at the time of CNS prophylaxis. Further evidence to support this finding was provided by Moore et al. (1986) who found that leukaemic subjects treated before 5 years of age performed worse on measures of intelligence and academic achievement than those who received the same therapy after that age. Moore et al. (1986) interpreted this result as being supportive of the hypothesis proposed by Dobbing (1968) that the brain is particularly vulnerable to biological insults during the period of rapid development.

Summary of Chemotherapy

In summary, the cerebral and cerebellar changes reported to follow CNS chemotherapy vary between studies in terms of the sites and types of damage, and the clinical presentations described. Alterations in the white matter of the cerebrum and cerebellum were documented by Smith (1975) while Skullerud and Halvorsen (1978) failed to detect central white matter abnormalities in a child with acute leukaemia. Clinical symptoms ascribed to the administration of chemotherapy (in particular, methotrexate) have included disorientation to time and place, gait disturbance, impaired reading and arithmetical abilities (Pizzo et al., 1976), progressive flaccid paresis, mental deterioration (Skullerud and Halvorsen, 1978), spastic quadriplegia or paraplegia, aphasia, slurred speech and a depressed level of responsiveness (Meadows and Evans, 1976). The cerebral and cerebellar damage reported, in association with the aphasia and dysarthria noted by Meadows and Evans (1976), suggests that both speech and language deficits may occur when cytotoxic drugs (in particular methotrexate) have been administered to the CNS. While some studies attribute the reported changes to methotrexate, two studies involved subjects who also received radiotherapy (Meadows and Evans, 1976; Smith, 1975). Isolating methotrexate as the sole cause of damage can be questioned in such cases. In addition, there are studies which failed to detect CNS changes in large groups of children who received chemotherapy but not radiotherapy (Ochs *et al.*, 1980; Tamaroff *et al.*, 1982). Such findings further question the validity of isolating methotrexate as the sole agent of damage when all or part of the subject group had irradiation in addition to chemotherapy.

Combined Radiotherapy and Chemotherapy

Overall, the CNS damage and deficits observed following combined radiotherapy and chemotherapy are similar to those reported when either treatment is administered alone and include focal lesions of the paraventricular white matter, ventricular dilation, cortical atrophy, basal ganglia calcifications, widespread calcium deposits in the subcortical white and grey matter, and in the cerebellar regions, demyelination, subcortical necrosis and cerebrovascular changes (Arnold *et al.*, 1978; Brouwers *et al.*, 1985; Di Chiro *et al.*, 1988; Giralt *et al.*, 1978; Mueller *et al.*, 1976; Norrell *et al.*, 1974; Packer *et al.*, 1986).

Clinical manifestations of CNS prophylaxis have included akinetic mutism, expressive aphasia (Norrell *et al.*, 1974), language deficits (Kramer *et al.*, 1988), word finding difficulties (Brouwers *et al.*, 1985; Meadows *et al.*, 1981), intellectual disabilities (Brouwers *et al.*, 1985; Duffner *et al.*, 1983; Eiser, 1978; Holmes and Holmes, 1975; Kramer *et al.*, 1988; Meadows *et al.*, 1981), learning disabilities (Duffner *et al.*, 1983; Holmes and Holmes, 1975; Kramer *et al.*, 1988; Meadows *et al.*, 1981; Moss *et al.*, 1981), and ataxia and other physical disabilities (Duffner *et al.*, 1983; Holmes and Holmes, 1975). Whether the deficits associated with combination radiotherapy and chemotherapy are of greater severity than those observed when only one form of treatment is used has not been addressed.

Thus, the data reported in the literature strongly suggest that children who receive any combination of radiotherapy and chemotherapy for CNS prophylactic treatment should be monitored closely for the appearance of CNS changes and/or decline in functional abilities.

References

ANSEL, S. and NABEMEZI, J. S. (1974) 'Two year survey of hematologic and malignancies in Uganda', *Journal of the National Cancer Institute*, **52**, pp. 1397–401.

ARNOLD, H., KUHNE, D., FRANKE, H. and GROSCH, I. (1978) 'Findings in computerized axial tomography after intrathecal methotrexate and radiation', *Neurology*, **16**, pp. 65–8.

AUR, R., SIMONE, J., HUSTE, D., RIVERA, G., DAHL, G., BOWMAN, P. and GEORGE, S. (1978) 'Multiple combination therapy for childhood acute lymphocytic leukaemia (ALL)', (Abstract), *Blood*, **52**(5) (Suppl. 1), Abstract No. 490, p. 238.

BAMFORD, F. N., MORRIS-JONES, P., PEARSON, D., RIBEIRO, G. G., SHALET, S. M. and BEARDWELL, C. G. (1976) 'Residual disabilities in children treated for intracranial space-occupying lesions', *Cancer*, **37**, pp. 1149–51.

BROADBENT, V. A., BARNES, N. S. and WHEELER, T. K. (1981) 'Medulloblastoma in childhood: Long-term results of treatment', *Cancer*, **48**, pp. 26–30.

BROUWERS, P., RICCARDI, R., FEDIO, P. and POPLACK, D. G. (1985) 'Long-term neuropsychologic sequelae of childhood leukemia: Correlation with CT brain scan abnormalities', *Journal of Pediatrics*, **106**, pp. 723–8.

BURNS, M. S. and BOYLE, M. (1984) 'Aphasia after successful radiation treatment: A report of two cases', (Letter to the Editor), *Journal of Speech and Hearing Disorders*, **49**, pp. 107–11.

CHESSELLS, J. M. (1985a) 'Cranial irradiation in childhood lymphoblastic leukaemia: Time for reappraisal?', *British Medical Journal*, **291**, p. 686.

CHESSELLS, J. M. (1985b) 'Risks and benefits of intensive treatment of acute leukaemia', *Archives of Disease in Childhood*, **60**, pp. 193–5.

CH'IEN, L. T., RHOMES, J. A., VERZOSA, M. S., COBURN, T. P., GOFF, J. R., HUSTU, H. O., PRICE, R. A., SEIFERT, M. J. and SIMONE, J. V. (1981) 'Progression of methotrexate-induced leukoencephalopathy in children with leukaemia', *Medical and Pediatric Oncology*, **9**, pp. 133–41.

COPELAND, D. R., FLETCHER, J. M., PFEFFERBAUM-LEVINE, B., JAFFE, N., REID, H. and MAOR, N. (1985), 'Neuropsychological sequelae of childhood cancer in long-term survivors', *Pediatrics*, **75**, pp. 745–3.

CURNES, J. T., LASTER, D. W., BALL, M. R., MOODY, D. M. and WITCOFSKI, R. L. (1986) 'MRI of radiation injury to the brain', *American Journal of Roentgenology*, **147**, pp. 119–24.

DANOFF, B. F., COWCHOCK, F. S., MARQUETTE, C., MULGREW, L. and KRAMER, S. (1982) 'Assessment of the long-term effects of primary radiation therapy for brain tumours in children', *Cancer*, **49**, pp. 1580–6.

DAVIES, J. N. P. (1965) 'Leukaemia in children in tropical Africa', *Lancet*, **ii**, pp. 65–7.

DAVIS, P. C., HOFFMAN, J. C., PEARL, G. S. and BRAUN, I. F. (1986) 'CT evaluation of effects of cranial radiation therapy in children', *American Journal of Roentgenology*, **147**, pp. 587–92.

DE REUCK, J. and VANDER EECKEN, H. (1975), 'The anatomy of the late radiation encephalopathy', *European Neurology*, **13**, pp. 481–94.

DEUTSCH, M. (1982) 'Radiotherapy for primary brain tumors in very young children', *Cancer*, **50**, pp. 2785–9.

DI CHIRO, G., OLDFIELD, W., WRIGHT, D. C., DE MICHELE, D., KATZ, D. A., PATRONAS, N. J., DOPPMAN, J. L., LARSON, S. M., ITO, M. and KUFTA, C. V. (1988) 'Cerebral necrosis after radiotherapy and/or intraarterial chemotherapy for brain tumours: PET and neuropathological studies', *American Journal of Roentgenology*, **150**, pp. 189–97.

DI LORENZO, N., NOLLETTI, A. and PALMA, L. (1978) 'Late cerebral radionecrosis', *Surgical Neurology*, **10**, pp. 281–90.

DOBBING, J. (1968) 'Vulnerable periods in the developing brain', in Davison A. N. and Dobbin, J. (Eds) *Applied Neurochemistry*, Oxford, Blackwell Scientific.

DOOMS, G. C., HECHT, S., BRANT-ZAWADZKI, M., BERTHIAUME, Y., NORMAN, D. and NEWTON, T. H. (1986) 'Brain radiation lesions: MR Imaging', *Radiology*, **158**, pp. 149–55.

DUFFNER, P. K., COHEN, M. E., and THOMAS, P. (1983) 'Late effects of treatment on the intelligence of children with posterior fossa tumours', *Cancer*, **51**, pp. 233–7.

DUFFNER, P. K., COHEN, M. E., THOMAS, R. M and LANSKY, S. B. (1985) 'The long-term effects of cranial irradiation on the central nervous system', *Cancer*, **56**, pp. 1841–6.

EDINGTON, G. M. and HENDRISKE, M. (1973) 'Incidence and frequency of lymphoreticular tumors in Ibadan and the western state of Nigeria', *Journal of the National Cancer Institute*, **50**, pp. 1623–31.

EISER, C. (1978) 'Intellectual abilities among survivors of childhood leukaemia as a function of CNS irradiation', *Archives of Disease in Childhood*, **53**, pp. 391–5.

EISER, C. (1980) 'Effects of chronic illness on intellectual development: A comparison of normal children with those treated for childhood leukaemia and solid tumours', *Archives of Disease in Childhood*, **55**, pp. 766–70.

EISER, C., and LANSDOWN, R. (1977) 'Retrospective study of intellectual development in children treated for acute lymphoblastic leukaemia', *Archives of Disease in Childhood*, **9**, pp. 429–38.

ESSELTINE, D. W., FREEMAN, C. R., CHEVALIER, L. M., SMITH, R., O'GORMAN, A. M., DUBE, J., WHITEHEAD, V. M. and NOGRADY, M. B. (1981) 'Computed tomography brain scans in long term survivors of childhood acute lymphoblastic leukaemia', *Medical and Paediatric Oncology*, **9**, pp. 429–38.

FARBER, S., DIAMOND, L. K., MERCER, P. D., SYLVESTER, R. F. and WOLFF, J. A. (1948) 'Temporary remissions in acute leukemia in children produced by folic acid antagonist, 4-aminopteroyl-glutamic acid (aminopterin)', *New England Journal of Medicine*, **238**, pp. 787–93.

FERNBACH, D. J., GEORGE, S. L., SUTOW, W. W., RAGAB, A. H., LANE, D. M., HAGGARD, M. E. and LONSDALE, D. (1975) 'Long-term results of reinforcement therapy in children with acute leukemia', *Cancer*, **36**, pp. 1552–9.

FREI, E. (1965) 'Progress in treatment for the leukemias and lymphomas', *Cancer*, **18**, pp. 1580–4.

GIRALT, M., GIL, J. L., BORDERAS, F., OLIVEROS, A., GOMEZ-PEREDA, R., PARDO, J., MARTINEZ-IBANEZ, F. and RAICHS, A. (1978) 'Intracerebral calcifications in childhood lymphoblastic leukemia: A new iatrogenic disease?' *Acta Haematology*, **59**, pp. 193–204.

GREEN, D. M., FREEMAN, A. I., SATHER, H. N., SALLAN, S. E., NESBIT, M. E. Jr., CASSADY, J. R., SINKS, L. F., HAMMOND, D. and FREI, I. (1980) 'Comparison of three methods of central-nervous-system prophylaxis in childhood acute lymphoblastic leukaemia', *Lancet*, **i**, pp. 1398–402.

HAGHBIN, M. (1976) 'Chemotherapy of acute lymphoblastic leukemia in children', *American Journal of Hematology*, **1**, pp. 201–9.

HODGES, S. and SMITHELLS, R. W. (1983) 'Intracranial calcification and childhood medulloblastoma' (Letter to the Editor). *Archives of Disease in Childhood*, **58**, pp. 663–4.

HOLLAND, J. F. and GLIDEWELL, O. (1972) 'Chemotherapy of acute lymphoblastic leukemia of childhood cancer', *Cancer*, **30**, pp. 1480–7.

HOLMES, H. A. and HOLMES, F. F. (1975) 'After ten years, what are the handicaps and lifestyles of children treated for cancer?' An examination of the present status of 124 such survivors', *Clinical Pediatrics*, **14**, pp. 819–23.

HUDSON, L. J., MURDOCH, B. E. and OZANNE, A. E. (1989) 'Posterior fossa tumours in childhood: associated speech and language disorders post-surgery', *Aphasiology*, **3**, pp. 1–18.

HUGHES, W. T., FELDMAN, S., AUR, R. J. A., VERZOSA, M S., HUSTU, O. and SIMONE, J. V. (1975) 'Intensity of immunosuppressive therapy and the incidence of pneumocystis carinii pneumonitis', *Cancer*, **36**, pp. 2004–9.

HUSTU, H. O. and AUR, R. J. A. (1978) 'Extramedullary leukemia', *Clinical Hematology*, **7**, pp. 313–37.

JACKEL, C. A., MURDOCH, B. E., OZANNE, A. E. and BUTTSWORTH, D. L. (in press) 'Language abilities of children treated for acute lymphoblastic leukaemia: Preliminary findings', *Aphasiology*.

JACQUILLAT, C., WEIL, M., GEMON, M. F., IZRAEL, V., SCHAISON, G., AUCLERC, G., ABLIN, A. R., FLANDRIN, G., TANZER, J., BUSSEL, A., WEISGERBER, C., DRESCH, C., NAJEAN, Y., GOUDEMARD, M., SELIGMANN, M., BOIRON, M. and BERNARD, J. (1973) 'Evaluation of 216 four-year survivors of acute leukemia', *Cancer*, **32**, pp. 286–93.

JANNOUN, L. (1983) 'Are cognitive and educational development affected by age at which prophylactic therapy is given in acute lymphoblastic leukaemia?' *Archives of Disease in Childhood*, **58**, pp. 953–8.

KALEITA, T. A. and AL-MATEEN, M. (1985) 'Subacute necrotizing leukoencephalopathy after treatment for acute lymphoctyic leukemia', (Letter to the Editor) *New England Journal of Medicine*, **312**, p. 317.

KAPLAN, H. S. (1975) 'Present status of radiation therapy of cancer: An overview', in Becker F. F. (Ed.) *Cancer: A Comprehensive Treatise: Vol. 6. Radiotherapy, Surgery and Immunotherapy*, New York, Plenum Press, pp. 3–38.

KEARSLEY, J. H. (1983) 'Late cerebrovascular disease after radiation therapy — Report of two cases and a review of the literature', *Australasian Radiology*, **27**, pp. 11–18.

KIM, T., NESBIT, M. E., D'ANGIO, G. D. and LEVITT, S. H. (1972) 'The role of central nervous system irradiation in children with acute lymphoblastic leukemia', *Radiology*, **104**, pp. 635–41.

KRAMER, J. H., NORMAN, D., BRANT-ZAWADZKI, M., ABLIN, A. and MOORE, I. M. (1988) 'Absence of white matter changes on magnetic resonance imaging in children treated with CNS prophylaxis therapy for leukemia', *Cancer*, **61**, pp. 928–30.

LEE, K. F. and SUH, J. H., (1977) 'CT evidence of grey matter calcification secondary to radiation therapy', *Computerized Tomography*, **1**, pp. 103–10.

LICHTOR, T., WOLLMAN, R. L. and BROWN, F. D. (1984) 'Calcified basal ganglionic mass 12 years after radiation therapy for medulloblastoma', *Surgical Neurology*, **21**, pp. 373–6.

LITTMAN, P., COCCIA, P., BLEYER, W. A., LUKENS, J., SIEGEL, S., MILLER, D., SATHER, H. and HAMMOND, D. (1987) 'Central nervous system (CNS) prophylaxis in children with low risk acute lymphoblastic leukaemia (ALL)', *International Journal of Radiation, Oncology, Biology, Physics*, **13**, pp. 1443–9.

LUDWIG, R., CALVO, W., KOBER, B. and BRANDEIS, W. E. (1987) 'Effects of local irradiation and i.v. methotrexate on brain morphology in rabbits: Early changes', *Journal of Cancer Research and Clinical Oncology*, **113**, pp. 235–40.

McCALLA, J. L. (1985) 'A multidisciplinary approach to identification and remedial intervention for adverse late effects of cancer therapy', *Symposium on Pediatric Oncology*, **20**, pp. 117–30.

McWHIRTER, W. R. and MASEL, J. P. (1987) *Paediatric Oncology: An Illustrated Introduction*, Sydney, Williams and Wilkins.

McWHIRTER, W. R., PEARN, J. H., SMITH, H. and O'REGAN, P. (1986) 'Cerebral astrocytoma as a complication of acute lymphoblastic leukaemia', *Medical Journal of Australia*, **145**, pp. 96–7.

MARKS, J. E., BAGLAN, R. J., PRASSAD, S. C. and BLANK, W. F. (1981) 'Cerebral radionecrosis: Incidence and risk in relation to dose, time, fractionation and volume', *International Journal of Radiation, Oncology, Biology, Physics*, **7**, pp. 243–52.

MARKS, J. E. and WONG, J. (1985) 'The risk of cerebral radionecrosis in relation to dose, time and fractionation', *Progress in Experimental Tumor Research*, **29**, pp. 210–18.

MARTINS, A. N., JOHNSTON, J. S., HENRY, J. M., STOFFEL, T. J. and DI CHIRO, G. (1977) 'Delayed radiation necrosis of the brain', *Journal of Neurosurgery*, **47**, pp. 336–45.

MEADOWS, A. T. and EVANS, A. E. (1976) 'Effects of chemotherapy on the central nervous system', *Cancer*, **37**, pp. 1079–85.

MEADOWS, A. T., KREIMAS, N. L. and BELASCO, J. B. (1980) 'The medical cost of cure: Sequelae in survivors of childhood cancer', in Sullivan M. P. and van Eys, J. (Eds) *Status of the Curability of Childhood Cancers*, New York, Raven Press, pp. 263–76.

MEADOWS, A. T., MASSARI, D. J., FERGUSON, J., GORDON, J., LITTMAN, P. and MOSS, K. (1981) 'Declines in IQ scores and cognitive dysfunctions in children with acute lymphocytic leukaemia treated with cranial irradiation', *Lancet*, **ii**, pp. 1015–18.

MILLER, D. R. (1980) 'Childhood acute leukaemia', in Conn, H. F. (Ed.) *Current Therapy*, 32nd Ed., St. Louis, Mosby, pp. 292–9.

MILLER, D. R. (1982) 'Acute lymphoblastic leukemia', in Tebbi, C. K., (Ed.) *Major Topics in Pediatric and Adolescent Oncology*, Boston, Hall Medical, pp. 2–43.

MOE, P. (1984) 'Recent advances in the management of acute lymphoblastic leukaemia', *European Paediatric Haematology and Oncology*, **1**, pp. 19–28.

MOORE, I. A., KRAMER, J. and ABLIN, A. (1986) 'Late effects of central nervous system prophylactic leukaemia treatment on cognitive functioning', *Oncology Nursing Forum*, **13**, pp. 45–51.

MOSS, H. A., NANNIS, E. D. and POPLACK, D. G. (1981) 'The effects of prophylactic treatment of the central nervous system on the intellectual functioning of children with acute lymphoblastic leukemia', *American Journal of Medicine*, **71**, pp. 47–52.

MUCHI, H., SATOH, T., KAYOKO, Y., KARUBE, T. and MIYOA, M. (1987) 'Studies on the assessment of neurotoxicity in children with acute lymphoblastic leukemia', *Cancer*, **59**, pp. 881–95.

MUELLER, S., BELL, W. and SEIBERT, J. (1976) 'Cerebral calcifications associated with intrathecal methotrexate therapy in acute lymphocytic leukemia', *Journal of Pediatrics*, **88**, pp. 650–3.

MULHERN, R. K., OCHS, J., FAIRCLOUGH, D., WASSERMAN, A. L., DAVIS, K. S. and WILLIAMS, J. M. (1987) 'Intellectual and academic achievement status after CNS relapse: A retrospective analysis of 40 children treated for acute lymphoblastic leukemia', *Journal of Clinical Oncology*, **15**, pp. 933–40.

NEGLIA, J. P. and ROBISON, L. L. (1988) 'Epidemiology of the childhood acute leukemias', *Pediatrics Clinics of North America*, **35**, pp. 675–92.

NGUYEN, T. D., PANIS, X., FROISSART, D., LEGROS, M., CONINX, P. and LOIRETTE, M. (1988) 'Analysis of late complications after rapid hyperfractionated radiotherapy in advanced head and neck cancers', *International Journal of Radiation, Oncology, Biology, Physics*, **14**, pp. 23–5.

NIGHTINGALE, S., DAWES, P. J. D. K. and CARTLIDGE, N. E. F. (1982) 'Early-delayed radiation rhombencephalopathy', *Journal of Neurology, Neurosurgery and Psychiatry*, **45**, pp. 267–70.

NORRELL, H., WILSON, C. B., SLAGEL, D. E. and CLARK, D. B. (1974) 'Leukoencephalopathy following the administration of methotrexate into the cerebrospinal fluid in the treatment of primary brain tumours', *Cancer*, **33**, pp. 923–32.

OCHS, J. J., BERGER, P., BRECHER, M. L., SINKS, L. F., KINKEL, W. and FREENAM, A. I. (1980) 'Computed tomography brain scans in children with acute lymphoblastic leukaemia receiving methotrexate alone as central nervous system prophylaxis', *Cancer*, **45**, pp. 2274–8.

OCHS, J. and MULHERN, R. K. (1988) 'Late effects of antileukemic treatment', *Pediatric Clinics of North America*, **35**, pp. 815–33.

OCHS, J., PARVEY, L. S. and MULHERN, R. (1986) 'Prospective study of central nervous system changes in children with acute lymphoblastic leukaemia receiving two different methods of central nervous system prophylaxis', *Neurotoxicology*, **7**, pp. 217–26.

OCHS, J. J., RIVERA, G., RHOMES, J. A., HUSTU, H. O., BERG, R. and SIMONE, J. V. (1985) 'Central nervous system morbidity following an initial isolated central nervous system relapse and its subsequent therapy in childhood acute lymphoblastic leukaemia', *Journal of Clinical Oncology*, **3**, pp. 622–6.

PACKER, R. J., ZIMMERMAN, R. A. and BILANIUK, L. T. (1986) 'Magnetic resonance imaging in the evaluation of treatment-related central nervous system damage', *Cancer*, **58**, pp. 635–40.

PAINTER, M. J., CHUTORIAN, A. E. and HILAL, S. K. (1975) 'Cerebrovasculopathy following irradiation in childhood', *Neurology*, **25**, pp. 189–94.

PEARSON, A. D. J., CAMPBELL, A. N., MCALLISTER, V. L. and PEARSON, G. L. (1983) 'Intracranial calcification in survivors of childhood medulloblastoma', *Archives of Disease in Childhood*, **58**, pp. 133–6.

PEYLAN-RAMU, N., POPLACK, D. G., PIZZO, P. A., ADORNATO, B. T. and DI CHIRO, G. (1978) 'Abnormal CT scans in asymptomatic children with acute lymphocytic leukaemia after prophylactic treatment of the central nervous system with radiation and intrathecal chemotherapy', *New England Journal of Medicine*, **298**, pp. 815–18.

PINKEL, D. (1979) 'Treatment of acute lymphocytic leukaemia', *Cancer*, **43**, pp. 1128–37.

PIZZO, P. A., BLEYER, W. A., POPLACK, D. G. and LEVENTHAL, B. G. (1976) 'Reversible dementia temporally associated with intraventricular therapy with methotrexate in a child with acute myelogenous leukaemia', *Journal of Pediatrics*, **88**, pp. 131–3.

PIZZO, P. A., POPLACK D. G. and BLEYER, W. A. (1979) 'Neurotoxicities of current leukaemia therapy', *American Journal of Pediatric Hematology and Oncology*, **1**, pp. 127–40.

POPLACK, D. G. and REAMAN, G. (1988) 'Acute lymphoblastic leukaemia in childhood', *Pediatric Clinics of North America*, **35**, pp. 903–32.

PRICE, R. A. and BIRDWELL, D. A. (1978) 'The central nervous system in childhood leukaemia: II. Mineralizing microangiopathy and dystrophic calcification', *Cancer*, **42**, pp. 717–28.

PRICE, D. B., HOTSON, G. C. and LOH, J. P. (1988) 'Pontine calcification following radiotherapy: CT demonstration', *Journal of Computed Assisted Tomography*, **12**, pp. 45–6.

RIVERA, G. K. and MAUER, A. M. (1987) 'Controversies in the management of childhood acute lymphoblastic leukaemia: Treatment intensification, CNS leukaemia, and prognostic factors', *Seminars in Hematology*, **24**, pp. 12–26.

ROWLAND, J., GLIDEWELL, O. and SIBLEY, R. (1982) 'Effect of cranial irradiation (CRT) on neuropsychologic function in children with Acute Lymphoblastic Leukaemia', *Proceedings of the American Society of Clinical Oncology*, **1**, p.123.

SAFDARI, H., FUENTES, J. M., DUBOIS, J. B., ALIREZAI, M., CASTAN, P. and VLAHOVITCH, B. (1985) 'Radiation necrosis of the brain: Time of onset and incidence related to total dose and fractionation of radiation', *Neuroradiology*, **27**, pp. 44–7.

SAID, J. A., WATERS, B. G. H., COUSENS, P. and STEVENS, M. M. (1987) 'Neuropsychological after-effects of central nervous system prophylaxis in survivors of childhood acute lymphoblastic leukaemia', in Gates G. R. (Ed.) Proceedings of the twelfth annual brain impairment conference, Armidale, Australian Society for the Study of Brain Impairment.

SILVERMAN, C. L., PALKES, H., TALENT, B., KOVNAR, E., CLOUSE, J. W. and THOMAS, P. R. M. (1984) 'Late effects of radiotherapy on patients with cerebellar medulloblastoma', *Cancer*, **54**, pp. 825–9.

SIMONE, J. V. (1976) 'Factors that influence haematological remission duration in acute lymphocytic leukaemia', *British Journal of Haematology*, **32**, pp. 465–72.

SKULLERUD, K. and HALVORSEN, K. (1978) 'Encephalomyelopathy following intrathecal methotrexate treatment in a child with acute leukaemia', *Cancer*, **42**, pp. 1211–15.

SMITH, B. (1975) 'Brain damage after intrathecal methotrexate', *Journal of Neurology, Neurosurgery and Psychiatry*, **38**, pp. 810–15.

SOUTHAM, C. M., CRAVER, F. L., DARGEON, H. W. and BURCHENAL, J. H. (1951) 'A study of the natural history of acute leukaemia with special reference to the duration of the disease and the occurrence of remissions', *Cancer*, **4**, pp. 39–59.

STEHBENS, J. A., KISKER, C. T. and WILSON, B. K. (1983) 'Achievement and intelligence test-retest performance in pediatric cancer patients at diagnosis and one year later', *Journal of Pediatric Psychology*, **8**, pp. 47–56.

TAMAROFF, M., MILLER, D. R., MURPHY, M. L., SALWEN, R., GHAVIMI, F. and NIR, Y. (1982) 'Immediate and long-term post-therapy neuropsychologic performance in children with acute lymphoblastic leukaemia treated without central nervous system radiation', *Journal of Pediatrics*, **101**, pp. 524–9.

TAMAROFF, M., SALWEN, R. and MILLER, D. R. (1985) 'Neuropsychological sequelae in irradiated (1800 rads (r) and 2400 r) and non-irradiated children with acute lymphoblastic leukaemia (ALL)', *Proceedings of the American Society of Clinical Oncology*. **4**, p. 165.

TAYLOR, H. G., ALBO, V. C. PHEBUS, C. K., SACHS, B. R. and BIERL, P. G. (1987) 'Postirradiation treatment outcomes for children with acute lymphocytic leukaemia: Clarification of risks', *Journal of Pediatric Psychology*, **12**, pp. 395–411.

TEBBI, C. K. (1982) *Major Topics in Pediatric and Adolescent Oncology*, Boston, Hall Medical Publishers.

TILL, M. M., HARDISTY, R. M. and PIKE, M C. (1973) 'Long survivals in acute leukaemia', *Lancet*, **i**, pp. 534–8.

TIVEY, H. (1952) 'Prognosis for survival in the leukaemias of childhood', *Pediatrics*, **10**, pp. 48–59.

TSURUDA, J. S., KORTMAN, K. E., BRADLEY, W. G., WHEELER, D. C., VAN DALSEM, W. and BRADLEY, T. P. (1987) 'Radiation effects on cerebral white matter: MR evaluation', *American Journal of Roentgenology*, **149**, pp. 165–71.

TWADDLE, V., BRITTON, P. G., CRAFT, A. C., NOBEL, T. C. and KERNAHAN, J. (1983) 'Intellectual function after treatment for leukaemia or solid tumours', *Archives of Disease in Childhood*, **58**, pp. 949–52.

WHITT, J. K., WELLS, R. J., LAURIE, M. M., WILHELM, C. L. and McMILLAN, C. W. (1984) 'Cranial irradiation in childhood acute lymphocytic leukaemia: Neuropsychologic sequelae', *American Journal of Disease in Childhood*, **138**, pp. 730–6.

WRIGHT, T. L. and BRESNAN, M. J. (1976) 'Radiation-induced cerebrovascular disease in children', *Neurology*, **26**, pp. 540–3.

YAMASHITA, J., HANDA, H., YUMITORI, K. and ABE, M. (1980) 'Reversible delayed radiation effect on the brain after radiotherapy of malignant astrocytoma', *Surgical Neurology*, **13**, pp. 413–17.

YOUNG, J. L. and MILLER, R. W. (1975) 'Incidence of malignant tumours in U.S. children', *Journal of Pediatrics*, **86**, pp. 254–7.

Chapter 10

Acquired Childhood Speech Disorders: Dysarthria and Dyspraxia

Bruce E. Murdoch, Anne E. Ozanne and Jill A. Cross

Introduction

Although the presence of an articulatory disturbance has often been noted in children with acquired aphasia (Alajouanine and Lhermitte, 1965; Ferro *et al.*, 1982; Van Hout *et al.*, 1985), it is typical that no indication is given as to whether this disturbance represents a form of dysarthria, dyspraxia or a phonological disorder. Consequently the literature on acquired speech disorders in children has little to offer the clinician in either the diagnosis or treatment of these children. While the difficulty of applying models and theories developed for adults with acquired neurological disorders to children, particularly those still acquiring language, is acknowledged, until more information becomes available to refute their appropriateness it appears that such models are all that is available, at this stage, to help clinicians in the assessment and treatment of children with acquired speech disorders.

Definition of Dysarthria and Dyspraxia

Dysarthria and dyspraxia of speech are both motor disorders involving disruption of the motor control of speech. According to Darley *et al.* (1975: 2), the term 'dysarthria' is 'a collective name for a group of related speech disorders that are due to disturbance in muscular control of the speech mechanism resulting from impairment of any of the basic motor processes involved in the execution of speech'. According to this definition, speech disorders resulting from either somatic structural abnormalities (e.g. cleft palate, congenitally enlarged pharynx, malocclusion etc.) or psychological disorders (e.g. psychogenic aphonia) are not classified as dysarthrias. Rather, the term 'dysarthria' is used only to describe those speech disorders that result from damage to either the central or peripheral nervous system. The present chapter will confine itself to a discussion of acquired neurogenic speech disorders occurring in children as a result of injury to the brain or peripheral nerves following head trauma, cerebrovascular accidents, neoplasms, anoxic episodes etc. Discussion of speech disorders associated with congenital conditions such as cerebral palsy will not be included.

Although classified as a motor speech disorder, dyspraxia of speech differs from dysarthria in several important ways. Whereas in dysarthria the speech disorder results from either paralysis, weakness or incoordination of the muscles of the speech mechanism, dyspraxia of speech is a disorder of motor speech programming in which the individual has difficulty speaking because of a cerebral lesion that prevents him/her executing voluntarily, or on command, the complex sequence of muscle contractions involved in speaking. In the dyspraxic speaker, the muscles of the speech mechanism are neither weak nor paralyzed, as can be demonstrated by the child's ability to carry out movements of the face, tongue etc. during reflex activities such as licking the lips to retrieve a crumb. The disorder of motor speech programming is manifest in the child's speech primarily by errors in articulation and secondarily by what are thought by many researchers to be compensatory alterations of prosody (e.g. pauses, slow speech rate, equalization of stress etc.). Although both developmental and acquired forms of dyspraxia of speech have been identified, the present chapter will deal only with the acquired form of dyspraxia of speech.

Acquired Dysarthria

Neuropathological Substrate of Acquired Dysarthria

Contraction of the muscles of the speech mechanism to produce speech is regulated by nerve impulses originating in the motor cortex which pass to the muscles by way of the descending motor pathways. Depending on where in the motor system the damage is located, acquired brain and peripheral nerve lesions can cause a variety of different types of dysarthria. Components of the neuromuscular system that can be affected include the lower motor neurons, upper motor neurons, extrapyramidal system, cerebellum and neuromuscular junction, as well as the muscles of the speech mechanism themselves.

On the basis of acoustic-perceptual judgements of speech and neuroanatomical data, Darley *et al.* (1969a,b) identified six different types of dysarthria in adults including: flaccid, spastic, hypokinetic, hyperkinetic, ataxic and mixed (e.g. spastic-ataxic dysarthria). In that the same components of the neuromuscular system can be affected by acquired neurological disorders in children as in adults, as pointed out above, it would seem appropriate that the dysarthria classification system devised by Darley *et al.* (1969a,b) be used to describe acquired dysarthrias in children in the same way as it is used to describe the equivalent speech disorders in adults.

Flaccid dysarthria (lower motor neuron dysarthria)

Damage to the motor cranial nerves and spinal nerves represent lower motor neuron lesions. These lesions interrupt the conduction of nerve impulses from the central nervous system (CNS) to the skeletal muscles. Where either the bulbar cranial nerves (V,VII,IX, X, XI and XII) and/or the spinal nerves that supply the muscles of respiration are involved, changes in speech collectively referred to as flaccid dysarthria may result. In the case of the bulbar cranial nerves, the damage may involve the nerves either in their peripheral course or in their nuclei in the brainstem.

Symptoms of lower motor neuron lesions include a loss of muscle tone, muscle weakness, a loss or reduction of muscle reflexes, atrophy of the muscles involved and fasciculations. The actual name, flaccid dysarthria, is derived from the major symptom of lower motor neuron damage, flaccid paralysis. The characteristics of the speech deficit exhibited by patients with flaccid dysarthria varies from case to case depending upon which particular nerves are affected.

In addition to lesions in the lower motor neurons themselves, flaccid dysarthria can also result from either impaired nerve impulse transmission across the neuromuscular junction (such as occurs in myasthenia gravis) or disorders which involve the muscles of the speech mechanism themselves (e.g. muscular dystrophy).

Neurological disorders associated with motor neuron lesions in childhood
The lower motor neurons that innervate the muscles involved in speech production can be damaged by a variety of neurological diseases, including viral infections (e.g. poliomyelitis), tumours, cerebrovascular accidents (e.g. embolization resulting from congenital heart disease), degenerative disorders and traumatic head injury. The general name applied to flaccid paralysis of the muscles supplied by nerves arising from the bulbar regions of the brainstem (which, with the exception of the respiratory muscles, include the muscles of the speech mechanism) is bulbar palsy. Bulbar palsy can be caused by pathological conditions which affect either the cell body of the lower motor neurons in the cranial nerve nuclei or the axon of the lower motor neuron as it courses through the peripheral nerve. In particular, damage to cranial nerves V (trigeminal), VII (facial), X (vagus) and XII (hypoglossal) in their peripheral course can lead to flaccid dysarthria.

Trigeminal nerve disorders. The trigeminal nerves supply the muscles of mastication (temporalis, masseter, pterygoids) which in turn regulate the movement of the mandible. In children with unilateral trigeminal lesions, the mandible deviates towards the paralyzed side when the child is asked to open his or her mouth widely. This deviation is brought about by the unopposed contraction of the pterygoid muscles on the active side (i.e. the side opposite to the lesion). In addition the child will show a loss or reduction of muscle tone and atrophy in the muscles of mastication on the side of the lesion. Only minor alterations in speech occur, however, as a result of unilateral trigeminal lesions, in that movements of the mandible are impaired to only a small extent. A much more devastating effect on speech occurs following bilateral trigeminal lesions, the muscles responsible for the elevation of the mandible being too weak in many cases to approximate the mandible and maxilla. This inability, in turn, may prevent the tongue and lips from making the necessary contacts with oral structures for the production of labial and lingual consonants and vowels. Unilateral trigeminal lesions in children may result from traumatic head injury and brainstem tumours involving the pons. Bilateral flaccid paralysis of the masticatory muscles, on the other hand, may be seen in bulbar poliomyelitis.

Facial nerve disorders. The muscles of facial expression (e.g. orbicularis oris, buccinator etc.) are supplied by the facial nerves. Unilateral facial nerve lesions cause flaccid paralysis of the muscles of facial expression on the same side as the lesion. Consequently, children with such lesions present with drooping of the mouth on the affected side and saliva may constantly dribble from the corner. In addition, as a result of loss of muscle tone in the orbicularis oculi muscle, the lower eyelid may also droop. During smiling the mouth is retracted on the active side but not on the child's affected side. Likewise, during frowning, the frontalis muscle on the side contralateral to the lesion will corrugate the forehead; however, on the side ipsilateral to the lesion no corrugation will occur. In cases of bilateral facial nerve paralysis, saliva may drool from both corners of the mouth and the lips may be slightly parted at rest.

Both unilateral and bilateral facial nerve lesions affect speech production. Children with facial nerve lesions are unable to seal their lips tightly and during speech air escapes between their lips during the build-up of intraoral pressure. Consequently, unilateral facial nerve lesions cause distortion of bilabial and labiodental consonants. Speech impairments associated with bilateral facial nerve lesions range from distortion to complete obliteration of bilabial and labiodental consonants.

A number of different acquired disorders can cause malfunctioning of the facial nerves in children. In some cases the facial palsy may have an idiopathic origin, such as in Bell's palsy. Bell's palsy usually causes unilateral facial paralysis. Prognostically, in the region of 80 per cent of Bell's palsy cases recover in a few days or weeks. Unilateral facial paralysis can also result from closed head injuries, damage to one or other facial nerve during the course of a forceps delivery, compression of the facial nerve by tumour (e.g. acoustic neuroma) and damage to the facial nucleus by brainstem tumours (e.g. glioma).

Bilateral facial paralysis may occur in idiopathic polyneuritis (Guillian-Barré syndrome). In addition, sarcoidosis, bulbar poliomyelitis and some forms of basal meningitis may also cause facial diplegia as can some congenital disorders such as congenital hypoplasia of the nuclei of the VIIth and VIth cranial nerves (Möbius syndrome).

Vagus nerve disorders. Among other structures, the vagus nerves supply the muscles of the larynx and the levator muscles of the soft palate. Lesions of the vagus nerves, therefore, can affect either the phonatory or resonatory aspects of speech production or both, depending upon the location of the lesion along the nerve pathway. Lesions which involve the nucleus ambiguus in the medulla (as occurs in lateral medullary syndrome following occlusion of the postero inferior cerebellar artery) or the vagus nerve near to the brainstem (e.g. in the region of the jugular foramen) cause paralysis of all the skeletal muscles supplied via the vagus. Children with this type of lesion present with a flaccid dysphonia characterized by moderate breathiness, harshness and reduced volume. Other voice problems that may also be present include diplophonia, short phrases and inhalatory stridor. These voice abnormalities result from paralysis of the vocal cord on the side of the lesion which tends to lie in a slightly abducted position. In addition to the voice problem, these children also present with hypernasality due to paralysis of the soft palate on the affected side.

Lesions of the vagus which involve the nerve at a point distal to the exit of the pharyngeal nerve (which supplies the levator of the soft palate) but proximal to the exit of the superior laryngeal nerve, have the same effect on phonation as brainstem lesions. These lesions, however, do not cause hypernasality since the functioning of the levator veli palatini is not compromised. In those cases where the recurrent laryngeal nerve is involved, dysphonia in the absence of hypernasality is also present. In these latter cases, however, the cricothyroid muscles (the principal tensor muscles of the vocal cords) are not affected and the vocal cords are paralyzed closer to the midline (the paramedian position). Consequently, although the voice is likely to be harsh and reduced in loudness, there is likely to be a lesser degree of the breathiness than is seen in those children with brainstem lesions involving the nucleus ambiguus. The recurrent laryngeal nerve can be injured during surgery to the neck (e.g. thyroidectomy) or occasionally during chest surgery, especially on the left side where the nerve loops around the aortic arch. Bilateral damage to the recurrent laryngeal nerves is rare.

Hypoglossal nerve disorders. With the exception of palatoglossus, all the extrinsic and all the intrinsic muscles of the tongue are controlled by the hypoglossal nerves. Unilateral hypoglossal nerve damage therefore, as might occur in either brainstem conditions such as medial medullary syndrome or peripheral nerve lesions such as submaxillary tumours which compress one or other hypoglossal nerves, is associated with flaccid paralysis, atrophy and fasciculations in the ipsilateral side of the tongue. On protrusion the tongue deviates to the affected side.

In bilateral hypoglossal involvement, both sides of the tongue may be atrophied and show fasciculations. Although in this case protrusion occurs in the midline, the degree of protrusion may be severely limited. In addition, elevation of the tip and body to contact the alveolar ridge or hard palate may be difficult or impossible.

Although both phonation and resonation remain normal, lesions of the hypoglossal nerves therefore cause disturbances in articulation by interfering with normal tongue movement. The articulatory imprecision occurs especially during production of linguodental and linguopalatal consonants. In the case of unilateral lesions the articulatory imprecision may be temporary in that most patients learn to compensate for unilateral tongue weakness within a few days. More serious articulatory impairments, however, are associated with bilateral hypoglossal nerve lesions. As indicated above, tongue movement in such cases may be severely restricted and speech sounds such as high front vowels and consonants that require elevation of the tongue tip to contact the upper alveolar ridge or hard palate (e.g. /t/, /d/, /l/ etc.). may be grossly distorted.

Hypoglossal nerve lesions are rare in children and more commonly result from damage to the hypoglossal nucleus in the brainstem than from damage to the peripheral nerve itself. Some isolated cases of damage to the hypoglossal nerve are seen as the result of the child falling with something (usually a pencil) in their mouth.

Multiple cranial nerve disorders. In addition to individual damage to each of the bulbar cranial nerves, flaccid dysarthria can also result from simultaneous damage to a number of cranial nerves. For example, lesions in the region of the jugular foramen (the exit point of the IXth, Xth and XIth nerves) can cause the concurrent dysfunctioning of the pharynx, soft palate and larynx. The nerves passing through the jugular foramen can be affected by disorders such as tumours within the jugular foramen (i.e. glomus jugulare tumours), metastases involving the base of the skull and sarcoidosis.

Spastic dysarthria (upper motor neuron dysarthria)

Persistent spastic dysarthria is caused by bilateral disrupton of the upper motor neuron supply to the bulbar cranial nerve nuclei. Lesions of upper motor neurons that can cause dysarthria may be located in the cerebral cortex, the internal capsule, the cerebral peduncles or the brainstem. Clinical signs of upper motor neuron lesions include: spastic paralysis or paresis of the involved muscles, little or no muscle atrophy, hyperactive muscle stretch reflexes (e.g. hyperactive jaw-jerk) and the presence of pathological reflexes (e.g. positive Babinski sign, positive rooting reflex etc.).

In that the majority of the cranial nerve nuclei receive a bilateral upper motor neuron innervation, in general bilateral corticobulbar lesions are required to produce a permanent and severe spastic dysarthria. Usually only a transient impairment in articulation occurs subsequent to unilateral corticobulbar lesions. Such lesions cause a spastic paralysis or weakness in the contralateral lower half of the face, but not the upper part of the face, which may be associated with a mild, transient dysarthria due to weakness of the orbicularis oris. There is, however, no weakness of the forehead, muscles of mastication, soft palate (therefore no hypernasality), pharynx (therefore no swallowing problems) or larynx (therefore no dysphonia). In addition to the lower facial weakness, however, unilateral upper motor neuron lesions may produce a mild weakness of the tongue on the side opposite the lesion.

The general name given to spastic paralysis of the bulbar musculature as a result of bilateral upper motor neuron lesions is pseudobulbar palsy (supranuclear palsy). Pseudobulbar palsy, which takes its name from its clinical resemblance to bulbar palsy, may be associated with a variety of neurological disorders which bilaterally affect the upper motor neurons anywhere from their cell bodies, located in the motor cortex, through to their synapses with the appropriate lower motor neurons. Bilateral cerebrovascular accidents, multiple sclerosis, motor neuron disease, extensive neoplasms, congenital disorders, encephalitis and severe brain trauma are all possible causes of this syndrome. All aspects of speech production, including phonation, resonation, articulation and respiration are affected in pseudobulbar palsy, but to varying degrees. Overall, pseudobulbar palsy is characterized by features such as bilateral facial paralysis, dysphagia, hypophonia, bilateral hemiparesis, incontinence and bradykinesia.

Hypoxic ischaemic encephalopathy is the most common cause of spastic dysarthria in childhood. In most cases this is associated with intrapartum asphyxia, although severe anoxic brain damage at any stage can cause the same disorder. Brainstem ischaemia with infarction resulting from embolization in association with congenital heart disease can also cause pseudobulbar palsy in children (as it can bulbar palsy). Spastic dysarthria may also be seen in children who have suffered head injuries with elevated intracranial pressure and a midbrain or upper brainstem shearing injury (as a result of a deceleration/acceleration type of injury). Although a common cause of pseudobulbar palsy in adolescents and young adults, disseminated sclerosis is not a common cause of spastic dysarthria in pre-pubertal children. Degenerative disorders, such as metachromatic leukodystrophy can also cause childhood pseudobulbar palsy.

Dysarthria associated with extrapyramidal syndromes

Diseases which selectively involve the extrapyramidal system without affecting the pyramidal pathways are referred to as extrapyramidal syndromes. Movement disorders are the primary features of extrapyramidal syndromes and, where the muscles of the speech mechanism are involved, disorders of speech may occur. The major pathological changes associated with extrapyramidal disorders are located in the basal ganglia and their related nuclei (e.g. the substantia nigra).

Extrapyramidal syndromes share a number of related symptoms which include: (1) hypokinesia (akinesia) — slowness and poverty of spontaneous movement, (2) hyperkinesia — abnormal involuntary movements, (3) rigidity of muscles, and (4) loss of normal postural reactions.

Hypokinetic dysarthria

The term 'hypokinetic dysarthria' was first used by Darley *et al.* (1969a,b) to describe the resultant complex pattern of perceptual speech characteristics associated with Parkinson's disease. Parkinsonism occurs most commonly in persons in their 50s and 60s. However, a syndrome which, like idiopathic Parkinson's disease in adults, is associated with either a reduced level of dopamine in the substantia nigra or blockage of the dopamine receptors in the basal ganglia, also occurs in childhood. This syndrome is referred to as hypokinetic dyskinesia. In addition, a number of other conditions also predispose to the occurrence of Parkinson's disease in childhood. Drug-induced parkinsonism, for instance, can occur at all ages and subacute meningitis, such as that seen in association with measles may also present with a parkinsonian-like picture. Further, in past years, postencephalitic parkinsonism secondary to epidemic encephalitis was common in children.

The clinical picture in Parkinson's disease consists of four major groups of symptoms: tremor, rigidity of the muscles, akinesia, and loss of normal postural fixing reflexes. According to Darley *et al.* (1975) features of the speech disorder seen in adult Parkinson's patients include: difficulty in initiating speech, once speech is started the speech becomes faster (festinant speech), reduced loudness, variable speech rate between subjects, some patients speaking at a slower than normal rate and others speaking at a slightly faster than normal rate, and disturbed prosody (e.g. monopitch, reduced stress, monoloudness).

Hyperkinetic dysarthria

A variety of extrapyramidal disorders may cause hyperkinetic dysarthria. Each of these disorders is characterized by the presence of abnormal involuntary muscle contractions of the limbs, trunk, neck, face etc. which disturb the rhythm and rate of normal, motor activities, including those involved in speech production. The major extrapyramidal disorders that cause hyperkinetic dysarthria include myoclonic jerks, tics, chorea, athetosis, dyskinesia and dystonia.

According to the nature of the abnormal involuntary movements, hyperkinetic disorders are divided into quick hyperkinesias (e.g. myoclonic jerks, tics and chorea) and slow hyperkinesias (e.g. athetosis, dyskinesia and dystonia). In quick hyperkinesias, the abnormal involuntary movements are rapid and either unsustained or sustained only very briefly and occur at random in terms of the body part affected. In contrast, the abnormal involuntary movements seen in slow hyperkinesias build up to a peak slowly and are sustained for at least one second or longer. Muscle tone waxes and wanes producing a variety of distorted postures.

Myoclonic jerks. These are abrupt, sudden, unsustained muscle contractions that occur irregularly. The muscles of the limbs as well as those of the speech mechanism can be affected. The muscles of the face, soft palate, larynx, diaphragm etc. may be either involved individually or in combination (e.g. palatopharyngolaryngeal myoclonus). Myoclonic jerks may be seen in children in association with diffuse metabolic, infectious or toxic disorders of the CNS such as diffuse encephalitis and toxic encephalopathies. In addition they are also associated with convulsive disorders (epilepsy).

Tics. Tics are recurrent, but brief, unsustained compulsive movements that involve a relatively small part of the body. One distinctive childhood disease characterized by the progressive development of tics involving the face, neck, upper limbs and eventually the entire body is Gilles de la Tourette's syndrome. In this condition, which usually has an onset between 2 and 15 years of age, uncontrolled vocalizations (e.g. grunting, coughing, barking, hissing and snorting) occur often as a result of involuntary contractions of the muscles of the speech mechanism. In addition stuttering-like repetitions, unintelligible sounds and echolalia are also present in some cases. The cause of the condition is unknown, although it has been suggested that the pathophysiological basis of the disease is increased dopamine activity.

Chorea. Slower than myoclonic jerks, choreic contractions involve a single, unsustained, isolated muscle action that produces a short, rapid, uncoordinated jerk of part of the body, such as the trunk, limb, face, tongue etc. These contractions are random in their distribution and their timing is irregular and unpredictable. When superimposed on the normal movements of the speech mechanism during speech production, choreiform movements can cause momentary disturbances to the course of contextual speech. In fact, all aspects of speech can be disrupted in patients with chorea and the hyperkinetic dysarthria of chorea is characterized by a highly variable pattern of interference with articulation, phonation, resonation and respiration.

There are two major diseases in which choreic movements are present: Sydenham's chorea and Huntington's chorea. The onset of Sydenham's chorea usually occurs between 5 and 10 years of age, females being affected more than males. In many instances, Sydenham's chorea appears to be associated with either streptococcal infections (strep-throat) or rheumatic heart disease. Huntington's chorea is an inherited disorder which, although it can manifest in childhood, usually has its onset in adult life.

Athetosis. Athetoid movements are characterized by a continuous, arrhythmic, slow, writhing-type of muscle movement. These movements are always the same in the same patient and cease only during sleep. Although athetoid movements primarily involve the limbs, the muscles of the speech mechanism, including the muscles of the face, tongue etc. may also be affected, causing facial grimacing, protrusion and writhing of the tongue and difficulty in speaking and swallowing. Athetoid movements disrupt these functions by interfering with the normal contraction of the muscles involved. In most cases athetosis forms part of a complex of neurological signs, including those of cerebral palsy, that result from disordered development of the brain, birth injury or other aetiological factors. The condition is usually associated with pathological changes in the corpus striatum and cerebral cortex.

Dyskinesia (lingual-facial-buccal dyskinesia). Miller and Keane (1978) defined dyskinesia as 'impairment of the power of voluntary movements'. Although, according to this definition, all involuntary movements could be described as dyskinetic, only two dyskinetic disorders are described under this heading: tardive dyskinesia and levodopa-induced dyskinesia. Tardive dyskinesia is a well recognized side-effect of long-term neuroleptic treatment (treatment with a pharmacological agent having an anti-psychotic action), while levodopa-induced dyskinesia results from the use of Levadopa in the treatment of Parkinson's disease. In that the muscles of the tongue, face and oral cavity are often most affected, these two disorders are also termed lingual-facial-buccal dyskinesias. In both conditions, the basic pattern of abnormal involuntary movement is one of repetitive, slow writhing, twisting, flexing and extending movements, often with a mixture of tremor.

Dystonia. Dystonia tends to involve large parts of the body. The abnormal involuntary movements are slow and sustained for prolonged periods of time and may produce grotesque posturing and bizarre writhing movements. Although these involuntary movements mostly involve the trunk, neck and proximal parts of the limbs, the muscles of the speech mechanism can also be affected. A variety of conditions lead to dystonia, including encephalitis, head trauma, vascular diseases and drug toxicity (especially the more potent tranquillizers).

Ataxic dysarthria

Ataxic dysarthria is a motor speech disorder associated with damage to the cerebellum or its connections, in which a breakdown in the articulatory and prosodic aspects of speech are the predominant features. Although the cerebellum itself does not initiate any muscle contractions it acts to coordinate muscle actions initiated by other parts of the brain (e.g. the motor cortex and basal ganglia) so that those movements are performed smoothly and accurately.

Damage to the cerebellum or its connections leads to a condition called ataxia in which movements performed by skeletal muscles become uncoordinated. If the muscles of the speech mechanism are involved, speech production may become abnormal leading to a cluster of deviant speech dimensions collectively called ataxic dysarthria. Clinically the signs of damage to the cerebellum include ataxia, dysmetria, decomposition of movement, dysdiadochokinesia, hypotonia, asthenia, tremor, rebound phenomena, disturbance of posture and gait, nystagmus and dysarthria.

As indicated above, breakdown in the articulatory and prosodic aspects of speech are the predominant features of ataxic dysarthria. The imprecise articulation results in improper formation and separation of individual syllables leading to a reduction in intelligibility, while the disturbance in prosody is associated with loss of texture, tone, stress and rhythm of individual syllables. The dysprosody results in slow, monotonous and improperly measured speech, often termed 'scanning speech'.

There are a number of different causes of acquired ataxia in childhood, including: posterior fossa tumours (e.g. medulloblastomas, cerebellar astrocytomas etc; see Ch. 8), traumatic head injury, infections (cerebellar abscess), degenerative disorders (e.g. metachromatic leukodystrophy), and toxic, metabolic and endocrine disorders (e.g. heavy metal poisoning etc.).

Mixed dysarthria

Some disorders of the nervous system affect more than one level of the neuromuscular system. Consequently, in addition to the more 'pure' forms of dysarthria outlined above, clinicians may also be confronted by patients who exhibit 'mixed dysarthrias'. These may be caused by a variety of conditions including cerebrovascular accidents, head trauma, brain tumours, inflammatory diseases and degenerative conditions. A mixed ataxic-hypokinetic-spastic dysarthria may be seen in children with Wilson's disease (see Ch. 6).

Clinical Characteristics of Acquired Childhood Dysarthria

Considering that dysarthria following mutism has been noted in children with acquired aphasia, from its earliest reports (Bernhardt, 1885; Freud, 1897) it is surprising that no further detail on the characteristics of this dysarthria has been available until this decade. Generally only the presence of dysarthria has been noted in case descriptions or in group studies without details regarding the nature of the dysarthria being provided.

Alajouanine and Lhermitte (1965) reported that dysarthria occurs frequently following the initial period of mutism in children with acquired brain lesions. Twenty-two of their 32 patients presented with dysarthria in the acute stages, at which time these authors also noted a close correlation between the presence of hemiplegia and the occurrence of dysarthria. Twenty of their 22 dysarthric patients also presented with a severe hemiplegia. In their discussion of dysarthria, Alajouanine and Lhermitte (1965) noted that both paralytic and dystonic forms existed but the paralytic form was 'most important' in the acute stage. Unfortunately, Alajouanine and Lhermitte (1965: 655) in their description of dysarthria referred to the disorders of articulation as 'always compris(ing) a phonetic disintegration'. Yet later in their paper they gave two separate incidence figures, one for articulation disorders (13 of 23 subjects) and one for phonetic disintegration (10 of 23 subjects) when discussing the incidence of symptoms in their cases over 10 years of age. All subjects (i.e. 9) under 10 years of age had disorders of articulation and phonetic disintegration. Alajouanine and Lhermitte (1965) never clarified the relationship between dysarthria, disorders of articulation and phonetic disintegration. After 6 months, however, only 11 of 22 subjects had an articulation disorder while seven children still had phonetic disintegration, which the authors claimed improved rapidly. Twelve months post-onset no mention was made of any subject still presenting with dysarthria.

The relationship between articulation disorders and dysarthria in children with acquired aphasia is also unclear in the article by Hécaen (1983), as he refers to articulation disorders in the tables and dysarthria in the text. Therefore we must assume that the two terms are synonymous. While Hécaen (1983) supported the findings of Alajouanine and Lhermitte (1965) that more children less than 10 years of age (i.e. 64 per cent) present with dysarthria than children over 10 years of age (i.e. 45 per cent), his findings were not statistically significant. Nor was there a significant difference in the incidence of dysarthria depending on the cause. Hécaen (1983) also did not find as high an incidence of dysarthria in children with acquired aphasia who had left hemisphere lesions (i.e. 52 per cent) as had been found by Alajouanine and Lhermitte (1965). Hécaen's most significant finding was a higher incidence of dysarthria following a fronto-Rolandic lesion (81 per cent) than following a temporal lesion (20 per cent).

Several case studies documenting both the site of lesion as determined by computed tomographic (CT) scan and the presence of dysarthria have been reported. Cranberg *et al.* (1987) noted a mild dysarthria in a child 7 months after head injury which resulted in a haemorrhage in the left basal ganglia extending minimally into the left temporal lobe. Another haemorrhage was evident in the posterior right thalamus. Mild dysarthria was also noted by Aram *et al.* (1989) in a child 5 years after a left middle cerebral artery occlusion. Magnetic resonance imaging (MRI) revealed a left subcortical lesion involving the head of the caudate, the anterior and posterior limbs of the internal capsule and the globus pallidus. Another case reported by Aram *et al.* (1983) with a subcortical lesion, this time involving the posterior aspect of the globus pallidus, the posteromedial aspect of the putamen, a portion of the posterior limb of the internal capsule and the body of the caudate, presented with a very mild dysarthria in the acute stage. The dysarthric symptoms included occasional cluster reduction and consonant omissions in multisyllabic words. One year post-onset no dysarthria was noted.

Dysarthria has also been noted in children following surgical removal of cerebellar tumours. Rekate *et al.* (1985) reported six cases who initially presented with muteness lasting from 3 weeks to 3 months. All six cases on resolution of the mutism presented with cerebellar (ataxic) dysarthria. The prognosis of the dysarthria varied. One case still presented with mild cerebellar dysarthria $2\frac{1}{2}$ years after surgery while another had regained normal speech within 6 months of surgery. Muteness resolving into a dysarthria characterized by a monotonous tone was also reported in one case by Volcan *et al.* (1986).

Mutism appeared to be a key factor in the development of ataxic dysarthria following surgery to remove a posterior fossa tumour in the cases described by Hudson *et al.* (1989). Based on their observation that the only two cases to present with ataxic dysarthria were also the only two subjects in their group who experienced a period of mutism after surgery, Hudson *et al.*, (1989) tentatively postulated a relationship between the occurrence of a period of mutism after surgery and the development of an ataxic dysarthria. One of the two cases presented with six of the ten features of ataxic dysarthria described by Darley *et al.* (1969a,b). These included imprecise consonants, excess and equal stress, harsh voice, prolonged phonemes, prolonged intervals and slow rate. Pitch breaks, variable pitch, a lack of volume control and explosive onsets were also evident as were slow oral movements which lacked control. The profile obtained on the Frenchay Dysarthria Assessment (Enderby, 1983) was consistent with the pattern characteristic of ataxic dysarthria given in the manual. The other case, who had received surgery at 2 years 7 months of age, presented with language and probably cognitive problems in addition to his dysarthria when tested at 8 years 8 months of age. Following surgery this latter case had a persistent left facial palsy. His profile on the Frenchay Dysarthria Assessment therefore indicated a mixed ataxic-flaccid dysarthria. Incoordination was apparent in the lip and tongue movements together with lack of laryngeal control. The presence of a left facial palsy resulted in lip and jaw asymmetry at rest and restricted the range of lip and jaw and tongue movements on the left side. Tongue movements were also restricted. A phonological analysis showed a number of inconsistent phoneme productions and the retention of the phonological processes of cluster reduction, syllable reduction, stopping, backing to velars, as well as progressive and regressive assimilation. Five of the ten ataxic dysarthric characteristics (Darley *et al.*, 1969a,b) were present including imprecise consonants, excess and equal stress, irregular articulatory breakdowns, prolonged phonemes and slow rate. A lack of volume control was also noted. Overall this case presented as largely unintelligible.

The features of dysarthria described by Darley *et al.* (1969a,b) have also been used by Bak and co-workers in two papers describing acquired dysarthria in children. Bak *et al.* (1983) reported the course of acquired dysarthria seen in a 6-year-old boy and related it to the recovery of his tongue and mouth movements. Initial CT scans in this case were normal but at a later stage a small infarct in the left thalamus was noted. In the acute stage the child presented as anarthric. Twelve days after admission the patient was difficult to understand. His speech contained 14 of the characteristics of dysarthric speech described by Darley *et al.* (1969a,b). Eight of these features were prominent.

These included imprecise consonants, distorted vowels, hypernasality, continuous and transient breathy voice, harsh pitch and monoloudness and monopitch. Three weeks after admission the breathiness had become less consistent but he interrupted polysyllabic words by breathing and swallowing. Rate of speech was slow. Five weeks post-onset considerable improvement had been noted in the hypernasality, breathiness and distorted vowels and consonants. On discharge the only abnormality was imprecise consonants. The authors concluded that there had been a remarkable improvement in the four main dysarthric features seen in this child but that no single feature contributed to the impairment of intelligibility. From documenting the recovery of mouth and tongue movements Bak *et al.* (1983) concluded that there is a relationship between the recovery of dysarthria and the recovery of movements of oral structures. For example, recovery of normal function of the vocal cords coincided with a decrease in breathiness after the third week while hypernasality was still noted when the gag reflex was still absent and the uvula still hanging.

While a relationship was evident between neurological signs and dysarthria in their second study (Van Dongen *et al.*, 1987), for some patients recovery from dysarthria preceded neurological recovery. In some cases patients with moderate neurological deficits recovered from anarthria with minimal change in their neurological status. In this latter article Van Dongen *et al.* (1987) presented the dysarthric features of four children with bilateral supranuclear facial palsy and four children with bilateral peripheral facial palsy. The children with peripheral lesions generally presented with a milder form of dysarthria. This is in contrast to adults presenting with similar lesions. The characteristics of the dysarthria seen in the children included weakened vowels and/or consonants and hypernasality. One of these cases (a dyspneic) with severe pharyngeal weakness also exhibited frequent inhalation, harsh voice and mild stress reduction. In contrast the children with the central lesion initially presented as anarthric. As this resolved the dysarthric characteristics included breathiness, reduced stress, weakened/dropped vowels and consonants, hypernasality and many pauses. Four patients recovered within 3 weeks while recovery in the other four took more than 6 weeks. The recovery period, however, was not related to the site of the lesion.

As with acquired childhood aphasia, it would appear that the recovery of dysarthria is greater in children than seen in adults. Preliminary evidence also suggests that the severity of the dysarthria may not be as great in children as seen in some similar lesions in adults. While the use of dysarthria types used with adult cases, such as those described by Darley *et al.* (1969a,b) may be debatable, it is clear that the features used to describe dysarthria in adults are appropriate to use with children if as Alajouanine and Lhermitte (1965: 655) suggest 'the phonetic development of the child at the onset is taken into account'.

Acquired Dyspraxia

Acquired verbal dyspraxia (dyspraxia of speech, articulatory dyspraxia) is a motor speech programming disorder characterized primarily by errors in articulation and secondarily by alterations in prosody. Although most of what we know about this disorder comes from studies on adult subjects, it has been speculated that acquired verbal dyspraxia can also occur in children with brain injuries. Unfortunately only scant information regarding the nature and occurrence of this disorder in childhood is available in the literature, with the presence of verbal dyspraxia occasionally being noted by authors as one of the speech/language disorders to occur amongst others following brain injury, but with few details being provided. As in adults, it appears that acquired verbal dyspraxia usually occurs in combination with an acquired aphasia and/or dysarthria. One possible reason for the lack of attention paid to acquired verbal dyspraxia in the literature is that the condition appears to resolve quickly.

This is true whether the dyspraxia is oral or verbal in nature. The only two articles which make reference to acquired dyspraxia in children either document its recovery or note its presence in the early stages post-onset. Aram *et al.* (1983) described the oral apraxia seen in a 7-year-old right-handed girl with acquired capsular/striatal aphasia. On day four after onset the child was totally mute and unable to produce non-speech oral movements on command but could produce them on imitation. Two days later these non-speech movements were initiated on command as was phonation. Within another two days a full range of tongue movements was possible and vowel sounds could be imitated. At this time two word phrases were spontaneously produced. Some weakness of the right facial muscles was present but no dysarthria was noticeable. No further mention of speech disturbances was made, although aphasic symptoms were still present.

Three out of the 15 cases of children with acquired aphasia described by Cooper and Flowers (1987) presented with dyspraxia one month after onset. One case was head-injured while two of the three cases had suffered haematomas. All 3 cases were communicating orally at the time the dyspraxia was noted. Therefore a verbal dyspraxia can be assumed. No information on the dyspraxia symptoms or their recovery was given. Therefore in the absence of detailed descriptions of dyspraxic symptoms in children one must again turn to the adult literature.

Features of dyspraxia of speech seen in adults include:

1   Visible and audible groping to achieve correct individual articulatory postures and sequence of postures to produce sounds and words.
2   Highly variable articulatory errors (e.g. /v/ may at different times be produced /v/, /z/, /p/, /f/, /r/, /b/, /h/ and /w/.
3   Based on perceptual analysis with the naked ear, articulatory errors appear to involve substitutions rather than distortions of individual phonemes as occurs in dysarthria.

4   A greater number of articulatory errors occur during repetition than during conversational speech.
5   The number of articulatory errors increases as the complexity of the articulatory exercise increases — few errors are made on single consonants while more errors occur on consonant clusters.
6   In addition to articulatory disturbances, as these patients speak, they slow down their rate of speech, space their words and syllables more evenly and stress them more equally.
7   Speech output is non-fluent because of pausing and hesitating while the individual gropes for articulatory placement and makes repeated efforts to produce words correctly.

A detailed case description of a child with acquired verbal dyspraxia is presented later in this chapter, illustrating the presence of a number of these features.

Assessment and Treatment of Motor Speech Disorders

The assessment and treatment techniques of acquired dysarthria and dyspraxia in children discussed in this chapter draw on knowledge gleaned from several sources: the literature describing adult motor speech disorders, cerebral palsy, the development of normal phonology and the distinctive features of phonemes. Assessment procedures are similar for dysarthria and dyspraxia and these two disorders, together with aphasia, often coexist. Particularly in the early stages post-onset, differential diagnosis may be difficult.

The concomitant problems associated with acquired aphasia may also be present in the child with acquired dysarthria and/or dyspraxia. These have been discussed in Chapter 2. Additional problems may include feeding difficulties and these may occur with both dysarthria and dyspraxia. However, the incidence of feeding problems and the persistence of these difficulties has not been documented. It would seem that in many children these problems resolve in the first few weeks of therapy. However, it appears that children with severe dysarthria and an associated quadriplegia may present with long-term feeding difficulties. It is not the purpose of this text to discuss the assessment and treatment of feeding difficulties. This area has been addressed by Ylvisaker and Logemann (1985) and Logemann (1983). The knowledge of the acquisition of oral feeding skills reported by Morris (1982) will also help the clinician in assessing and treating difficulties in this area.

Phonological delays and articulation problems unrelated to a neurological cause may also be present (e.g. those articulation problems associated with oral structural abnormalities). Differential diagnosis of acquired motor speech problems, articulation difficulties and phonological delays is important if appropriate treatment goals are to be formulated.

Assessment of Acquired Motor Speech Disorders in Children

The assessment of acquired motor speech disorders should involve the gathering of relevant information, the observation of the child's abilities in a variety of settings and the systematic testing, combined with an objective evaluation scale, of the speech mechanism during non-speech and speech activities with attention being paid to the involuntary and voluntary control of the speech mechanism. The information should include a description of the child's phonological system before the lesion and a neurological report on the site of the brain lesion and the nature of the neurological impairment.

Several assessment tools designed for the adult client (e.g. Frenchay Dysarthria Assessment (Enderby, 1983), Working with Dysarthrics (Robertson and Thomson, 1986), and the Apraxia Battery for Adults (Dabul, 1979) may be used successfully with children although some modification may be necessary. These modifications may include the simplification of instructions, the use of play situations when asking the child to sustain a sound (e.g. 'Let's see how long you can sound the siren on your fire engine.') or the substitution of a child-oriented articulation test and a selection of multisyllabic words of increasing complexity all of which would be in the child's receptive vocabulary. The Nuffield Centre Dyspraxia Programme (The Nuffield Hearing and Speech Centre, 1985) designed primarily for the child with developmental dyspraxia is also a useful assessment and treatment tool with children with acquired motor speech disorders.

The tools mentioned above represent a systematic approach to the assessment of the child's speech mechanism but no assessment would be complete without an analysis of the child's functional speech and non-speech activities. Judgments need to be made on how well the child is understood at home, in school, with peers and in the community. If the child's message breaks down, why does it fail? An analysis of a speech sample should follow a similar systematic approach to that detailed in the assessment profiles (e.g. Respiration: How does the child's respiratory cycle affect his speech? Is his/her breath control poor? Prosody: Does the child phrase incorrectly so that the meaning of the utterance is lost? Is his/her rate of speech too slow?). Included in these observational sessions would also be a judgement of the child's eating skills.

As mentioned previously the classification system for the dysarthrias — flaccid, spastic, ataxic, hypokinetic, hyperkinetic and mixed — proposed by Darley *et al.* (1975) for adults with acquired dysarthria, would seem appropriate for use with children as long as the clinican takes into consideration the child's phonological development. Darley *et al.* (1975) suggested five parameters requiring assessment when diagnosing motor speech disorders.

Respiration: the volume and control of the exhaled air
Phonation: the quality, harshness, duration, pitch, steadiness and loudness of the voice

Resonance: the hypernasality or hyponasality of voice. The testing for nasal emission of the airstream during speech

Articulation: the precision of isolated sounds, sound combinations, single words and phrases

Prosody: the rate, intonation, stress and other suprasegmental features of oral communication and overall intelligibility

Robertson and Thomson (1986), basing their assessment profile on Darley and co-workers' parameters, divided their assessment tool into eight areas including the five mentioned above and the following:

Facial Musculature: the function of jaws, lips, tongue and palate during speech

Diadochokinesis: the rate and precision of repetitive movement using speech sounds and oral movements

Reflexes· the presence of drooling during eating or speech, the cough reflex, chewing and swallowing of liquids and solids

Intelligibility: the overall integration and coordination of all motor speech processes.

The most important pragmatic skills to assess in a child with a motor speech disorder are the paralinguistic features and the non-verbal behaviours that the child uses in a communicative act. Is the child able to convey his/her attitudes or emotions by changes in intonation, pitch, stress or emphasis? Can he/she alter the meaning of an utterance by using suprasegmental devices to signal the change rather than by altering the form? Are the child's facial expressions appropriate to the situations or is his/her face 'masklike' so that the listener is unable to read the non-verbal cues? Is pause time too great leaving the dialogue partner wondering whether the listener is ignoring them, does not know the answer or is thinking? With some children, even though the formal assessment reveals near-normal motor speech skills, effective communication is hampered by their problems with some paralinguistic and non-verbal behaviours.

For example, Carol, a 12-year-old girl, who had been injured in a motor vehicle accident, was shown to have made a good recovery when a dysarthric assessment was administered 12 months after the injury. However, pragmatic problems were evident in conversation. Her volume was soft, articulation imprecise, although she had demonstrated good intelligibility with single words and sentences in the formal testing situation, and her face lacked mobility so that it was hard to tell what she might be thinking. Inclusion in a pragmatics group with her peers, which addressed these specific problems in functional situations, helped modify her behaviour.

Within applicable parameters the salient features of neuromuscular function in the articulators should be assessed at rest, during involuntary movement and during voluntary movement.

These are:

the strength of muscular contraction
the speed of movement
the accuracy of movement
the range of excursion of the muscle
the steadiness of the contraction
the tone of the muscle

However, the clinician must not automatically assume that any abnormality observed during the assessment procedure is directly attributed to dysarthria or dyspraxia (e.g. a harsh or husky voice may be the result of endotracheal intubation). Some symptoms may need further investigation.

The assessment for dyspraxia may follow similar parameters to dysarthria but particular attention is paid to the following:

any observable difference between involuntary and voluntary movement
the ability of the child to sequence sounds (e.g./p/,/t/, and /p/, /t/, /k/)
his/her ability to repeat the sequence of sounds several times
his/her ability to repeat minimal pairs using manner and place contrasts (e.g. bow, toe and pea, bee)
his/her ability to articulate words of increasing complexity (e.g. butter, topcoat, crocodile, kangaroo)

Dyspraxia may be present when:

involuntary movement of the articulators appears superior to volitional movement
inconsistent errors are demonstrated during repetitive oral movements and speech production of phonemes, words and phrases
deterioration in performance is observed as the word length increases
automatic speech is more intelligible than propositional speech
searching behaviours, similar to those observed in adults with acquired dyspraxia, are present in the child's speech
the child's facial expression seems to suggest that he/she is puzzled about how to use his/her muscles of articulation to make the required sound
some alteration in prosody is observed (e.g. rate of speech)

Inconsistent errors are frequently heard in children who are still developing their phonological system so differential diagnosis between normal phonological processes (e.g. assimilation, final consonant deletion etc.) and the inconsistent errors (e.g. phonemic anticipatory errors, transpositions, voicing errors, omissions) heard in the speech of a dyspraxic child is important when assessing children with acquired motor speech disorders. A knowledge of the child's speech development before his/her brain lesion is necessary to make this clinical judgement.

Treatment of Acquired Motor Speech Disorders in Children

Basic principles of therapy

Darley *et al.* (1975) proposed five basic principles of therapy for motor speech disorders in adults with acquired problems: compensation, purposeful activity, monitoring, an early start and motivation. These basic principles also apply to children.

1 Compensation — the ability of the individual to maximize their remaining potential. Children have a great capacity to compensate perhaps because speech patterns, particularly in children who are still acquiring phonemes, are not as well established as those in adults. Effective compensation may rely on adequate monitoring skills and this skill may be difficult to establish in some children.

2 Purposeful activity — the child must become aware of how their articulators work and what is important in the communicative act to make it intelligible to the listener. They must not only think of what they wish to say but how they are going to say it.

3 An early start — the earlier the child becomes aware of the 'how' of communication the better before poor habits hinder rehabilitation efforts. There is also a greater chance that the monitoring skills necessary to maintain intelligibility become ingrained and are automatically applied in communicative situations.

4 Monitoring — the ability of the individual to constantly check that his/her communication is intelligible. Children may find this skill difficult to learn, particularly paralinguistic features which change constantly depending on the length and intent of the utterance. This skill may be taught as a strategy. If the listener does not understand, then the child remembers, when repeating, to take a deep breath, not to say too many words on the one breath and to clearly pronounce clusters and final consonants. When they are older perhaps another burst of therapy may be in order to reinforce these principles.

5 Motivation — the desire of the child to embrace the above principles. Children need to understand the importance of the techniques they are learning and wish to put them into practice if therapy is to succeed. A pragmatic approach, where the child can learn the consequences of both poor and intelligible communication, may reinforce the child's desire to communicate effectively. Many children make an excellent recovery with only mild difficulties with their muscles of articulation, yet subtle problems

remain causing their speech to sound imprecise and monotonous. If the child does not have the motivation (see case study on Gary following) to monitor his/her speech, then intelligibility may remain a problem in many situations.

Treatment in the early stage

In the early stage of recovery in dysarthria and dyspraxia, treatment may be focused on feeding difficulties and graded oral and facial stimulation. It is only when the child is aware and ready to take an active interest in learning that specific therapy on communication skills can start.

The literature describing recovery from dysarthria and that documenting recovery from dyspraxia frequently mention an initial period of mutism. During this time and until a child's speech becomes functional it is essential that the child has some form of communication. A reliable signal for 'yes' and 'no' is one of the early treatment goals. Some children may initiate their own communication by using gesture or pantomime and this needs to be encouraged by all persons caring for them.

> For example, Barry, 14 years of age, had sustained a severe head injury and was quadriplegic and anarthric. In the early stage of his recovery he had very little movement and only differentiated vocalization. He introduced his own 'yes' and 'no' communication. For 'yes' he cocked the index finger of his left hand and for 'no' he blinked twice.

A simple picture board, Blissymbols (Hehner, 1979, 1984) or Compic (Anderson *et al.*, 1986) communication board may be the most appropriate form of augmentative communication to introduce, particularly as many children have physical disabilities which would hamper their use of a signing system. However, the system chosen depends on the child's cognitive, receptive language, perceptual and motor abilities and their desire to interact with others.

The introduction of an augmentative communication system may facilitiate the return of verbal communication. However, some children are unable to phonate either because they have a severe motor involvement or because they have an apraxia of phonation. This condition may resolve spontaneously or may require specific treatment. Many of these children vocalize spontaneously in play situations, during other therapy sessions or in emotional situations such as laughing when watching television. All of the team members involved with the care of the child need to bring these vocalizations to their attention when they occur. The speech and language clinician may find it beneficial to share some treatment sessions with other team members and therefore to be on hand to shape these vocalizations. The literature documenting the treatment of voice problems, particularly the techniques for facilitating voice in vocal cord paralysis (Boone, 1971; Greene, 1957) has suggestions which may be adapted and used with these children.

Children with a severe involvement and poor prognosis for recovery may require a more sophisticated communication device such as a voice output device or a computer-based system with environmental control options. There is a considerable body of knowledge on augmentative communication systems regarding how to choose the appropriate one for the client and how to facilitate the client's use of his/her communication device (De Ruyter and La Fontaine, 1987; Dowden *et al.*, 1986; Odor *et al.*, 1986; Behrmann, 1984; Scheifelbusch, 1980; Vanderheiden and Grilley, 1977).

Treatment of Acquired Dysarthria

Articulation

Treatment of acquired dysarthria in children must be functional and pragmatically appropriate. Many of the treatment goals may be achieved through direct work on the child's articulation. Compensation techniques may be necessary if tongue or lip movements remain restricted (the blade of the tongue may be used instead of the tongue tip for sounds such as /l/, /n/, /t/, or /d/). A knowledge of the distinctive features of phonemes is an advantage when alternative tongue or lip movements are required. If sounds are correctly produced then hypernasality and/or hyponasality may be effectively reduced and nasal emission eliminated without introducing any exercises specifically designed for work on resonance. If, as articulation improves, there is little reduction in hypernasality then the child's velopharyngeal competence must be questioned and an appropriate referral initiated. Correct vocal attack may also be incorporated into articulation work. When formulating articulation goals consideration must be given to the developmental acquisition of sounds. However, it is usually best to choose a sound that the child is able to imitate and which will make the greatest difference to his/her intelligibility (e.g. the /s/ sound or in some instances /s/ clusters).

Drooling

Drooling also seems to improve as articulation improves. However, gentle reminders to swallow during treatment sessions are often all that is needed to stop drooling. If not, then a behaviour management programme may need to be implemented. A baseline may be taken over a few sessions and then goals for the subsequent sessions formulated with cooperation from the child. The reward system may be tokens or stars which, when the child collects a certain number, enables him/her to buy something from the 'Therapy Shop' such as a balloon, colouring-in book or a fancy sticker. A promise to use the computer was a very successful reward with one young child seen in our clinic.

Wendy, a 4-year-old, had been kicked in the head by a horse. The resulting brain damage left her with a right-sided hemiparesis, dysarthria and verbal dyspraxia. Wendy drooled excessively and the front of her dress at the neck line was constantly wet and grubby. A programme using operant conditioning techniques was implemented with little success at first until the computer was used as a reward. She was told she could not play on the computer unless she stopped drooling because she would break the computer if the workings were wet. This reward was used in speech and language treatment times, in occupational therapy and at school. After being denied use of the computer a few times, she ceased drooling and this behaviour carried over to non-computer situations.

Prosody

Prosodic difficulties may be treated using language activities (e.g. the Fokes Sentence Builder (Fokes, 1976) designed to teach correct syntax, may be used to help children phrase appropriately and not try to say too may words on one breath if their respiratory control is poor). The teaching method that Fokes uses is concrete, i.e. a number of boxes representing 'who', 'is doing', 'what', 'where' and 'which' and a sentence is generated using the boxes, 'The boy/is stopping/the big bus/on the road'. This approach seems to help children, particularly the younger ones, to understand the concept of correct phrasing. Older children may be helped through oral reading with the clinician at first marking acceptable phrasing. The child is encouraged to take a breath at the end of a phrase group. Often the use of carrier phrases in games may facilitate correct articulation and phrasing (e.g. When playing 'Fish', the child may be encouraged to ask, 'May I have the car, please?', or 'Can I have the picture that goes with the lock?'). The extension of the exercises into conversational speech is necessary and a tape recording of the child's speech may help the child make objective judgements about his/her communication and assist him/her to change. Some older children have enjoyed reading and/or acting simple plays. Tasks involving volume, stress, emphasis and intonation may be incorporated naturally into the activity. Younger children enjoy improvizations (see Creative Dramatics in Ch. 2) and similar goals may be formulated for them.

Pragmatics

Inclusion in a group where the emphasis is on pragmatic skills may be beneficial, particularly if video recording is available. Role playing activities which allow the child to practice the skills learned in individual sessions may be designed and these activities recorded and rated by his/her peers. The activities may involve daily living skill tasks (e.g. buying something at a shop, asking directions or giving information to someone) and the individual must remember appropriate volume, pitch, emphasis and articulation. Non-verbal behaviours such as eye contact, physical proximity, body posture, gestures and facial expression may also be discussed and modified if necessary.

Some children who lack a variety of facial expressions may need to be encouraged to use head nodding or vocal fillers such as 'um' to let the speaker know they are actively listening. The speech and language clinician and the occupational therapist may plan a joint outing to a community facility (e.g. shopping centre or restaurant) where the individuals may put into practice therapy goals. This activity has proved beneficial and enjoyable with all ages but has had excellent results with adolescents who suddenly realize how important it is to achieve treatment goals if they are to become independent and accepted by the community.

It is only in severe cases of dysarthria which do not respond to the above procedures that gross motor exercises to strengthen muscles and Proprioceptive Neuromuscular Facilation (PNF) (Robertson and Thomson, 1986) may be employed. In most cases of children with acquired dysarthria, it would seem that the most appropriate way to work on gross movements is during feeding and swallowing therapy and that gross motor exercises be used only when all else has failed to achieve the desired results.

Treatment of acquired dyspraxia

There is little reported literature on the manifestation and recovery of acquired dyspraxia in children. It would seem that most often dyspraxia coexists with either acquired aphasia and/or acquired dysarthria. Acquired dyspraxia also seems to resolve either spontaneously or with intervention in the first year after the brain lesion.

Treatment techniques

Many of the treatment techniques which have been developed for the developmentally dyspraxic child may be useful in the child with acquired dyspraxia. However, the difficulties experienced by the child with the acquired disorder appear to resolve at a much greater pace than those of the developmentally dyspraxic child and this must be a consideration in therapy. Oral dyspraxia if present with verbal dyspraxia appears to resolve first and basic oral motor work is mostly unnecessary unless it serves as an introduction to verbal dyspraxic therapy or is combined with feeding therapy. Treatment goals for children with acquired dyspraxia may best be met by working on the child's articulation. Initially, visual and tactile cueing may be needed to help the child approximate the sound. The younger child benefits from some form of visual representation of the sound (e.g. the picture of a snail for 's' or if they are reading, the letter). Some children benefit from working in front of a mirror, in others this activity only seems to confuse them. These latter children have better success when watching the clinician make the sound after she/he has explained the placement of the articulators. Phonetic cueing as described by Vaughan and Clark (1979) and the cued articulation (Passy, 1985) method of helping individuals remember by using simple hand signs and how to pronounce and/or sequence the consonant sounds of English, may also serve as useful treatment procedures. However, the clinician's own knowledge of distinctive features of the phonemes will help him/her develop appropriate treatment techniques. There are also those children who require a 'hands on' approach (e.g. the clinician helps the child with lip closure for 'm') if they are to succeed in making the required sound.

Treatment of acquired dyspraxia may involve the following steps:

Imitation of single sounds starting with those that the child finds the easiest (vowels and consonants)

Repetition of these sounds (e.g. /m/, /m/, /m/)

Repetition of a sequence of sounds, first two and then three (e.g./m/, /b/, /m/, /b/ and /p/, /t/, /k/)

Combining of these sounds into consonant-vowel, vowel-consonant, consonant-vowel-consonant and consonant-vowel-consonant-vowel.

Using the words in pragmatically appropriate situations (e.g. asking for more of something)

Contrasting words by place, voice and manner (e.g. tar, car; poo, boo; taw, saw)

Disyllabic words (e.g. puppy, pudding)

Use of the child's expressive vocabulary in phrases and simple sentences (this work could be incorporated into language work if the child also has acquired aphasia)

Selection of polysyllabic words which the child may have found difficult in the treatment session, at home or in the classroom. Team members can be alerted to listen for difficult words and record them for the speech and language clinician who can help the child with them in a later session.

Many of these activities will be used simultaneously (e.g. imitation of the single sounds which may have proved difficult for the child and the combination of established sounds in monosyllabic and disyllabic words). If the child has prosodic or pragmatic difficulties then the activities outlined in the section on dysarthria may be used.

The suggestions for assessment and treatment of acquired motor speech disorders in children outlined above are not conclusive. More research into the area of these acquired disorders is necessary if the most appropriate assessment and treatment procedures are to be developed.

Summary

The reports in the literature have little to offer the clinician in either the diagnosis or treatment of acquired motor speech disorders in children. The available models for assessment and treatment of motor speech disorders have been developed for adults and until more research into acquired motor speech disorders in children is forthcoming, these models are all that is available to help the clinician with the assessment and treatment of the acquired disorders in childhood.

With acquired motor speech disorders in children ten parameters — respiration, phonation, resonance, articulation, prosody, facial musculature, diadochokinesis, reflexes, intelligibility and pragmatics — are assessed. In each applicable parameter the salient neuromuscular functions involved in motor speech disorders (strength, speed, range and accuracy of movement, steadiness of the contraction and tone) are analyzed at rest, with voluntary and with involuntary movement. Differences between dysarthria and dyspraxia are mainly seen in the parameters of articulation, facial musculature with voluntary and involuntary movement and diadochokinesis.

Treatment goals for acquired motor speech disorders in children should be, when possible, functional and pragmatically appropriate. These goals may best be met by direct work on articulation. If children have prosodic difficulties then inclusion in a group where pragmatic problems are addressed seems beneficial. Finally, further research into the manifestation and recovery of children with acquired motor speech disorders will assist the clinician with the assessment and treatment of these children.

Case Reports

Case 1 — Dysarthria

The patient, Gary, was a 13-year-old, right-handed male who sustained brain damage following cerebral anoxia caused by suffocation. On admission to hospital he was described as drowsy, though orientated and easily rousable. Spasms involving his lower limbs and hyperactive reflexes were noted. Some ankle clonus was also evident. Fundoscopy at this time was normal.

One month after the accident he was still aphemic, showed profuse myoclonus, marked bilateral hand tremor, a severe spastic gait and was emotionally labile. While in hospital he received intensive rehabilitation from all three therapies as well as psychiatric help for his extreme anxiety. He had one grand mal convulsion but was not on any anticonvulsant therapy. Agitation and worry about having a fit would occasionally cause him to hyperventilate. An EEG performed after the seizure was normal. He had been in the first year of high school when the accident occurred. The history of his academic skills and behaviour before the injury indicated that he was a slow learner and impulsive.

Neurological examination

A neurological examination carried out 5 weeks post-onset showed some mildly abnormal cranial nerve function, especially involving the facial nerves. Generalized increased muscle tone with brisk reflexes, especially in the lower limbs, was noted. There was a marked clonus of both ankles and the patient appeared to have added choreiform movements. Other general examination was normal.

Neuroradiological examination

A CT scan performed 5 weeks post-onset demonstrated the presence of a slightly dilated ventricular system and hypodense changes laterally in the territories of the lateral striate and medial striate arteries. The hypodense areas involved the lenticular nucleus and head of the caudate nucleus on each side and were consistent with cerebral anoxia. The lesions also possibly involved the anterior and posterior limbs of the internal capsule to some extent.

Speech and language recovery

During the 3 months following the accident Gary's speech abilities showed a considerable recovery. Initially he was mute but used a letter board to communicate. Receptive language appeared intact. Some feeding problems were also present. At 7 weeks post-onset he could vocalize in single words but these were difficult to understand mainly because of poor lip movement. A week later he was speaking in short sentences but the overall intelligibility of his speech remained poor. The Frenchay Dysarthria Test was administered and results indicated that his main difficulties were reduced strength, range, speech and accuracy of his lip and palate movements. Some difficulty was observed with alternate tongue movements. Generally, his communication was characterized by imprecise consonants, particularly bilabial sounds, a slow and laboured rate of speech which would increase in rate towards the end of the phrase and a prosodic impairment. No apraxic element was revealed. On discharge from the hospital to a Rehabilitation Community Agency, 3 months post-onset, his speech showed signs of hypokinetic dysarthria with some difficulty initiating speech movements.

Assessment

Concomitant Problems
Gary walked with a spastic gait and was fitted with boots and a calliper to his right leg. His dynamic balance was unreliable, particularly when moving. Increased tone and bilateral intention tremor in his upper limbs caused significant problems with writing so typing was introduced as a faster alternative for written communication at school.

Gary viewed himself as a failure because he was repeating Grade 8 and was self-conscious about his appearance and unhappy about wearing the calliper. At home he had frequent mood swings, bouts of depression and impulsive behaviour which his mother found difficult to control. He showed little insight into his own part in the constant fighting at home.

Language
While in hospital the Western Aphasia Battery (WAB) was administered and no aphasic element was revealed. Although his language results were within the normal range, reports from his teachers indicated some difficulties in acquiring new knowledge and definite academic concept and skills deficits. Gary's pragmatic language skills were poor. Using the Clinical Discourse Analysis (Damico, 1985) results indicated difficulties with revision behaviour, specific vocabulary, giving and asking for information and poor eye contact. As a conversational partner he was passive and did little to maintain the conversation. It is probable that his language deficits existed before his accident and that they were exacerbated by the injury.

Speech
Three months post-onset the Frenchay Dysarthria Test was readministered and spontaneous speech samples in different situations were taken. The test revealed mild problems with lips, palate and tongue

movements in speech. These results indicated a good prognosis. Although he could achieve variations in pitch and volume during the test procedure his voice remained monotone and quiet in conversation. Word and sentence stress and emphasis were even, with little variety, intonation patterns flat and breath groupings often inappropriate. His conversational speech was frequently unintelligible and sounded monotonous.

Therapy

Individual therapy sessions concentrated on phoneme production in words, phrases, sentences and paragraphs, with particular emphasis on final consonants. As the precision of his articulation improved, stress, emphasis, intonation patterns and breath groupings were explained and practised. Articulation and prosody practice were integrated. A computer proved a motivating therapy tool and software designed for reading, especially programs in a game format, were used. Gary would read the passages aloud initially trying to achieve clear articulation. When he had improved, correct word stress, breath groupings as well as variety of emphasis and intonation patterns were introduced. The passages were taped and then rated by Gary and the clinician. A chart was kept of his progress. He also attended a group with four other boys his own age who had similar pragmatic problems. The treatment goals formulated in his individual sessions were transferred to the group situation. The group played numerous card and board games, planned outings, discussed films and television programmes and role-played various situations. During the last 15 minutes of the session individual and group goals were discussed and decisions made as to whether these goals had been met. Gary made good progress. In both individual and group sessions his speech was intelligible with only mild prosodic problems. However, his motivation to monitor his own speech outside the structured environment of the treatment sessions and the on-site school was poor.

Conclusion

Eighteen months after the accident Gary was discharged to attend high school near his home. On discharge there were still mild problems with the strength, range and accuracy of lip and tongue movements but the intelligibility of his speech both in the testing situation and from informal observation in other therapies and school was good. He expressed concern at returning to a new High School. His self-image was still poor and although some counselling had been suggested it was rejected because of the distance he would need to travel to receive the help. He continued to be reviewed at the rehabilitation centre for a further 12 months until his family discontinued contact. The last time he was assessed the results on the Frenchay Dysarthria Test were similar to those on discharge but the intelligibility and prosody of this speech had deteriorated. He was unhappy at home and at school and his motivation to continue to monitor his speech was poor. When asked about his speech, he shrugged and said 'he got by'.

Summary — Case 1

Gary was a 13-year-old boy who suffered brain damage as a result of cerebral anoxia. Before the accident he was reported to be a slow learner and impulsive. Intention tremor was present in his upper limbs and his gait was spastic. Initially after the accident he was mute and used a letter board but no aphasia was apparent. Seven weeks after the accident he was saying single words but these were difficult to understand mainly because of poor lip movement. By 8 weeks he had progressed to short sentences but intelligibility remained poor. His speech was diagnosed as hypokinetic dysarthria. At 3 months after the accident a Frenchay Dysarthria Assessment revealed only mild problems in the articulators. However, Gary viewed himself as a failure and his motivation was poor. Prosodic problems persisted although he was able to modify these behaviours in treatment sessions but he lacked the desire to monitor himself outside the treatment room. Treatment goals were functional and gross motor work was carried out mainly at mealtimes. Individual therapy goals concentrated on articulation in words, phrases, sentences and spontaneous speech. Group goals involved work on paralinguistic features and pragmatic functions. Despite making a good neurological recovery, Gary's speech remained 'slurred' and monotonous, primarily because he lacked the desire to monitor his communication.

Case 2 — Dyspraxia

Nicola, at 6 years 3 months of age, suffered an embolic cerebrovascular accident of the left middle cerebral artery during the peri-operative period after the repair of anomalous pulmonary venous drainage. Before the neurological episode she had been developing normally and was in first grade at school.

Neurological history

Initially, Nicola presented with a dense right hemiparesis which was generally hypotonic in both upper and lower extremities. Her arm was more severely affected than her leg, her right hand having no functional grasp and release. There was no apparent primitive reflex activity or obvious motor planning problems. Her general awareness of her right hand and arm was poor. She was unable to walk without assistance and her protective reactions were sluggish. Her visual perceptual abilities were affected, particularly figure-ground, visual memory and visual sequential memory. She also had a severe oral and verbal dyspraxia with a suspected expressive dysphasic component.

Eight months after the insult, Nicola was walking with the aid of a below-knee calliper and was using her left hand for writing. Sensation was generally intact on the right side but she continued to neglect her right arm and had to be reminded to use it in bilateral activities. Visual perception was age appropriate. Some inattention to task and poor concentration was still noted in her behaviour.

Assessment

One week after the cerebrovascular accident, Nicola was informally assessed. She presented with a right upper motor neuron weakness with associated drooling from the right side of her mouth. Her lips drooped on the right but the range of movement when she puckered was only mildly reduced. Her range of tongue movement appeared adequate for eating and speech. When she was required to imitate oral movements, gross attempts and groping movements were noted. She was unable to repeat single sounds. Her spontaneous output consisted of an undifferentiated vowel and an attempt at 'no'. Informal assessment indicated adequate auditory comprehension skills; she responded appropriately to conversation and was able to follow 4-stage commands. An expressive dysphasia was suspected. Nicola used facial expression, gross gestures and vowel sounds for expressive communication. A Blissymbol communication board was introduced.

One month after the accident, Nicola's muscle weakness was resolving with only some occasional drooling. Informal testing revealed that the range and strength of lip movements were mildly reduced on the right side with a mild oral dyspraxia persisting. She had no eating or drinking difficulties. Nicola was able to imitate /b,m,p,n,d,t,s/ in consonant-vowel combinations. Her spontaneous verbalizations included consonant-vowel and consonant-vowel-consonant syllables as word approximations. She continued to use a Blissymbol communication board for expressive communication.

Two months after onset, Nicola presented with moderate verbal dyspraxia. An informal assessment using elicited single words revealed the following errors — stopping of liquids and affricates, inconsistent stopping of fricatives, fricative simplification, cluster reduction and simplification, inconsistent deletion of unstressed syllables and inconsistent assimilation. A spontaneous speech sample showed she also had difficulty with velar phonemes as well as the above errors. Repetition of phoneme sequences and syllable sequences was marked by substitutions, transposition errors, delayed responses and visual and audible searching. Speech was intelligible if the listener had some contextual cues. A moderate prosodic impairment, i.e. a reduced rate of speech and reduced modulation of pitch and duration was present.

Nicola's expressive language at this time was functional and the use of the communication board was discontinued. However, the Boston Diagnostic Aphasia Examination (Goodglass and Kaplan, 1983), administering only the Responsive Naming and Visual Confrontation Naming subtests, indicated significant word-finding difficulties. From a language sample it was noted that her utterances were characterized by restricted syntactic constructions with many phrase structure elements (determiners, prepositions, pronouns, copula, auxiliary verbs) and morphological inflections (irregular plurals, 'ing', 'ed', 3rd person singular 's') omitted. She responded to semantic and phonetic cueing. Verbal paraphasias were present in her language and made up half of all error responses. Her receptive language, using the Reynell Developmental Language Scale — Revised (Reynell, 1977), comprehension scale only, revealed a mild difficulty. On the Token Test for Children (Di Simone, 1978), Nicola's score on subtests II, III, IV and V were below one and two standard deviations. On subtest I she was average. These scores confirmed observations that she was having difficulty with instructions of increasing length and complex linguistic concepts.

Eight months after the accident, Nicola's speech was intelligible in all situations. The Nuffield Centre Dyspraxia Programme (Nuffield Hearing and Speech Centre, 1985) was administered. Nicola could not volitionally elevate her tongue tip but when eating a biscuit she cleaned her top lip without effort. Imitations of single sounds revealed only an inability to make voiced and voiceless /the/ and mild distortions of /l/ and /r/. An analysis of a video tape recording of Nicola before the cerebrovascular accident showed no difficulties in her phonological system. Cluster simplification, involving these same phonemes (e.g. /fl/ became /fw/ and /br/ and /bw/) as well as fricative simplification /the/voiceless became /f/, was present. Repetition of phoneme sequences and syllable sequences were still marked by delayed responses and slow rate of repetition with some visible searching behaviours but these problems did not seem to hamper her functional communication. Repetition of contrasting consonant-vowel structures (e.g. bee, me) were accurate and slow but not effortful. A mild prosodic impairment, mainly a reduced rate of speech, was present when her syntactic construction was complex or when a polysyllabic word she used was new to her vocabulary. Word retrieval and syntactic difficulties exacerbated this problem. There was little detectable muscle weakness.

Her language abilities improved daily. In 5 months Nicola progressed from using single words to phrases and syntactically correct simple sentences. Language testing on the TOLD-2 Primary (Newcomer and Hammill, 1988) placed her in the below average range on most subtests except the vocabulary subtests which were in the average range. On the Peabody Picture Vocabulary Test (Dunn, 1965) she scored at the 70th percentile. Spontaneous language samples revealed that verbal paraphasias had decreased and rarely occurred in conversational speech. Word-retrieval difficulties were still apparent but only when the linguistic demands in the situation increased, e.g. with narrative tasks or when she was explaining something that had happened at school and the information she was giving was new to the listener. Her utterances had increased in length and she was using 'and', 'and then', and 'because' as conjunctions as well as 'who', 'what', 'where' and 'why' questions. Embedded clause structures were not used consistently.

Nicola had returned to school 7 weeks post-onset. Her teacher reported that she was coping with the work in Grade 1 and was just a little below average in a class of 25. She was to go into Grade 2 in the new school year.

Treatment

Nicola's treatment was intensive, daily at first and then three times per week when she returned to school. It was also as functional as possible. Blissymbols were introduced 2 weeks post-onset and she learned to use approximately 90 symbols in one and two symbol constructions. Intensive articulation therapy was carried out beginning with the imitation of single phonemes, using visual and tactile cueing. The sounds which were the easiest for her to imitate were incorporated into consonant-vowel combinations and if these made words or approximations of words, e.g. 'more' or 'ba' for 'ball' they were then used in pragmatically appropriate situations. For example, the physiotherapist often played ball with Nicola who loved this activity, and she would require Nicola to request the game.

The Nuffield Centre Dyspraxia Programme was used successfully with Nicola who loved the pictures representing the sounds and sound sequencing exercises. However, as soon as Nicola was able to produce monosyllabic words as consonant-vowel or vowel-consonant they were introduced into early verbal expressive language therapy. Within 2 months of her cerebrovascular accident, most dyspraxic therapy goals were met in language activities, e.g. playing a game of 'Fish' with contrasting /sh/ and /ch/ sounds. Treatment goals required her to ask the question and to pronounce correctly the 'sh' or 'ch' sound. As her articulation improved no specific speech goals were formulated. Polysyllabic words which gave her trouble during language activities were noted and her mother also noted the ones with which she had problems at home. They were then worked on directly in therapy and incorporated into some language activity. Very little basic motor work was necessary as her oral dyspraxia resolved quickly and she had no eating or drinking difficulties.

Conclusion

At 8 months post-onset, Nicola was still in the active recovery phase. Her right lower facial muscle weakness had resolved. Oral and verbal dyspraxia was mild with her expressive dysphasia being her main problem. Speech and language therapy would continue.

Summary - Case 2

Nicola made an excellent recovery of communicative abilities since she first presented with a severe oral and verbal dyspraxia. Initially, a Blissymbol communication board was used to give her some form of communication but this was discontinued after approximately 2 months when her verbal expression was functional. Treatment involved imitation and repetition of single phonemes, consonant-vowel, vowel-consonant, consonant-vowel-consonant combinations, minimal pairs, disyllabic and polysyllabic words. As Nicola's articulation improved, an expressive dysphasic component became apparent and subsequent treatment incorporated dyspraxic therapy and language therapy. Eight months after the cerebrovascular accident, Nicola presented with a mild dyspraxia which did not hamper her functional communication and a mild to moderate expressive dysphasia. Therapy would continue.

References

ALAJOUANINE, T. and LHERMITTE, F. (1965) 'Acquired aphasia in children', *Brain*, **88**, pp. 653–62.

ANDERSON, K., BLOOMBERG, K., DUNNE, L., JONES, P. and SNELLERMAN, J. (1986) *Computer Pictographs for Computer Communication*, Victoria, Swinburne Ltd.

ARAM, D. M., EKELMAN, B. L. and GILLESPIE, L. L. (1989) 'Reading and lateralized brain lesions', in Von Euler, K. (Ed.) *Developmental Dyslexia and Dysphasia*, Hampshire, England, Macmillan Press.

ARAM, D. M., ROSE, D. F., REKATE, H. L. and WHITAKER, H. A. (1983) 'Acquired capsular/striatal aphasia in childhood', *Archives of Neurology*, **40**, pp. 614–17.

BAK, E., VAN DONGEN, H. R. and ARTS, W. F. M. (1983) 'The analysis of acquired dysarthria in childhood', *Developmental Medicine and Child Neurology*, **25**, pp. 81–94.

BEHRMANN, M. M. (1984) *Handbook of Microcomputers in Special Education*, San Diego, College-Hill Press.

BERNHARDT, M. (1885) 'Ueber die spastiche cerebral paralyse im kinder satter (hemiplegia spastica infantalis), nebst einem excurse uber: Aphasie bei kindern', *Archiv für Pathologische Anatomie und Physiologie und für Klinische Medecin*, **102**, pp. 26–80.

BOONE, D. R. (1971) *The Voice and Voice Therapy*, Prentice Hall, New Jersey.

COOPER, J. A. and FLOWERS, C. R. (1987) 'Children with a history of acquired aphasia: Residual language and academic impairments', *Journal of Speech and Hearing Disorders*, **52**, pp. 251–62.

CRANBERG, L. D., FILLEY, C. M., HART, E. J. and ALEXANDER, M. P. (1987) 'Acquired aphasia in childhood: Clinical and CT investigations', *Neurology*, **37**, pp. 1165–72.

DABUL, B. (1979) *Apraxia Battery for Adults*, Oregon, C.C. Publications Inc.

DAMICO, J. S. (1985) 'Clinical discourse analysis. A functional language assessment technique', in Simon, C.S. (Ed.) *Communication Skills and Classroom Success: Assessment of Language-Learning Disabled Students*, San Diego, College-Hill Press.

DARLEY, F. L., ARONSON, A. E. and BROWN, J. R. (1969a) 'Different diagnostic patterns of dysarthria', *Journal of Speech and Hearing Disorders*, **12**, pp. 246–69.

DARLEY, F. L., ARONSON, A. E. and BROWN, J. R. (1969b) 'Clusters of deviant speech dimensions in the dysarthrias', *Journal of Speech and Hearing Research*, **12**, pp. 462–96.

DARLEY, F. L., ARONSON, A. E. and BROWN, J. R. (1975) *Motor Speech Disorders*, Philadelphia, W. B. Saunders.

DE RUYTER, F. and LA FONTAINE, L. M. (1987) 'The non-speaking brain-injured: A clinical and demographic database report', *Augmentative and Alternative Communication*, **3**, pp. 18–25.

DI SIMONE, F. (1978) *The Token Test for Children*, Hingham, Mass, Teaching Resources.

DOWDEN, P. R., HONSINGER, M. J. and BEUKELMAN, D. R. (1986) 'Serving non-speaking patients in acute care settings: An intervention approach', *Augmentative and Alternative Communication*, **2**.

DUNN, L. M. (1965) *Peabody Picture Vocabulary Test*, Circle Pines, MN, American Guidance Service.

ENDERBY, P. (1983) *Frenchay Dysarthria Assessment*, San Diego, College-Hill Press.

FERRO, J. M., MARTINS, I. P., PINTO, F. and CASTRO-CALDAS, A. (1982) 'Aphasia following right striato-insular infarction in a left handed child: A clinico-radiological study', *Developmental Medicine and Child Neurology*, **24**, pp. 173–82.

FOKES, J. (1976) *Fokes Sentence Builder*, USA, DLM Teaching Resources.

FREUD, S. (1897) *Infantile Cerebral Paralysis*, trans. by L. A. Russin, 1968, Coral Gables, University of Miami.

GOODGLASS, H. and KAPLAN, E. (1983) *The Assessment of Aphasia and Related Disorders*, Philadelphia, Lea and Febiger.

GREEN, M. C. L. (1957) *The Voice and Its Disorders*, New York, Macmillan.

HÉCAEN, H. (1983) 'Acquired aphasia in children: revisited', *Neuropsychologia*, **21**, pp. 581–7.

HEHNER, B. (1979) *Blissymbols for Use*, Toronto, Blissymbolics Communication Institute.

HEHNER, B. (1984) *A Supplement to Blissymbols for Use*, Toronto, Blissymbols Communication Institute.

HUDSON, L. J., MURDOCH, B. E. and OZANNE, A. E. (1989) 'Posterior fossa tumours in childhood: Associated speech and language disorders post-surgery', *Aphasiology*, **3**, pp. 1–18.

LOGEMANN, J. (1983) *Evaluation and Treatment of Swallowing Disorders*, San Diego, College Hill Press.

MILLER, B. F. and KEANE, C. B. (1978) *Encyclopedia and Dictionary of Medicine, Nursing and Allied Health*, Philadelphia, W. B. Saunders.

MORRIS, S. E. (1982) *The Normal Acquisition of Oral Feeding Skills: Implications of Assessment and Treatment*, New York, Therapeutic Media Inc.

NEWCOMER, P. L. and HAMMILL, D. D. (1988) *Test of Language Development-2 Primary*, Austin, Pro-Ed.

Nuffield Centre Dyspraxia Programme (1985) London, Nuffield Hearing and Speech Centre.

ODOR, P., MAXWELL, C., MILLAR, S., MILNE, M., NISBET, P. and SMITH, D. (1986) 'Communication aids and computer based learning assessment techniques and related developments for communication impaired learners', University of Edinburgh, CALL Project.

PASSEY, J. (1985) *Cued Articulation*, Victoria, J. Passy.

REKATE, H. L., GRUBB, R. L., ARAM, D. M., HAHN, J. F. and RATCHESON, R. A. (1985) 'Muteness of cerebellar origin', *Archives of Neurology*, **42**, pp. 697–8.

REYNELL, J. (1977) *Reynell Developmental Language Scales—Revised*, Oxford, NFER Publishing Company Ltd.

ROBERTSON, S. J. and THOMSON, F. (1986) *Working with Dysarthrics: A Practical Guide to Therapy for Dysarthria*, Winslow, Winslow Press.

SATZ, P. and BULLARD-BATES, C. (1981) 'Acquired aphasia in children', in Sarno, M.T. (Ed.), *Acquired Aphasia*, New York, Academic Press.

SCHEIFELBUSCH, R. L. (1980) *Nonspeech Language and Communication: Analysis and Intervention*, Baltimore, University Park Press.

VANDERHEIDEN, G. C. and GRILLY, K. (Eds.) (1977) *Non-vocal Communication Techniques and Aids for the Severely Physically Handicapped*, Baltimore, University Park Press.

VAN DONGEN, H. R., ARTS, W. F. M. and YOUSEF-BAK, E. (1987) 'Acquired dysarthria in childhood: An analysis of dysarthric features in relation to neurologic deficits', *Neurology*, **37**, pp. 296–9.

VAN HOUT, A., EVRARD, P. and LYON, G. (1985) 'On the positive semiology of acquired aphasia in children', *Developmental Medicine and Child Neurology*, **27**, 231–341.

VAUGHAN, G. R. and CLARK, R. M. (1979) *Speech Facilitation: Extraoral and Intraoral Stimulation Technique for Improvement of Articulation Skills*, Springfield, Charles C. Thomas.

VOLCAN. I., COLE, G. P. and JOHNSTON, K. (1986) 'A case of muteness of cerebellar origin', *Archives of Neurology*, **43**, pp. 313–14.

YLVISAKER, M. and LOGEMANN, J. (1985) 'Therapy for feeding and swallowing disorders following head injury', in Ylvisaker, M. (Ed.) *Head Injury Rehabilitation: Children and Adolescents*, London, Taylor and Francis, pp. 195–215.

Index